Tumors of the Kidney, Bladder, and Related Urinary Structures

Atlas of Tumor Pathology

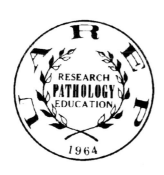

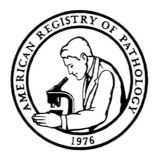

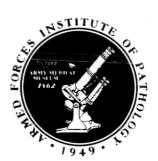

ATLAS OF TUMOR PATHOLOGY

Third Series
Fascicle 11

TUMORS OF THE KIDNEY, BLADDER, AND RELATED URINARY STRUCTURES

by

WILLIAM M. MURPHY, M.D.*
Professor of Pathology and Urology
University of Tennessee
and Midsouth Pathology Group
Memphis, Tennessee 38146

J. BRUCE BECKWITH, M.D.
Professor of Pathology and Laboratory Medicine
Head of Division of Pediatric Pathology
Loma Linda University School of Medicine
Loma Linda, California 92350

GEORGE M. FARROW, M.D.
Professor of Pathology
Mayo Medical School
Consultant, Department of Pathology
Rochester, Minnesota 55905

* Currently, Department of Pathology and Laboratory Medicine
University of Florida College of Medicine
Gainesville, Florida 32610

Published by the
ARMED FORCES INSTITUTE OF PATHOLOGY
Washington, D.C.

Under the Auspices of
UNIVERSITIES ASSOCIATED FOR RESEARCH AND EDUCATION IN PATHOLOGY, INC.
Bethesda, Maryland
1994

Accepted for Publication
1993

Available from the American Registry of Pathology
Armed Forces Institute of Pathology
Washington, D.C. 20306-6000
ISSN 0160-6344
ISBN 1-881041-15-8

ATLAS OF TUMOR PATHOLOGY

EDITOR
JUAN ROSAI, M.D.
Department of Pathology
Memorial Sloan-Kettering Cancer Center
New York, New York 10021-6007

ASSOCIATE EDITOR
LESLIE H. SOBIN, M.D.
Armed Forces Institute of Pathology
Washington, D.C. 20306-6000

EDITORS' NOTE

The Atlas of Tumor Pathology has a long and distinguished history. It was first conceived at a Cancer Research Meeting held in St. Louis in September 1947 as an attempt to standardize the nomenclature of neoplastic diseases. The first series was sponsored by the National Academy of Sciences-National Research Council. The organization of this Sisyphean effort was entrusted to the Subcommittee on Oncology of the Committee on Pathology, and Dr. Arthur Purdy Stout was the first editor-in-chief. Many of the illustrations were provided by the Medical Illustration Service of the Armed Forces Institute of Pathology, the type was set by the Government Printing Office, and the final printing was done at the Armed Forces Institute of Pathology (hence the colloquial appellation "AFIP Fascicles"). The American Registry of Pathology purchased the Fascicles from the Government Printing Office and sold them virtually at cost. Over a period of 20 years, approximately 15,000 copies each of nearly 40 Fascicles were produced. The worldwide impact that these publications have had over the years has largely surpassed the original goal. They quickly became among the most influential publications on tumor pathology ever written, primarily because of their overall high quality but also because their low cost made them easily accessible to pathologists and other students of oncology the world over.

Upon completion of the first series, the National Academy of Sciences-National Research Council handed further pursuit of the project over to the newly created Universities Associated for Research and Education in Pathology (UAREP). A second series was started, generously supported by grants from the AFIP, the National Cancer Institute, and the American Cancer Society. Dr. Harlan I. Firminger became the editor-in-chief and was succeeded by Dr. William H. Hartmann. The second series Fascicles were produced as bound volumes instead of loose leaflets. They featured a more comprehensive coverage of the subjects, to the extent that the Fascicles could no longer be regarded as "atlases" but rather as monographs describing and illustrating in detail the tumors and tumor-like conditions of the various organs and systems.

Once the second series was completed, with a success that matched that of the first, UAREP and AFIP decided to embark on a third series. A new editor-in-chief and an associate editor were selected, and a distinguished editorial board was appointed. The mandate for the third series remains the same as for the previous ones, i.e., to oversee the production of an eminently practical publication with surgical pathologists as its primary audience, but also aimed at other workers in oncology. The main purposes of this series are to promote a consistent, unified, and biologically sound nomenclature; to guide the surgical pathologist in the diagnosis of the various tumors and tumor-like lesions; and to provide relevant histogenetic, pathogenetic, and clinicopathologic information on these entities. Just as the second series included data obtained from ultrastructural (and, in the more recent Fascicles, immunohistochemical) examination, the third series will, in addition, incorporate pertinent information obtained with the newer molecular biology techniques. As in the past, a continuous attempt will be made to correlate, whenever possible, the nomenclature used in the Fascicles with that proposed by the World Health Organization's International Histological Classification of Tumors. The format of the third series has been changed in order to incorporate additional items and to ensure a consistency of style throughout. This includes the dropping of the 's possessive in eponymic terms, in accordance with the WHO and the International Nomenclature of Diseases. Close cooperation between the various authors and their respective liaisons from the editorial board will be emphasized to minimize unnecessary repetition and discrepancies in the text and illustrations.

To its everlasting credit, the participation and commitment of the AFIP to this venture is even more substantial and encompassing than in previous series. It now extends to virtually all scientific, technical, and financial aspects of the production.

The task confronting the organizations and individuals involved in the third series is even more daunting than in the preceding efforts because of the ever-increasing complexity of the matter at hand. It is hoped that this combined effort—of which, needless to say, that represented by the authors is first and foremost—will result in a series worthy of its two illustrious predecessors and will be a suitable introduction to the tumor pathology of the twenty-first century.

Juan Rosai, M.D.
Leslie H. Sobin, M.D.

PREFACE AND ACKNOWLEDGMENTS

This Atlas was created as a standard reference text for individuals interested in tumors of the kidneys, bladder, and urinary collecting system. Realizing that readers have varying levels of prior knowledge of the subject, we have emphasized diagnostic features as they appear through the light microscope. Knowledge in this area continues to evolve and areas of controversy are unavoidable. In such cases, we have attempted to clarify the issues and provide a point of view. Emerging information is included in separate sections on Special Techniques. Since most readers will use this Atlas as an encyclopedia, referring to individual sections rather than an entire chapter, we have not hesitated to be repetitious when reiterations add clarity and perspective. References have been selected and cited for the convenience of the reader. Review articles and the current literature have been emphasized. We claim no personal priority to the knowledge base and apologize if seminal contributions have been overlooked.

Any work of this scope reflects the collective efforts of investigators whose thoughts have directly contributed to the literature, and pathologists whose consultation material has enriched the perspectives of the authors. We are especially grateful to those individuals whose contributions have made this particular text possible. They include colleagues and fellows such as Drs. Mark S. Soloway, George F. Bale, Nigel Palmer, Nancy Kiviat, Jeffrey Bonadio, Douglas Weeks, Craig Zuppan, Paulo Faria, Kiran Mishra, and Michael Lieber. The constant support and encouragement of our colleagues at Baptist Memorial Hospital (BMH), Loma Linda University (LLU), and Mayo Clinic and Foundation (MCF) have allowed us the freedom to pursue this work. We are indebted to the reviewers, those anonymous experts whose efforts added perspective and clarity to the final product. A great deal of effort has been expended to create high quality illustrations and for this we are grateful to Ms. Rebecca Rodgers (BMH) and Ms. Mary Metzler (LLU). Professional library support was extended by Ms. Nancy Smith (BMH). Manuscripts of this magnitude require more than just typing. The entire work was most ably coordinated by Ms. Linda Bryant (BMH) with contributions from Nancy Browning, M.S. (NWTS Pathology Center) and Ms. Cindy Miller (MCF). Support from these and all others who have helped is gratefully acknowledged.

William M. Murphy, M.D.
J. Bruce Beckwith, M.D.
George M. Farrow, M.D.

Permission to use copyrighted illustrations has been granted by:

American Medical Association:
    Arch Pathol 1963;76:277–89. For figure 1-2.

American Society of Clinical Pathologists Press:
    Atlas of Bladder Carcinoma, 1986. For figures 2-48 and 2-69.

Chapman & Hall:
    A Textbook of Histology. 8th ed. 1962. For figure 1-3.

JB Lippincott Company:
    Cancer 1968;22:545–50. For figures 1-250, 1-251, 1-255, 1-256, and 1-258.
    Cancer 1968;22:551–5. For figures 1-291, 1-293, and 1-296.
    Cancer 1968;22:556–63. For figure 1-175.
    Cancer 1968;22:564–70. For figures 1-263, 1-268, and 1-275.
    Cancer 1972;29:1597–605. For figure 1-16.
    Cancer 1984;53:1555–65. For Table 2-4.
    Manual for Staging of Cancer, 1992. For Table 1-25.

John Wiley & Sons:
    Med Pediatr Oncol 1993;21:158–68. For figures 1-69, 1-73.

Radiology Society of North America:
    Radiology 1977;125:633–5.

Raven Press:
    Diagnostic Surgical Pathology, 1994. For figure 1-7.

Springer-Verlag, New York, Inc.:
    TNM Atlas: Illustrated Guide to the TNM/pTNM-Classification of Malignant
        Tumours, 1989. For figure 1-196.
    World J Urol 1987;5:71–9. For Tables 1-27 and 1-28.

WB Saunders:
    Renal Carcinoma, 1967. For figure 1-10.
    Urological Pathology, 1989. For figures 1-127, 1-131, 1-133, 1-134, 1-138, 1-139, 1-142,
        1-148, 1-149, 1-156, 1-174, 1-191, 1-192, 1-209, 1-238, 1-245, 1-254, 1-269, 1-273, 1-276,
        1-290, 1-299, 2-40, 2-61, 3-1, 4-3, and Tables 2-5 and 2-7.

Williams & Wilkins Company:
    J Urol 1968;100:420–3. For Table 1-22.
    J Urol 1969;101:297–301. For Table 1-24.
    J Urol 1982;127:1090–1. For Table 1-26.
    Lab Invest 1966;15:1357–94. For figures 1-11 and 1-12.
    Pathology and Pathobiology of the Urinary Bladder and Prostate, 1992. For Table 2-3.

TUMORS OF THE KIDNEY, BLADDER, AND RELATED URINARY STRUCTURES

Contents

TUMORS OF THE KIDNEY, BLADDER, AND RELATED URINARY STRUCTURES

1
TUMORS OF THE KIDNEY

NORMAL ANATOMY

Since the anatomy of the kidney has been detailed in several publications, only those features particularly relevant to the understanding of the development of renal tumors are emphasized here (2,6,11,12,14). The human kidney is derived from the nephric ridge, a longitudinal protrusion of primitive mesenchyme situated just lateral to the somites. Three successive stages are recognized in the embryonic development of renal tissue: pronephros, mesonephros, and metanephros. The pronephros is transient and important in humans only because its proximal portion forms the mesonephric duct. The mesonephros develops as a series of solid cords which canalize to form tubules and enter the mesonephric duct. The proximal portion of each primitive tubule indents and receives a branch from the aorta to form a glomerulus. These nephrons first appear rostrally and progressively add new units caudally. Ultimately, the primitive mesonephros regresses, preserved only as rudimentary parovarian tubules in females and components of the excretory duct system of the testis in males.

The human kidney is formed from the metanephros. It begins as a ureteric bud which emerges from the dorsal side of the caudal end of the mesonephric duct on about day 28 of gestation (fig. 1-1). As the ureteric bud grows into the caudal region of the nephric ridge, a condensed cap of mesenchymal tissue, the nephrogenic blastema, appears at its apex. The nephrogenic blastema forms most of the structures of the kidney and the ureteric bud gives rise to the ureter, renal pelvis, calices, and renal collecting ducts. Since the ureteric bud and nephrogenic blastema are both of mesodermal origin, the kidney is an entirely mesodermal organ.

The path of ascent of the kidney as it moves from the caudal region of the embryo toward its eventual position in the abdomen determines the position of the future ureter. The advancing end of the ureteric bud, with its cap of blastemal cells, dilates and undergoes a series of dichotomous branchings, which form the pelvicaliceal system. The first three to five branches are reabsorbed to form the pelvis and calices (fig. 1-2). Subsequent branches extend into the metanephric blastemal region, forming the precursors of the future collecting ducts. As each branch of the ureteric bud advances, its lumen dilates to form an ampulla and the apical blastema elongates

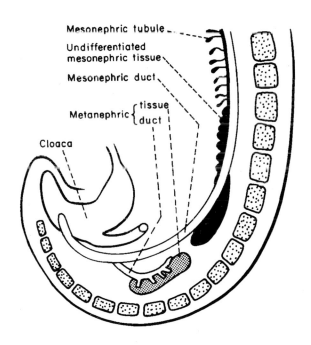

Figure 1-1
DEVELOPMENT OF THE METANEPHRIC KIDNEY
The ureteric bud arises from the caudal end of the mesonephric duct and gives rise to the ureter, renal pelvis, calices, and collecting ducts. The metanephric blastema, shown in fine gray stippling, is induced by the ureteric bud to form the nephrons and renal stroma. (Fig. 1 from Fascicle 12, 2nd Series.)

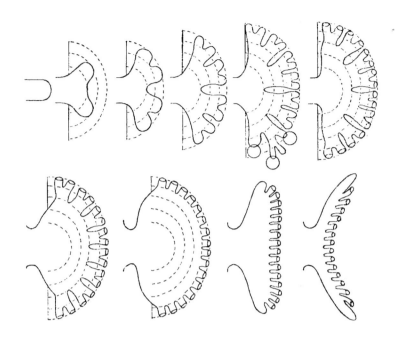

Figure 1-2
DEVELOPMENT OF RENAL
PELVIS, CALICES, AND PAPILLAE
Coalescence of the third to fifth generations of branches of the ureteric bud forms the renal pelvis and primary calices. (Fig. 10 from Osathanondh V, Potter EL. Development of human kidney as shown by microdissection. Arch Pathol 1963;76:277–89.)

and folds to form a tubular structure in the shape of the letter S. The proximal portion of this developing nephron connects to the adjacent ampulla to establish a collecting duct while the remaining blastema differentiates into other parts of the renal tubule (fig. 1-3). The lobar pattern created by the branching ureteric bud is established early in renal development (fig. 1-4) (5). Approximately 12 generations of nephrons form between the 8th and 34th weeks of gestation; this constant elongation and branching pushes the blastemal cells to the periphery of the lobes (fig. 1-5) (12). When new nephrons cease to generate, at about the 34th gestational week, blastemal cells are no longer apparent in the normal kidney, and no new glomeruli or tubules can be formed. All renal growth from this point onward is the result of the enlargement of existing structures.

The mature human kidney is a bean-shaped organ located in the lumbar peritoneal space opposite vertebrae T-12 to L-3 (2,6,11,14). On average, each adult kidney is 12 cm in length, 6 cm in width, and 2.5 cm in thickness. In men, the average weight is 125 to 170 g whereas in women it is 115 to 155 g. The kidney comprises 8 to 18 independently functional units fused together to form lobes, each composed of a medullary pyramid and the adjacent cortical mantle. This lobar structure is usually prominent on the external

surface of the kidney in newborns. These "fetal lobations" occasionally remain in adults but differential growth of nephrons usually obliterates them and the surface of the normal adult kidney is ordinarily smooth.

The convex outer surface of the kidney is invested with a capsule composed of a thin fibroblastic layer which is difficult to dissect from the underlying nephrons, and an outer, thicker layer easily stripped by blunt dissection (fig. 1-6). The renal capsule is covered by fat, which is in turn surrounded by a condensation of retroperitoneal connective tissue, the perirenal fascia of Gerota. Gerota fascia may be in direct contact with the renal capsule anteriorly, where perirenal fat is scanty.

An important, but rarely emphasized component of the kidney, is the renal sinus (figs. 1-7–1-9). Located on the medial aspect of the kidney, this concave structure is a major pathway of tumor dissemination and an important landmark for evaluating tumor extension. The renal sinus contains the renal calices, variable portions of the pelvis, and the major vascular and neural structures that supply the kidney. These structures are surrounded by richly vascularized connective tissue contiguous to the perirenal fat. The most distinguishing feature of the renal sinus in histologic sections is its lack of a capsule (figs. 1-7, 1-9). This contrasts with the thick fibrous capsule

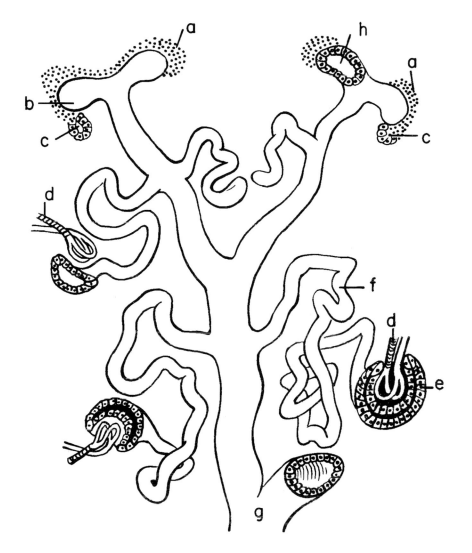

Figure 1-3
DIAGRAM OF NEPHRON
DEVELOPMENT IN THE
METANEPHRIC KIDNEY
a: Metanephrogenic tissue
capping ampulla of collecting
tubule. b: Enlarged blind end
of ampulla. c: Primordium of
uriniferous tubule just formed
from metanephrogenic tissue.
d: Vessel which forms the glomerulus. e: Bowman capsule
cut open. f: Uriniferous tubule
in later stage of development.
g: Collecting tubule formed
from ureteric bud of the mesonephric duct. h: Ampulla of collecting tubule cut open. (Fig.
28-22 from Bloom W, Fawcett
DW. A textbook of histology.
8th ed. New York: Chapman &
Hall, 1962 [Modified from
Corning].)

that covers the convex portion of the renal cortex and the pelvicaliceal system within the sinus (fig. 1-8). Other important features of the renal sinus in histologic sections include the presence of large blood vessels, pelvicaliceal structures, and adjacent medullary pyramids.

The vascular supply of the normal kidney is variable. Most kidneys receive a single renal artery and vein which arborize in the renal sinus and supply the parenchyma in such a way that each nephron is a self-contained functioning unit with its own blood supply and filtration system. Lymphatics are numerous in the renal cortex but are absent in the medulla (7,10). They drain via the renal sinus into hilar and regional lymph nodes adjacent to the aorta and vena cava. Since

true hilar lymph nodes (defined as nodes on the renal side of the hilar plane) are rarely present, the distinction between hilar and para-aortic nodes is arbitrary.

The kidney is supplied with adrenergic nerve fibers from the celiac plexus (9). Most nerves reach the renal parenchyma via the renal sinus and arborize with the vascular system.

The gross appearance of the mature human kidney hemisected in the frontal plane is distinctive. The cortex is 0.7 to 1.0 cm in thickness and is easily distinguished from the medulla by its configuration, position, and color. Cortical tissue extending between medullary pyramids is vari-ably shaped but usually referred to as the columns of Bertin. Closer inspection reveals radially

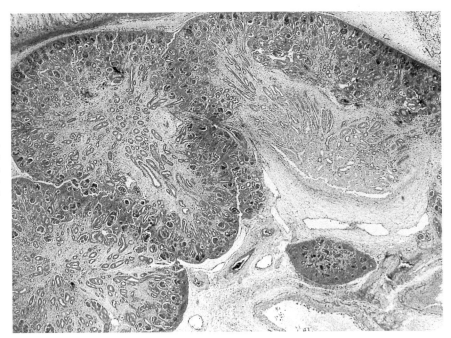

Figure 1-4
DEVELOPING KIDNEY IN
A 21-WEEK FETUS
The lobar pattern is well established, with blastemal cells concentrated at the cortical periphery. The first generations of cortical nephrons are situated at the cortico-medullary junction.

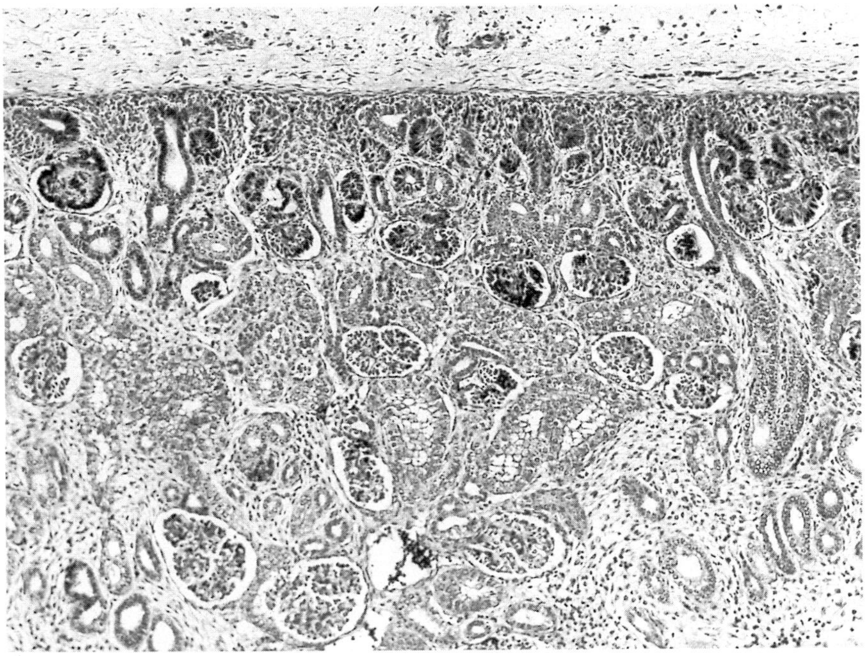

Figure 1-5
DEVELOPING KIDNEY
AT 21 WEEKS
Blastemal cells and early glomerular development are seen at the lobar periphery of the above specimen.

arranged medullary rays extending from the cortex into the medulla. These rays comprise collecting ducts, straight segments of proximal and distal tubules, and straight blood vessels. Each kidney contains 1 to 2 million nephrons, the glomerular portions of which can often be seen with the unaided eye.

Histologically, the normal renal parenchyma consists of four parts: blood vessels, glomeruli, tubules, and interstitium. Excellent reviews of the microscopic anatomy are available and only the most pertinent features are described here (2,6, 12,14). The renal blood vessels are structurally similar to those in other body sites. Glomeruli

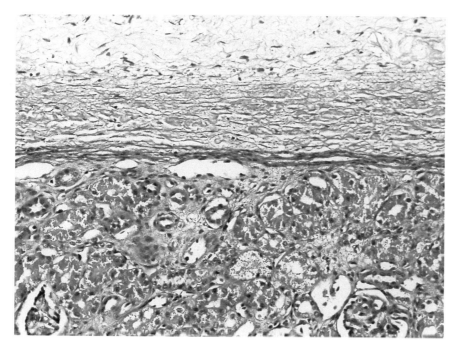

Figure 1-6
RENAL CAPSULE
A discrete layer of fibroblasts is seen adjacent to the cortex, with a condensed collagenous layer above.

Figure 1-7
KIDNEY SEEN IN CROSS SECTION
The renal sinus in this adult specimen is filled with fat, which surrounds the major renal vessels and pelvicaliceal system. (Fig. 4 from Beckwith JB. Renal neoplasms in childhood. In: Sternberg SS, ed. Diagnostic surgical pathology. New York: Raven Press 1994: 1741–66.)

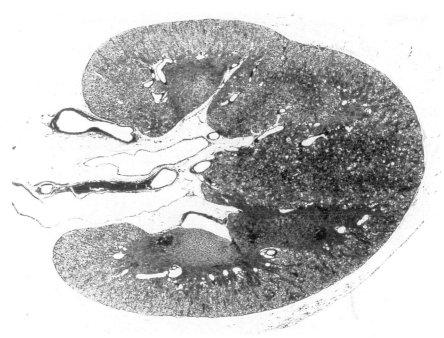

are complex structures composed of specialized endothelial, epithelial, and mesangial cells arranged around a relatively thick basement membrane. They manifest a variety of antigenic determinants, many of which are shared by the proximal tubules (1,4,8). The juxtaglomerular apparatus, a structure composed of vascular smooth muscles, granular and agranular cells of the extraglomerular mesangium, and the macula densa of the distal tubule, occupies a portion of the vascular pole of the glomerulus. A complex tubular system begins at the urinary pole and extends to the renal papilla. This system is traditionally divided into the proximal tubule, loop

Figure 1-8
KIDNEY IN
CROSS SECTION

Drawing of specimen shown in figure 1-7. The renal capsule, shown as a thick black line, surrounds the convex surface of the kidney, but disappears from the cortical surface as it enters the renal sinus. Cortical surfaces lining the sinus lack a capsule. The capsule surrounding the pelvicaliceal system is shown by crosshatched markings. This may extend over adjacent medullary pyramids but does not cover cortical structures.

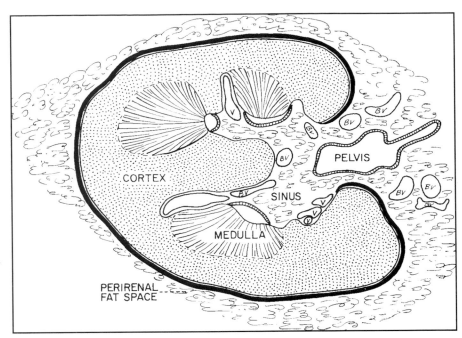

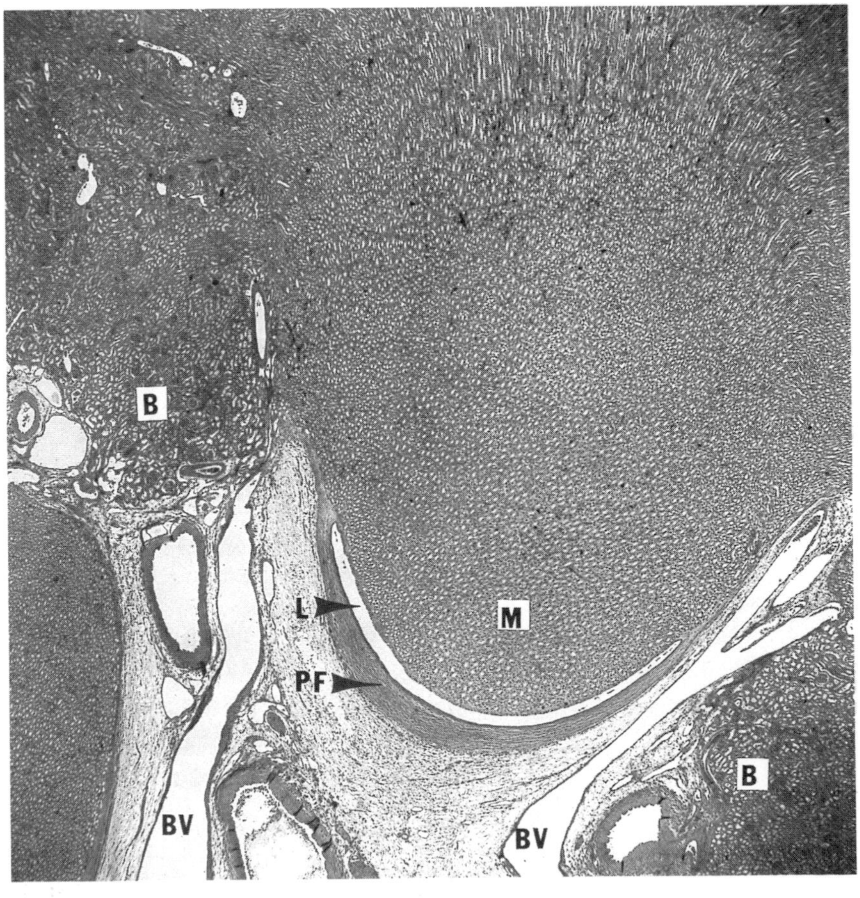

Figure 1-9
RENAL SINUS

This low-power photomicrograph shows the capsular tissue surrounding the pelvicaliceal system and the lack of capsule over cortical tissues of the sinus. B: Cortex surrounding renal sinus; BV: branches of renal vein; PF: fascial layer surrounding pelvicaliceal system; M: medullary pyramid; L: caliceal lumen.

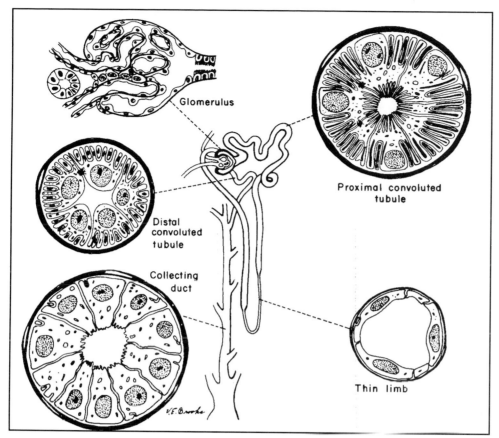

Figure 1-10
GENERAL HISTOLOGIC FEATURES OF THE NEPHRON

Cross sections of the various segments of the tubule roughly indicate the cellular morphologic features and the relative size of cells and tubules at these sites. (Fig. 1-5 from Bennington JL, Kradjian R. Renal carcinoma. Philadelphia: WB Saunders, 1967.)

of Henle, distal tubule, and collecting duct, although each consists of distinctive subunits (fig. 1-10). The proximal tubule is composed of convoluted and straight portions, lined by tall columnar cells with acidophilic cytoplasm rich in structures necessary for active fluid transport: densely packed microvilli and basal undulations, endocytic vacuoles, and mitochondria (figs. 1-11, 1-12). The loop of Henle has thin descending and thick ascending portions lined by cuboidal and columnar cells with variable expressions of microvilli and cytoplasmic organelles (fig. 1-13). Tamm-Horsfall protein is an antigenically recognizable substance produced by these cells (13). The distal tubule is narrower and shorter than the proximal tubule and has fewer microvilli and organelles. It contains specialized cells and the macula densa of the juxtaglomerular apparatus. Collecting ducts consist of cuboidal cells with pale acidophilic cytoplasm and centrally placed nuclei. Cytoplasmic lipofuscin granules may be prominent. Collecting duct cells have been subtyped according to their electron density (light

and dark) as well as the length and density of their microvilli (fig. 1-14) (14). All types may have single central cilia best demonstrated by scanning electron microscopy. Collecting ducts coalesce to form the terminal ducts of Bellini; 10 to 25 terminal ducts open into the area cribrosa at the tip of a medullary papilla. The interstitium is more easily conceptualized as a space than a structure; it is usually visualized only when abnormal. It contains specialized interstitial cells and connective tissue elements.

Immunohistochemical observations indicate that the antigenic composition of the nephron varies in different regions (1,3). Antibodies to glycoproteins of various molecular weights can distinguish proximal from distal tubules and collecting ducts. Identification of these areas is not yet exact but may be helpful in determining the origin and differentiation of certain renal neoplasms. Collecting ducts, for example, react strongly with antibodies to high molecular weight cytokeratins whereas proximal and distal tubules are ordinarily nonreactive.

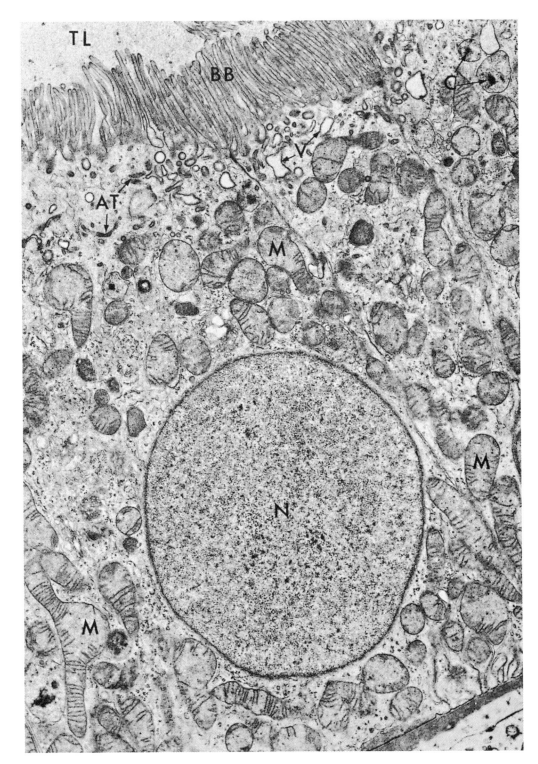

Figure 1-11
PROXIMAL CONVOLUTED TUBULAR CELL

The apical part of the proximal convoluted tubular cell is covered by tightly packed microvilli forming the brush border (BB). In the apical cytoplasm, apical tubules (AT), vacuoles (V), and cytosomes (C) are evident. The mitochondria (M), tubular lumen (TL), and nucleus (N) are also indicated (X9300). (Fig. 5 from Tisher CC. Human renal ultrastructure. I. Proximal tubule of healthy individuals. Lab Invest 1966;15:1357–94.)

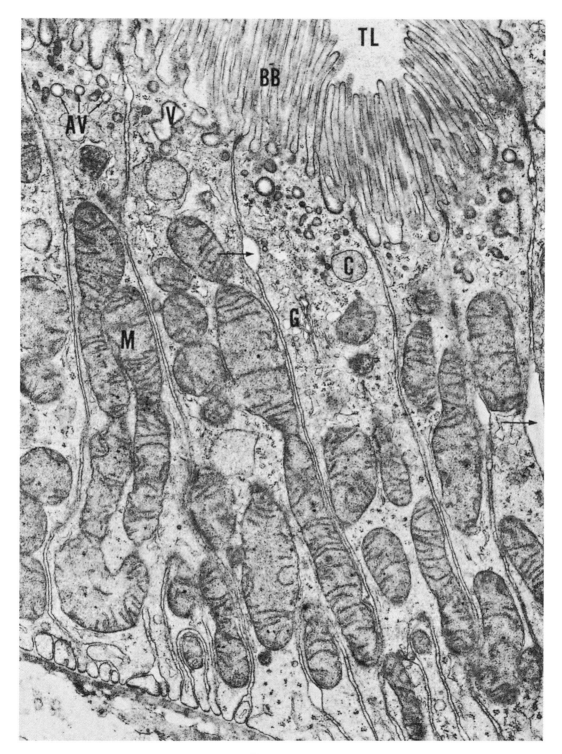

Figure 1-12
PROXIMAL CONVOLUTED TUBULAR CELL

In the proximal convoluted tubular cells, the mitochondria (M) are often elongated and tortuous. Deep invaginations of the apical cell membrane form apical tubules, vesicles (AV), and vacuoles (V). Note the dense homogenous material in some apical vacuoles and similar dense bodies in the apical cytosomes (C). The golgi (G), brush border (BB), and tubular lumen (TL) are also indicated (X18,800). (Fig. 7 from Tisher CC. Human renal ultrastructure. I. Proximal tubule of healthy individuals. Lab Invest 1966;15:1357–94.)

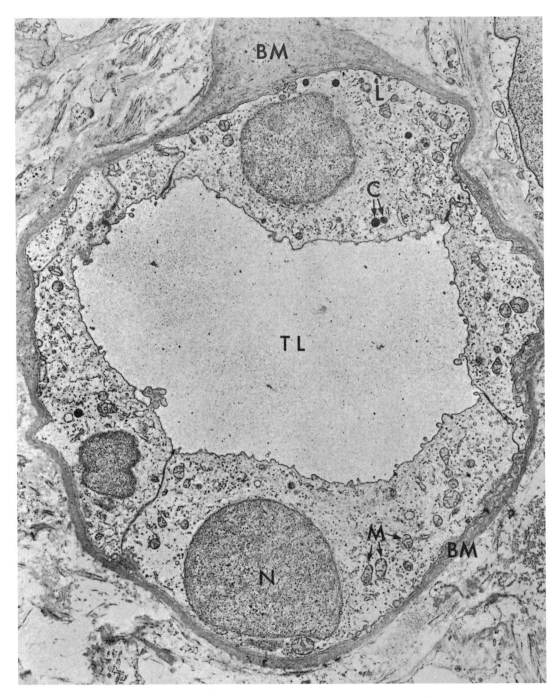

Figure 1-13
LOOP OF HENLE

In the thin limb of the loop of Henle, the cells assume a more squamoid configuration with nuclei (N) that often display infolding. Basal and lateral cell interdigitations are infrequent. The basement membrane (BM) is often quite variable in thickness. Occasional small mitochondria (M), cytosomes (C), and droplets of lipid (L) are present. The tubular lumen (TL) is also indicated (X6700). (Fig. 10 from Fascicle 12, 2nd Series.)

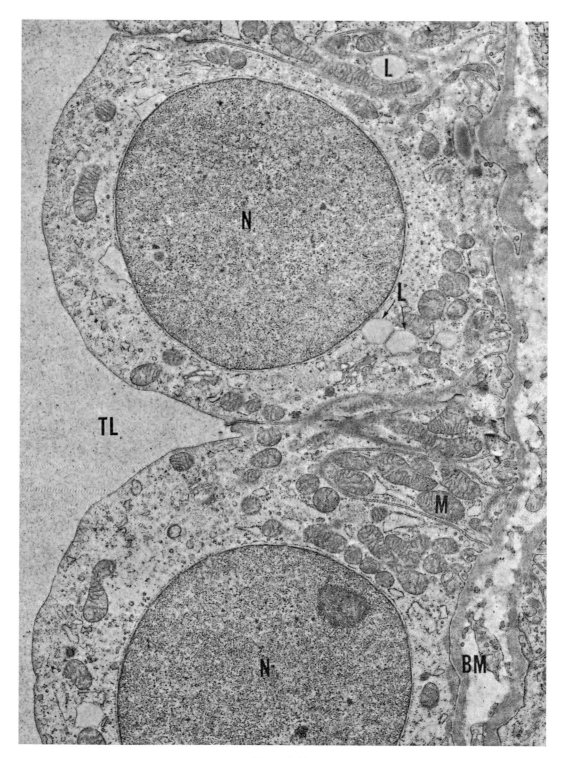

Figure 1-14
CORTICAL COLLECTING TUBULE CELLS

Note the relative paucity of organelles as compared to proximal tubular cells. Cortical collecting ducts often have a relatively smooth apical surface, though short plicae may be seen, and are more prominent in medullary collecting duct cells along with microvilli on some cells. A single cilium is usually present in the apex of the collecting duct cell, best shown with scanning electron microscopy. Membrane bound lipid (L) is present in the basal cytoplasm. The tubular lumen (TL), nucleus (N), and basal lamina (BM) are also indicated. (Courtesy of Dr. C. Craig Tisher, Durham, NC.)

TUMORS OF
INFANCY AND CHILDHOOD

Most renal tumors evolve along histogenetic pathways dictated by patient age at onset. Tumors arising in infants and children are almost exclusively neoplasms that manifest substantial mesenchymal differentiation, often reminiscent of embryonal tissue. Renal tumors appearing in adults are more varied, may not be neoplastic, and usually have characteristics of epithelial differentiation. Even so, distinctions based upon age rather than histology are arbitrary: embryonal cancers can occur in adults and typical renal carcinomas may arise in children.

CLASSIFICATION

Kidney tumors arising in infants and children are described using the classification shown in Table 1-1.

NEPHROBLASTOMA (WILMS TUMOR)

Definition. Nephroblastoma is an embryonal neoplasm derived from nephrogenic blastemal cells (21,24,45,69,73,75,80). Several lines of differentiation, including blastemal, epithelial, and stromal, are usually expressed and many nephroblastomas replicate the histology of developing kidneys. Essentially monomorphous tumors may arise and when this occurs, the cells are usually of blastemal or embryonal tubular differentiation. Although not preferred, the eponymic designation Wilms tumor is commonly used, despite the fact that Wilms was not the first to describe this entity (84). Following a general trend toward eliminating the possessive form of eponyms in medical nomenclature, we recommend that when the preferred term nephroblastoma is not used, the alternate term be expressed as "Wilms tumor" (34).

General Features. Nephroblastoma is usually diagnosed in young children and is uncommon in neonates and infants (fig. 1-15) (16,18,28,30,50). The mean age at diagnosis for males is 36.5 months and for females 42.5 months. Over 90 percent of cases have appeared in patients under 6 years of age; nephroblastomas have occurred occasionally in adults.

With the exception of patients having certain developmental disorders, the etiology and pathogenesis of nephroblastoma are unknown. The

Table 1-1

CLASSIFICATION OF KIDNEY TUMORS
IN INFANTS AND CHILDREN

Nephroblastoma (Wilms tumor)
    Unfavorable histology
    Favorable histology

Cystic nephroma and cystic, partially differentiated
    nephroblastoma

Mesoblastic nephroma

Clear cell sarcoma

Rhabdoid tumor

Rare tumors

relatively stable incidence of disease in all geographic regions suggests that environmental factors do not play a major role (33). There is no striking sex predilection. The variation in incidence among different racial groups, however, indicates a genetic predisposition. Whereas the general risk is approximately 1 in 8 to 10,000 live births among whites, the incidence among blacks is higher and the frequency among Orientals is lower. These incidences do not seem to be affected by immigration patterns, so that black and oriental Americans have the same relative frequency of disease as Africans and Asians.

The increased frequency of nephroblastoma in patients with several uncommon developmental disorders led to the discovery of specific genetic loci predisposing to this condition (Tables 1-2, 1-3) (46). The first genetic locus was identified in patients with the Wilms-Aniridia genital anomaly–retardation syndrome (WAGR) (71). These patients have a consistent deletion in chromosome 11p13 of their somatic cells. A similar deletion occurring in nephroblastoma cells of some patients without a constitutional anomaly in this region led to the suspicion that a gene important in the pathogenesis of nephroblastoma resided in the p13 region of chromosome 11. In 1990, the gene was cloned and designated WT1 (31,44). This gene encodes a zinc finger transcription factor that is expressed in the early development of the kidney and genital system (47). Abnormalities involving WT1 are consistently found in the tumors of WAGR patients as well as in those with Denys-Drash syndrome (glomerulonephritis, pseudohermaphroditism, and nephroblastoma), but are present in some patients with sporadic nephroblastomas.

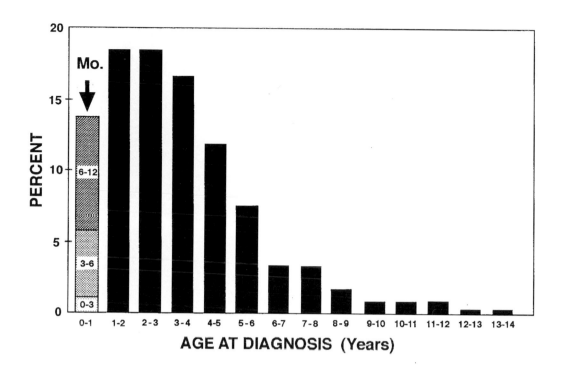

Figure 1-15
NEPHROBLASTOMA
Age distribution, based on 2500 NWTS cases.

Table 1-2

**CONDITIONS ASSOCIATED WITH
DEFINITE INCREASED RISK OF
NEPHROBLASTOMA**

Wilms-Aniridia genital anomaly-retardation
(WAGR) syndrome

Beckwith-Wiedemann syndrome

Hemihypertrophy

Denys-Drash syndrome

Familial nephroblastoma

Table 1-3

**CONDITIONS ASSOCIATED WITH
POSSIBLE INCREASED RISK OF
NEPHROBLASTOMA**

Renal malformations

Genital malformations

Cutaneous nevi, angiomas

Trisomy 18

Klippel-Trenaunay syndrome

Neurofibromatosis

Bloom syndrome

Cerebral gigantism

The recognition that genes other than WT1 could be involved in the pathogenesis of nephroblastoma led to the discovery of a second candidate gene, located in the distal region of the short arm of chromosome 11 (11p15.5) and designated WT2 (47,52). Several laboratories are currently attempting to clone this gene. The preferential loss of maternal alleles on chromosome 11 in cases of sporadic nephroblastoma suggests that

genomic imprinting is involved in the pathogenesis of this lesion (68). Abnormalities of chromosomes other than 11 are commonly observed, most often including chromosomes 1, 12, and 8, but also involving other chromosomes as well (74). Recent attention has also been directed toward a relatively high prevalence of abnormalities of 16q and it is suggested that a third nephroblastoma locus may reside in this region (63).

The occurrence of familial nephroblastoma further supports a genetic basis for the disease, at least in some individuals. Many families have more than one affected member (62). Among individuals registered in the National Wilms Tumor Study (NWTS) (30), approximately 1 percent have a positive family history for the same neoplasm. Most pedigrees suggest autosomal dominant transmission with variable penetrance and expressivity. It is important to emphasize that the fraction of nephroblastomas that may be due to heritable factors is low. In the small series reported to date, few cases have been observed in the offspring of nephroblastoma survivors (55). Evidence for genetic abnormalities notwithstanding, it is apparent that nephroblastoma can be initiated by more than one factor and that a simplistic, unitarian hypothesis of origin cannot account for all cases of this complex neoplasm.

Almost all nephroblastomas arise in the kidney, where they usually appear as unicentric tumors. However, multicentric masses in a single kidney are not uncommon and bilateral primary lesions have been observed in 5 percent of cases. Extrarenal nephroblastomas adjacent to the kidney may arise by exophytic growth from a narrow renal pedicle or from neoplastic transformation of an afferent branch of the ureteric bud (17,79). Inguinal, gonadal, or juxtagonadal nephroblastomas, thought to be derived from mesonephric remnants, have been recorded (67). The immature masses of nephrogenic tissue occasionally found in proximity to a neural tube defect in the lumbosacral region might be related to displacement of nephrogenic mesenchyme as part of the dysraphic process (69).

Clinical Features. Nephroblastoma is the most common genitourinary cancer in children, accounting for 80 percent of such tumors in patients less than 15 years of age (21,24,80). It is most common in children aged 1 to 3 years; 98 percent of cases have occurred in individuals under 10 years of age. Tumors occur with equal frequency in both kidneys. Most often, the diagnosis results from recognition of an abdominal mass although pain, hematuria, hypertension, and symptoms related to traumatic rupture are common. Imaging studies usually reveal one or more intrarenal masses but are not ordinarily helpful in distin-

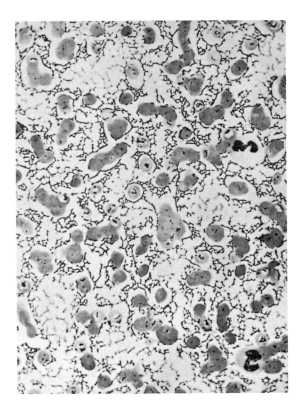

Figure 1-16
NEPHROBLASTOMA
This peripheral blood smear from a patient with nephroblastoma shows a characteristic precipitate. The larger, globular, pale-staining structures are erythrocytes; two neutrophilic leukocytes are included. (Wright-Giemsa stain) (Fig. 3 from Powars DR, Allerton SE, Beierle J, Butler BB. Wilms' tumor clinical correlation with circulating mucin in three cases. Cancer 1972;29:1597–605.)

guishing nephroblastomas from other pediatric renal neoplasms. Ultrasonography is especially effective for evaluating cystic components and in demonstrating extension of the tumor into the venous system. Computed tomography (CT) and magnetic resonance imaging (MRI) are especially useful for detecting small lesions and metastases. The demonstration of bilateral or multicentric tumors, a feature not observed in most other renal tumors of childhood, can be helpful in the clinical differential diagnosis.

Although several potential tumor marker substances have been associated with nephroblastoma, to date, no marker has been shown to be consistently present (33). Some patients have circulating serum mucin, which stains as blue granular material on conventionally prepared blood smears (fig. 1-16). An increased level of

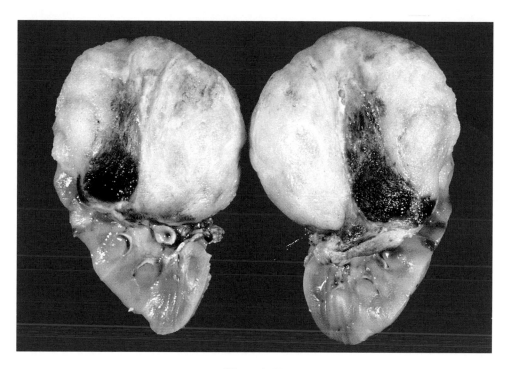

Figure 1-17
NEPHROBLASTOMA
Gross appearance. (Courtesy of Dr. Atilano G. Lacson, Halifax, Canada.)

hyaluronic acid, apparently resulting from increased activity of hyaluronic acid stimulating factor, is frequently present in the blood (57,76). Acquired von Willebrand factor has been observed in a few patients, where it has been associated with severe coagulopathies (35). Inactive renin may be a potentially useful marker for nephroblastoma (51,77). Serum levels of erythropoietin may be increased but the prevalence of this finding is probably no higher in patients with renal neoplasms than in other individuals (65). Neither urinary cytology nor aspiration cytology has been of particular value (57).

Pathologic Findings. Grossly, nephroblastomas are usually solitary, rounded masses sharply defined from the adjacent renal parenchyma by a pseudocapsule. Their size is extremely variable. The combined weight of tumor and kidney in the NWTS ranged from 60 to 6350 g, with a median of 550 g. Lesions tend to bulge from the sectioned surfaces and usually have a uniform, pale gray or tan appearance and a soft consistency (fig. 1-17). The sectioned surface may appear firm and whorled if a large fraction of the lesion is composed of mature stromal elements (fig. 1-18). The extremely soft consistency and friable texture of most nephroblastomas make them difficult to section without extensive displacement of tumor cells, an artifact that often complicates pathologic staging of the lesion. Nephroblastomas are often subdivided by prominent septa, imparting a distinctly lobulated appearance (figs. 1-17, 1-18). Polypoid protrusions of tumor into the pelvicaliceal system may occur (fig. 1-18). Some authors have recognized a resemblance to botryoid rhabdomyosarcoma (60). Pedunculated tumors arising from superficial cortex are rare and may account for some examples of pararenal disease. Cystic spaces may be a prominent feature (fig. 1-19). Hemorrhage and necrosis are often present but rarely prominent unless there was abdominal trauma prior to nephrectomy. Calcification is uncommon. Multicentric and bilateral tumors have been recorded in 7.0 and 5.4 percent of cases in the NWTS (fig. 1-20) (30). Nephroblastomas may originate anywhere in the kidney.

Nephroblastomas are usually demarcated by a dense tumor capsule composed of portions of renal capsule fused to intrarenal and perirenal

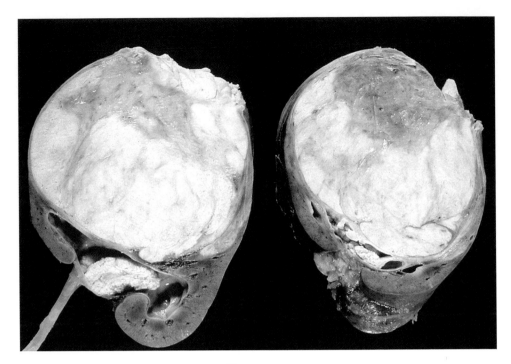

Figure 1-18
NEPHROBLASTOMA
Note the prominent septa subdividing the sectioned surface and the protrusion of tumor into the renal pelvis, resembling botryoid rhabdomyosarcoma.

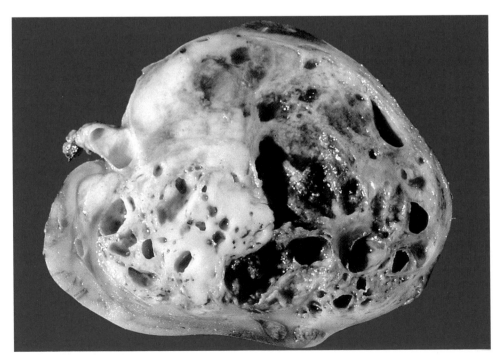

Figure 1-19
NEPHROBLASTOMA
Prominent cysts are seen. (Courtesy of Dr. Frederic A. Askin, St. Louis, MO.)

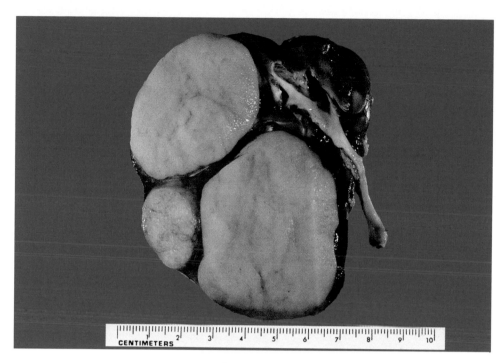

Figure 1-20
MULTICENTRIC NEPHROBLASTOMA
(Courtesy of Dr. David M. Parham, Memphis, TN.)

pseudocapsules. The line of demarcation is commonly obscured by inflammation, especially in association with hemorrhage and necrosis. The tumor may adhere to adjacent organs. Local extension into the renal vein and metastases to regional lymph nodes are common. Extensive permeation of intrarenal blood and lymphatic vessels may produce a false impression of multicentricity. These features are most commonly observed in predominantly blastemal tumors.

Microscopically, nephroblastomas rival teratomas in the diversity of their histologic patterns. A variety of cell types differentiating toward blastema, epithelium, and stroma are present in most lesions. The relative proportions of each cell or tissue type vary from specimen to specimen and the diverse cell types may express various degrees of differentiation, resulting in an almost infinite variety of potential patterns. Triphasic patterns, containing blastemal, stromal, and epithelial cell types, are the most characteristic but biphasic and monophasic lesions have often been observed (figs. 1-21, 1-22). For the sake of clarity, the various histologic components are described individually. Most of these

components represent various stages in normal or abnormal nephrogenesis, although some, such as skeletal muscle, represent potentialities of nephrogenic precursor cells best referred to collectively as heterologous elements.

The *blastemal pattern* resembles the condensed mesenchyme from which the kidney develops. Blastemal cells are small, closely packed, and mitotically active with minimal evidence of differentiation into recognizable epithelial or stromal structures. Blastema is present in most nephroblastomas and it may be the only element in the tumor. Blastemal cells occur in several distinctive patterns including diffuse, serpentine, nodular, and basaloid. More than one pattern is often found in the same tumor. Recognition of these patterns can facilitate differential diagnosis, especially of tumors at metastatic sites.

In the *diffuse pattern*, the blastema forms large sheets of small, densely packed cells (figs. 1-23–1-25). In some specimens, there is a general lack of cellular cohesiveness and an aggressive pattern of invasion into adjacent connective tissues and vessels. Tumors with this histologic pattern usually extend beyond the kidney and

17

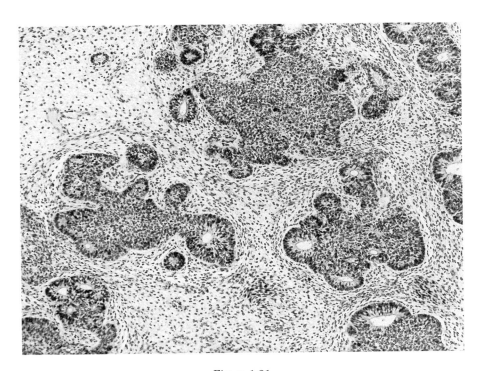

Figure 1-21
NEPHROBLASTOMA
Triphasic pattern, with prominent stromal, blastemal, and tubular elements.

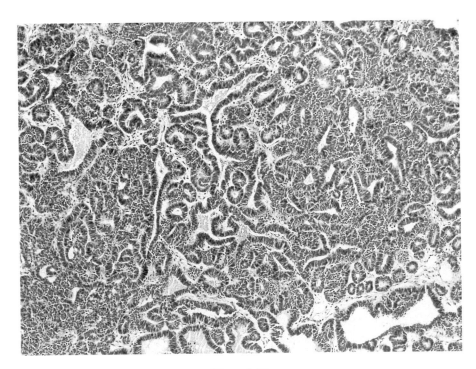

Figure 1-22
NEPHROBLASTOMA
Monophasic epithelial pattern is predominant.

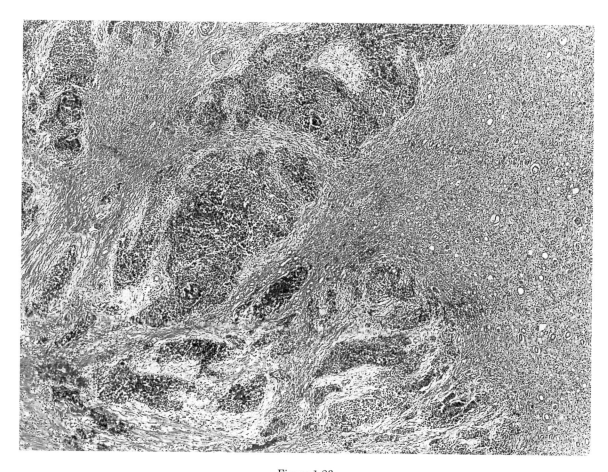

Figure 1-23
NEPHROBLASTOMA
Invasive diffuse blastemal pattern.

seem diffusely infiltrative rather than sharply circumscribed (fig. 1-23). Nevertheless, such lesions generally respond to current therapeutic regimens and are not classified among those with unfavorable histology. Most often, nephroblastomas composed of blastemal cells without distinct aggregation patterns have a more cohesive appearance (fig. 1-25). These lesions often have a rich vascular supply and are less aggressively invasive on histologic sections. Vague hints of tubular formation may be present. The blastemal cells of this pattern are usually rounded or polygonal but may be slightly elongated (fig. 1-25). Their nuclei are relatively small and regular, with round or oval shapes predominating. Chromatin tends to be slightly coarse but evenly distributed and nucleoli are usually small. It should be noted that details of nuclear structure may vary markedly under differing conditions of fixation. Delayed fixation often produces coarse clumping and cross-linking fixatives can make the chromatin appear quite delicate. Cytoplasm is scanty and usually does not stain well with hematoxylin and eosin (H&E) although granular, brightly acidophilic cytoplasmic staining may be observed in some regions. Cytoplasmic acidophilia is usually accompanied by nuclear pyknosis and is a degenerative phenomenon. Cell borders are often indistinct especially when formalin fixation is used. Mitotic figures are extremely numerous in most specimens.

The *serpentine blastemal pattern* is one of the most frequently encountered components of nephroblastomas (figs. 1-26, 1-27). It is characterized by undulating cords of blastemal cells set in a loose, myxoid or fibromyxoid stroma. The cords are relatively even, with frequent anastomoses. This

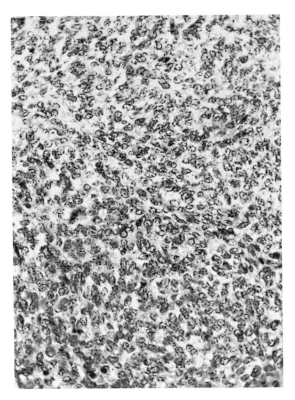

Figure 1-24
NEPHROBLASTOMA

When the diffuse, noncohesive pattern of blastema pre-dominates, it may be confused with other small cell tumors of childhood (X265). (Fig. 43 from Fascicle 12, 2nd Series.)

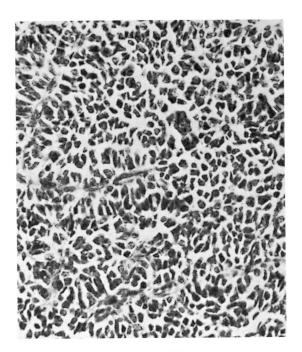

Figure 1-25
NEPHROBLASTOMA

Diffuse blastemal pattern with cohesive cells showing evidence of early tubulogenesis. (Fig. 48 from Fascicle 12, 2nd Series.)

pattern tends to be cohesive and usually lacks the aggressive invasiveness characterizing some diffuse blastemal nephroblastomas. The blaste-mal cords are sharply defined. The serpentine pattern of blastemal nephroblastoma is rarely confused with other primitive neoplasms of childhood and is virtually diagnostic. Even so, some specimens contain areas of progressive widening of the cell cords with gradual transition toward the cohesive type of diffuse blastemal pattern (fig. 1-27).

The *nodular blastemal pattern* resembles the serpentine pattern except that the blastemal islands are rounded and presumably spherical if seen three dimensionally (fig. 1-28). The stroma is similar to that of the serpentine pattern. Well-defined tubules may be present centrally in some nodules, a configuration reminiscent of the con-densations of blastema around the ampullary ends of the branching ureteric buds in the devel-oping kidney.

A *basaloid blastemal pattern* results when the serpentine or nodular patterns are outlined in a distinctive epithelial layer (fig. 1-29).

Most nephroblastomas have an *epithelial component* of differentiation. In some lesions, this is rare rosettes that are barely recognizable as early tubular forms; other nephroblastomas are composed predominantly or exclusively of easily recognizable tubular or papillary ele-ments (figs. 1-30, 1-31) (40). Most epithelial structures recapitulate various stages of normal nephrogenesis: tubules usually resemble devel-oping collecting ducts or nephrons in the fetal kidney; other epithelial structures resemble var-ious stages of glomerulogenesis (figs. 1-32, 1-33); and some glomerular structures closely resem-ble those of normal kidneys. Although glomeru-lar structures in nephroblastomas usually lack capillaries, many exceptions exist. The degree of differentiation in the nephronic elements varies greatly. Foci of mature cell types with low mitotic rates may represent evolution toward a benign state, a process comparable to the maturation of

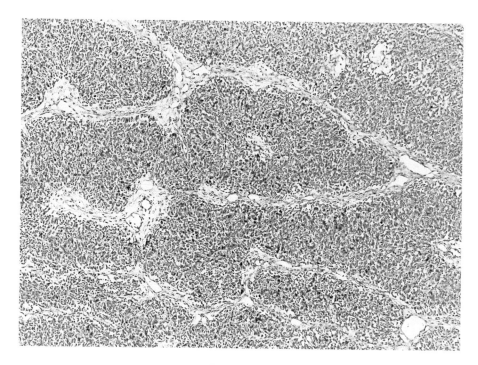

Figure 1-26
NEPHROBLASTOMA
Serpentine blastemal pattern.

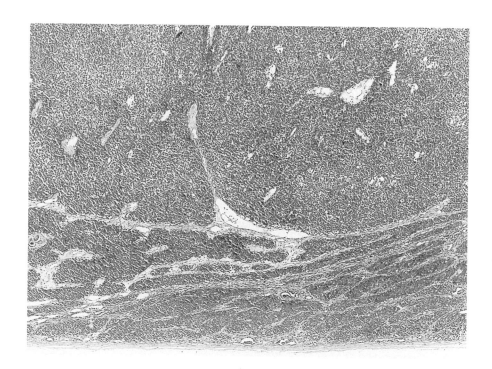

Figure 1-27
NEPHROBLASTOMA
Serpentine and diffuse blastemal patterns.

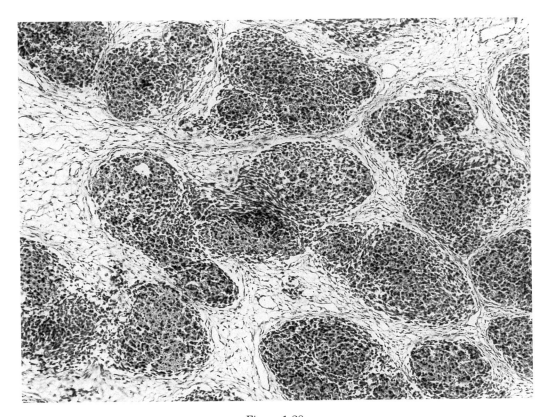

Figure 1-28
NEPHROBLASTOMA
Nodular blastemal pattern.

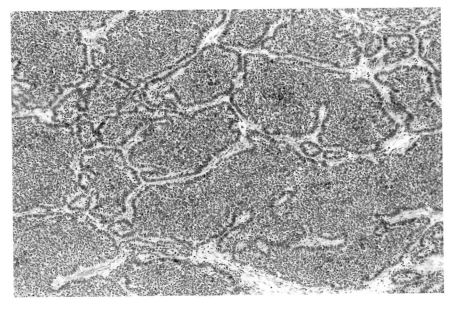

Figure 1-29
NEPHROBLASTOMA
Basaloid blastemal pattern.

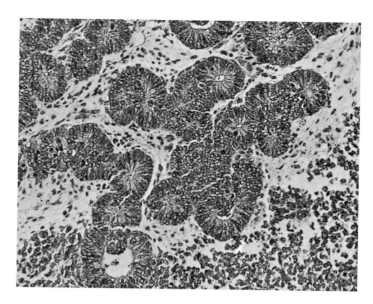

Figure 1-30
NEPHROBLASTOMA
Embryonal tubular pattern, with tall columnar cells and small lumina. (Fig. 50 from Fascicle 12, 2nd Series.)

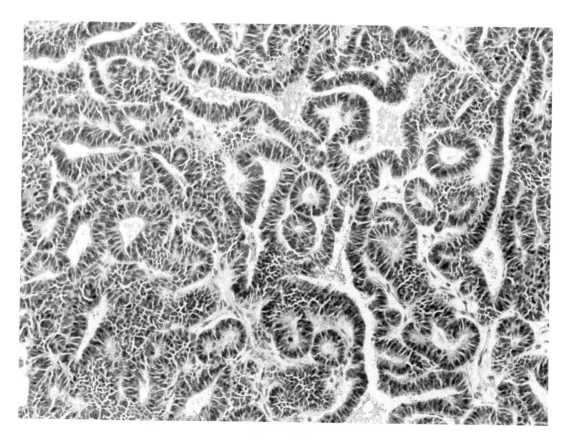

Figure 1-31
NEPHROBLASTOMA
Tubular structures predominate in this lesion.

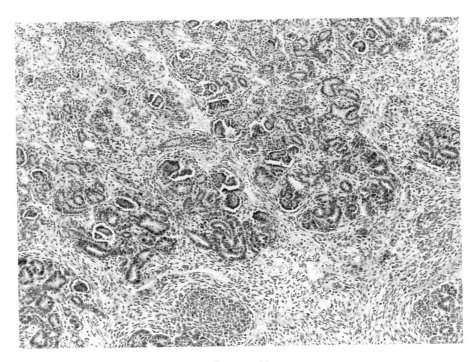

Figure 1-32
NEPHROBLASTOMA
Various stages of tubular and glomerular differentiation can be seen.

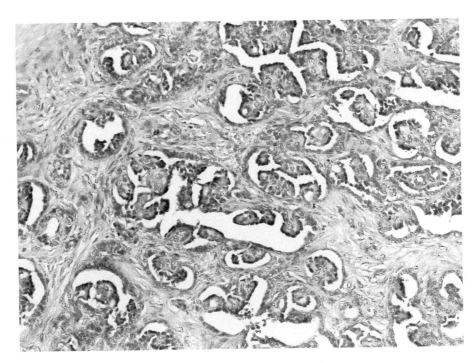

Figure 1-33
NEPHROBLASTOMA
Relatively mature glomeruli predominate in this field.

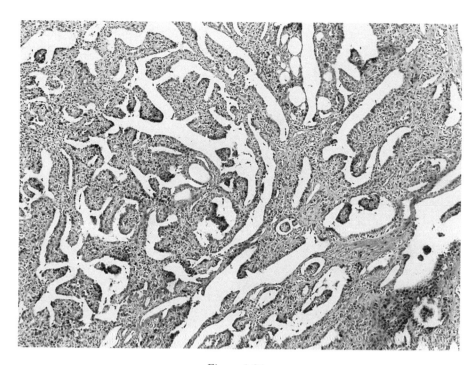

Figure 1-34
NEPHROBLASTOMA
Mature tubulopapillary pattern with low cell density and sparse to absent mitotic figures.

neuroblastomas into ganglioneuromas (figs. 1-33–1-35). Heterologous epithelial differentiation may occur, the most common elements being mucinous and squamous epithelium (figs. 1-36, 1-37). Occasionally, ciliated epithelium is present (fig. 1-38).

A variety of *stromal patterns* may occur. Myxoid and spindle cells resembling embryonic mesenchyme are found in nearly all specimens, where they form the matrix for most of the blastemal and epithelial foci. Smooth muscle and mature fibroblasts may be present. Skeletal muscle is the most common heterologous stromal cell type and large fields of the tumor often contain this pattern (fig. 1-39). Cells with cross-striations and central nuclei are present in many nephroblastomas. More primitive myoblastic elements can also be found, including the condensed mesenchyme characteristic of the "cambium layer" of botryoid embryonal rhabdomyosarcomas (fig. 1-40).

Almost any type of stromal differentiation, including adipose tissue, cartilage, bone and osteoid, mature ganglion cells, and neuroglial tissue, may be observed in nephroblastomas (figs. 1-41–1-44) (56,59,61). The heterogeneity may be so prominent as to suggest a teratoma and most lesions reported in the literature as renal teratoma are probably nephroblastomas. Terms such as "fetal rhabdomyomatous nephroblastoma" and "teratoid nephroblastoma" have been suggested for lesions with prominent heterologous differentiation (41,60,78,83). The structural diversity inherent in the nephroblastoma spectrum could engender an endless proliferation of descriptive terms and we do not encourage the use of subdesignation based upon morphology alone. Only those subtypes with important and consistent clinical implications should be considered in categories with separate names.

Recognition of histologic diversity in nephroblastomas is important primarily in achieving the correct diagnosis. The effect of current therapy is such that the majority of tumors, regardless of their heterogeneity, can be considered in the so-called "favorable" group. Nevertheless, a small percentage of nephroblastomas are associated with an adverse outcome and most of these

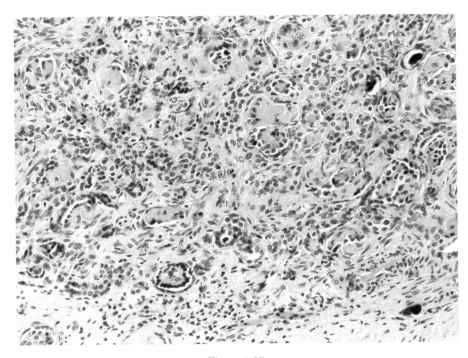

Figure 1-35
NEPHROBLASTOMA
Mature pattern with glomerular, tubular, and stromal cells showing little or no proliferative activity.

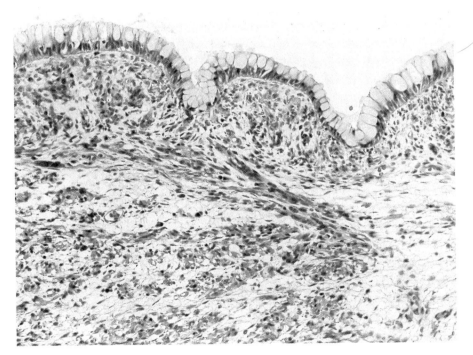

Figure 1-36
NEPHROBLASTOMA
Mucinous epithelium is sometimes a prominent feature.

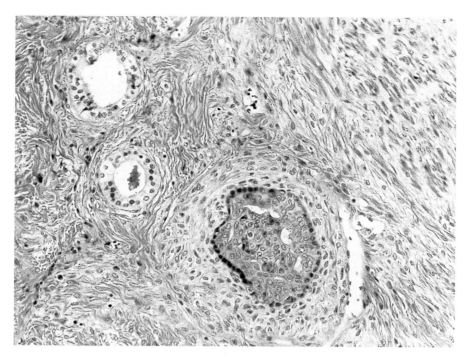

Figure 1-37
NEPHROBLASTOMA
A squamous epithelial focus.

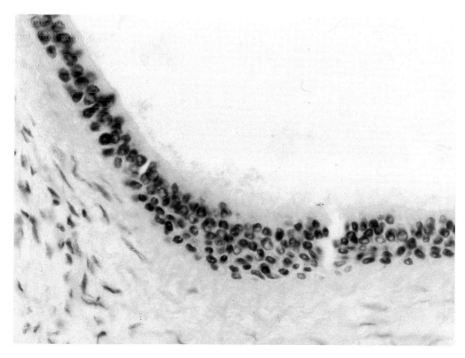

Figure 1-38
NEPHROBLASTOMA
Ciliated epithelium is occasionally encountered in a teratoid nephroblastoma.

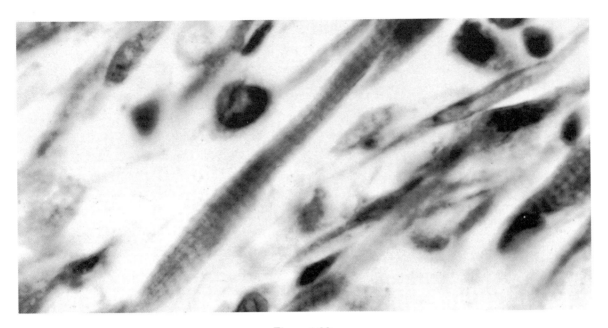

Figure 1-39
NEPHROBLASTOMA
Skeletal muscle is a commonly encountered element. (Fig. 58 from Fascicle 12, 2nd Series.)

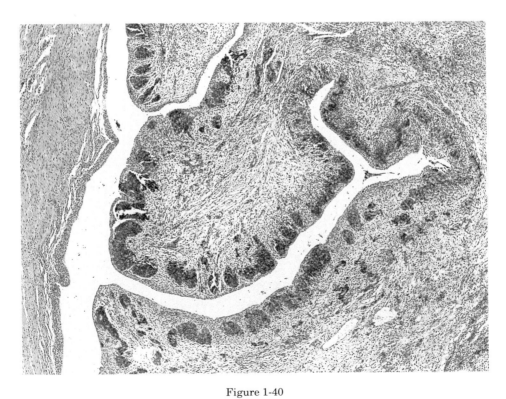

Figure 1-40
NEPHROBLASTOMA
Botryoid protrusions of tumor cells into lumen of the pelvicaliceal system. (See figure 1-18 for the gross appearance.)

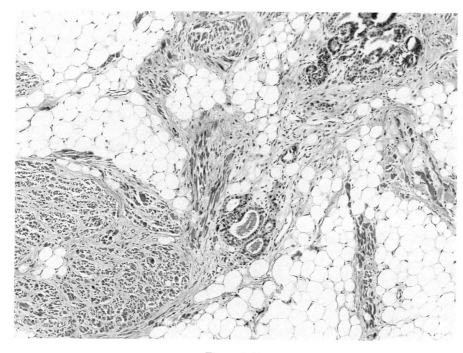

Figure 1-41
NEPHROBLASTOMA
Example showing adipose differentiation. The nodule of skeletal muscle seen near the left edge of the field is usually found in association with adipose elements.

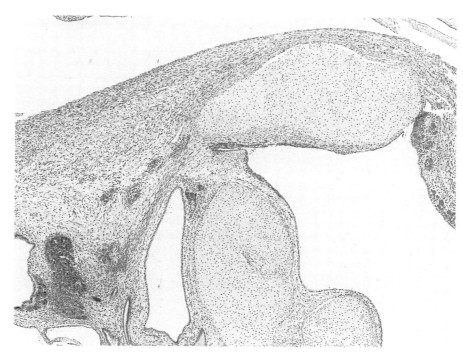

Figure 1-42
NEPHROBLASTOMA
Cartilage formation is evident.

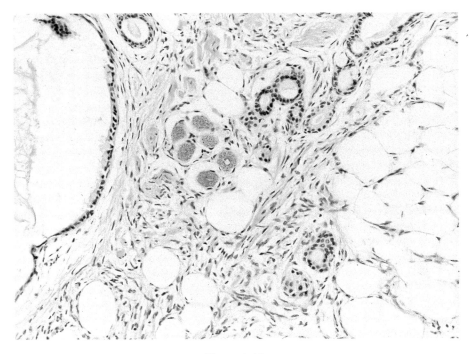

Figure 1-43
NEPHROBLASTOMA
A cluster of six mature ganglion cells is present near the center, along with other mature tubular and stromal elements in this teratoid nephroblastoma.

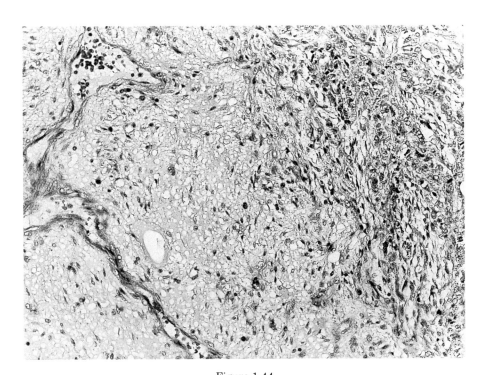

Figure 1-44
NEPHROBLASTOMA
A focus of neuroglial differentiation was confirmed by strongly positive staining for glial fibrillary acidic protein (GFAP).

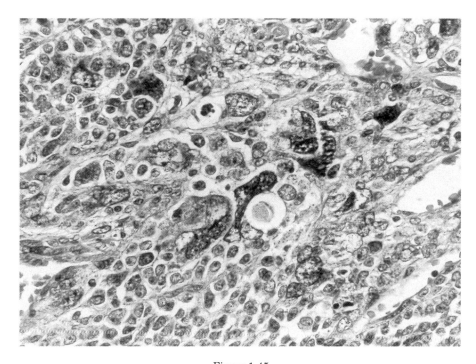

Figure 1-45
ANAPLASTIC NEPHROBLASTOMA
This field shows the huge, irregular-shaped nuclei that are a major criterion for recognition of anaplasia.

are recognized pathologically because of their "unfavorable" histology: areas of nuclear anaplasia or, rarely, foci of high-grade renal cell carcinoma (15,21,23,29,32,85).

As defined by the NWTS pathology center, anaplasia refers to extreme nuclear atypia rather than lack of cellular differentiation and presumably represents the presence of hypertetraploid DNA content. Histologic confirmation requires: 1) the presence of multipolar mitotic figures, and 2) marked nuclear enlargement with the major dimension of affected nuclei being at least three times that of apparently nonanaplastic nuclei in other areas of the specimen (figs. 1-45–1-48) (85). Nuclear enlargement should involve all diameters of the nucleus and should not be confused with simple elongation. The mitotic abnormalities must be of a type that indicates unequivocal increases in the total amount of DNA. Simple lagging of chromosomes on an anaphase spindle, for example, although constituting an "abnormal mitosis," should not be a criterion for anaplasia. Uneven separation of a diploid metaphase plate can produce an X- or Y-shaped mitotic figure mimicking tripolar or tetrapolar mitoses, but the

total length of the X or Y figure approximates that of a normal-appearing metaphase (fig. 1-49). In a true multipolar mitotic figure, each component is as large, or larger, than a normal metaphase (fig. 1-48). Multipolar mitotic figures are required for the diagnosis of anaplasia although in a limited sample, such as a small biopsy, marked nucleomegaly alone may be sufficient to suggest this change. Anaplasia is most consistently associated with poor prognosis when it is diffusely distributed (40). Focal anaplasia, recently redefined as the presence of one or a few sharply localized regions in a primary tumor, the majority of which contain no nuclear atypia, is associated with a prognosis approximating that for lesions of favorable histology (40). It is important to note that focal anaplasia as now defined, requires that the anaplastic changes be confined to intrarenal tumor sites. This determination is best achieved if at least one generous section is prepared for each centimeter of tumor dimension. In multicentric neoplasms, each individual tumor should be sampled using this criterion. Even so, anaplasia has no effect on prognosis for nephroblastomas confined to the kidney, i.e., stage I lesions (85). This and other evidence

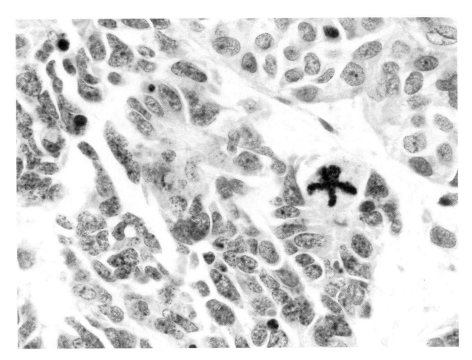

Figure 1-46
ANAPLASTIC NEPHROBLASTOMA
Note the multipolar mitotic figure.

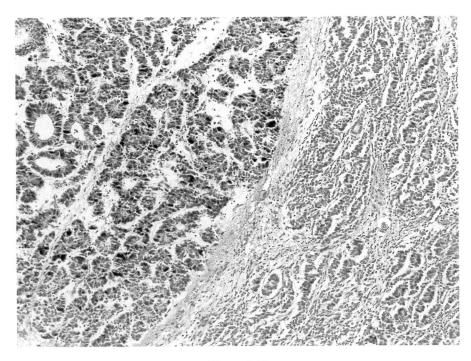

Figure 1-47
NEPHROBLASTOMA WITH FOCAL ANAPLASIA
A sharply demarcated nodular region at the left of this field was the only site of anaplasia in this tumor. The size discrepancy between nuclei in the two halves of this field is apparent even under low magnification.

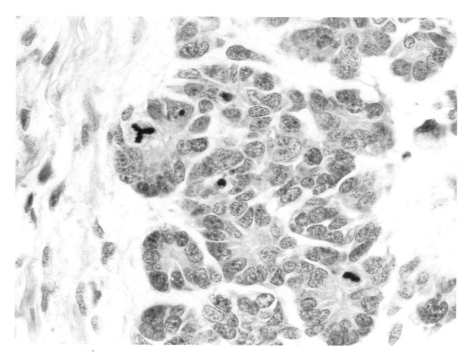

Figure 1-48
ANAPLASTIC NEPHROBLASTOMA

In a true tripolar mitosis, as seen toward the left edge, each limb is nearly the size of a more normal metaphase plate, as seen near the right lower corner. (Compare with figure 1-49.)

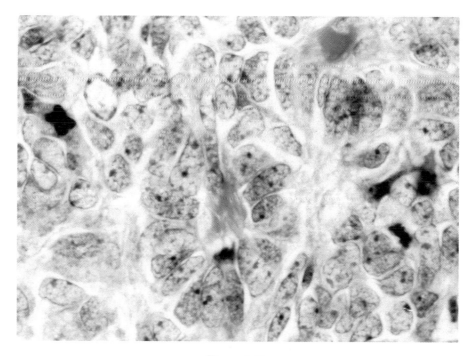

Figure 1-49
NEPHROBLASTOMA

An X-shaped mitotic figure, seen near the left upper corner, is approximately the same size as the apparently normal-sized metaphase plate near the right lower corner. This appearance can result from uneven separation of a normal metaphase, and should not be confused with truly multipolar mitotic figures. (Compare with figure 1-48.)

suggest that anaplasia is a marker of increased resistance to current therapy rather than a sign of increased tumor aggressiveness. Therefore, stage I nephroblastomas are treated similarly whether or not they contain cells with anaplasia.

In the NWTS, histologic anaplasia was observed in only 4.5 percent of nephroblastomas. Anaplasia is rare in neoplasms diagnosed during the first 2 years of life, increases in prevalence to approximately 10 percent by age 6 years, and remains at this level in tumors detected through the remainder of childhood and adolescence. Limited experience with adult nephroblastomas suggests that anaplasia has the same prognostic significance as in children. The rate of anaplasia is two to three times greater in blacks than whites.

Current efforts to refine the definition of unfavorable histology in nephroblastomas using quantitative cytometric techniques have yielded conflicting results. Flow cytometry is less effective than conventional histology in identifying those tumors associated with a poor prognosis, although flow cytometry in combination with high resolution karyotypic analysis is more sensitive (38–44,46,47–54,66). Image analysis is a more promising approach, with abnormalities of nuclear shape correlated with adverse outcome (42).

Foci of renal cell carcinoma within otherwise characteristic nephroblastomas are rare (15,21). When carcinomatous regions are of high cytologic grade, they confer an aggressive behavior and an adverse prognosis similar to that of a high-grade carcinoma in adults. This histologic pattern could be added to anaplastic nuclear changes as an indicator of unfavorable histology in nephroblastoma, but it remains to be determined how much of this change is required in order to confer an unfavorable prognosis.

Immunohistochemical studies have a limited role in the pathologic evaluation of nephroblastomas. The results reflect the cell types and levels of differentiation present in the lesion: skeletal muscle fibers, neural elements, and tubular formations show the immunohistochemical characteristics of these cell types (39,82). Structures in nephroblastomas that resemble components of the developing kidney have the same immunohistochemical features as their normal counterparts. The blastemal cells of nephroblastomas regularly express vimentin but other differentiation markers are usually absent (82). No single immunohistochemical reaction has been diagnostic for nephroblastoma.

Ultrastructural studies are usually not required for the diagnosis of nephroblastoma but can be helpful when a predominantly blastemal tumor must be differentiated from other "small blue cell tumors" such as lymphoma or neuroblastoma. Electron microscopy is of value if only a small amount of tissue is available. Ultrastructurally, nephroblastoma cells closely resemble those of the developing metanephros (64). The findings are dependent upon the cell types present and their degree of differentiation (fig. 1-50). The loosely aggregated, myxoid-appearing stroma seen with the light microscope appears more primitive ultrastructurally than the closely packed cells termed blastema. Primitive blastemal cells have sparse, poorly developed organelles; numerous free ribosomes; and a moderate number of mitochondria. Many cells interpreted as blastemal with the light microscope exhibit well-developed cell junctions and numerous organelles. A layer of thick, flocculent, electron-dense material frequently adheres to the cell surface. Microvilli are variable in number and prominence. Phagolysosomes and lipid droplets may occur.

Ultrastructural features that may be helpful in confirming the diagnosis in monophasic, poorly differentiated nephroblastomas include well-developed desmosomes and the characteristic flocculent coating. Cilia are more numerous than in other childhood tumors. Paired, confronting cisternae in mitotically active blastemal cells are usually a more prominent feature than in most other pediatric renal neoplasms (64).

Differential Diagnosis. Nephroblastomas must be distinguished from other pediatric renal tumors and neoplasms composed of so-called small blue cells. Table 1-4 represents an estimate of the likelihood of each tumor in childhood as a whole; these estimates do not reflect the likelihood of each neoplasm during various periods of childhood. Mesoblastic nephromas and rhabdoid tumors are far less common than nephroblastomas but occur more frequently during infancy than adolescence. Conversely, anaplastic nephroblastoma is virtually never encountered in infants. The differential diagnosis between nephroblastoma and other primary renal neoplasms of infancy and childhood is considered in detail in the sections describing those lesions.

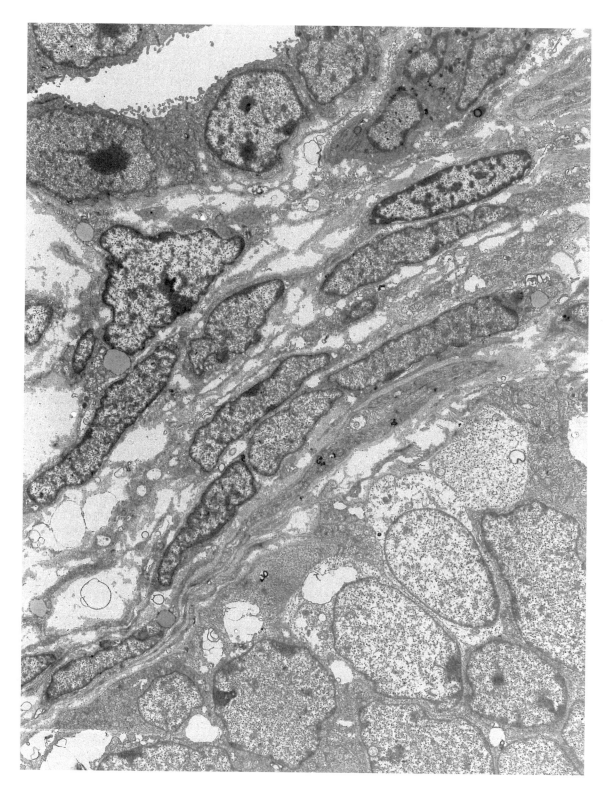

Figure 1-50
NEPHROBLASTOMA
Ultrastructural appearance of a triphasic specimen, with epithelial differentiation near the top of the field, stromal cells near the center, and blastemal cells near the bottom. (Courtesy of Dr. Gary W. Mierau, Denver, CO.)

Table 1-4

DIFFERENTIAL DIAGNOSIS OF PEDIATRIC RENAL NEOPLASMS

Neoplasm	Estimated Relative Frequency (%)
Nephroblastoma (nonanaplastic)	80
Nephroblastoma (anaplastic)	5
Mesoblastic nephroma	5
Clear cell sarcoma	4
Rhabdoid tumor	2
Miscellaneous	4
Neurogenic tumors	
Renal carcinoma, oncocytic tumors	
Angiomyolipoma	
Lymphoma	
Other rare neoplasms	

Nephroblastomas can resemble other poorly differentiated neoplasms of childhood. The differential diagnosis is especially important in abdominal tumors so large that the origin cannot be established clinically or at metastatic sites in cases of disseminated disease. Perhaps the most frequently encountered differential diagnostic problem is distinguishing nephroblastoma and neuroblastoma. Clinical features favoring neuroblastoma include elevated levels of catecholamine metabolites; stippled calcification on imaging studies; and widespread metastases to organs other than lung, liver, and lymph nodes. Histologically, the rosettes of some neuroblastomas or primitive neuroepithelial tumors may resemble the nascent tubular formations of tubular nephroblastoma (fig. 1-51). Tubulogenesis in a nephroblastoma is usually characterized by a single layer of nuclei arranged in parallel while the classic Homer Wright rosette of a neuroblastoma tends to have a zone of nuclear concentration around a central fibrillary core, without the formation of a distinct layer of parallel nuclei. Immunohistochemical studies and electron microscopy are sometimes required to resolve difficult cases.

The cells of a lymphoma occasionally resemble the diffuse blastemal pattern of a nephroblastoma but immunohistochemical phenotyping usually resolves the problem.

A nephroblastoma with heterologous patterns may resemble a mesothelioma, synovial sarcoma, hepatoblastoma, or pancreatoblastoma. Immunohistochemistry may be helpful in selected cases. The recently described intra-abdominal desmoplastic small round cell tumor should be added to the list (43). The bands of small blue cells alternating with desmoplastic zones seen in this tumor can resemble the serpentine blastemal pattern of nephroblastoma, however, the stroma of nephroblastoma is rarely rich in collagen. The small cell component of desmoplastic small cell tumor for neural and muscle markers is strongly positive. A distinctive 11:22 reciprocal translocation was found in one case of desmoplastic small cell tumor (72).

Mode of Dissemination. Nephroblastomas generally have a restricted pattern of extension (29). The most common sites of metastasis are regional lymph nodes, lungs, and liver (fig. 1-52). Metastatic sites other than these are unusual and should always suggest alternative diagnoses. Bony metastases, for example, occur in less than 1 percent of nephroblastomas. Unusual sites include the spinal epidural space and mediastinal lymph nodes following pulmonary metastasis (25). Tumors that rupture before or during nephrectomy may become implanted widely in the flank or peritoneum.

Staging. The most widely accepted staging system for nephroblastomas is that of the NWTS (Table 1-5) (36). Stage I tumors are contained within the renal capsule. This seemingly simple criterion can be difficult to assess when the renal capsule is part of a composite tumor capsule, which in some instances consists of fused intrarenal, renal, and perirenal connective tissue. It is possible for a tumor to extend into the perirenal fat, form a pseudocapsule, and appear to be encapsulated by the renal capsule when the invaded fat disappears (81). This progression from stage I to stage II can sometimes be detected by sampling the tumor capsule at its intersection with the renal capsule. In this region, one can sometimes track laterally from the deepest level of tumor penetration and demonstrate that tumor cells are in the same plane as perirenal fat (fig. 1-53).

Nephroblastomas are often surrounded by a layer of active granulation tissue (fig. 1-54). These inflammatory pseudocapsules are usually associated with perirenal hemorrhage or extensive

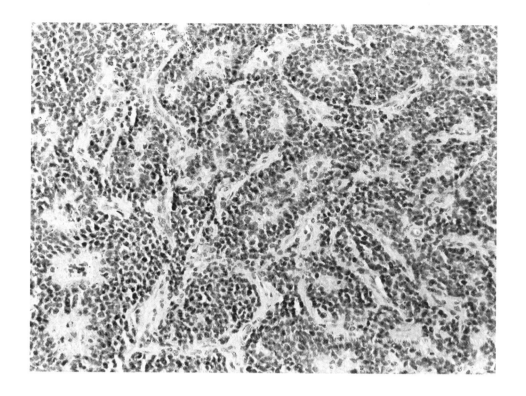

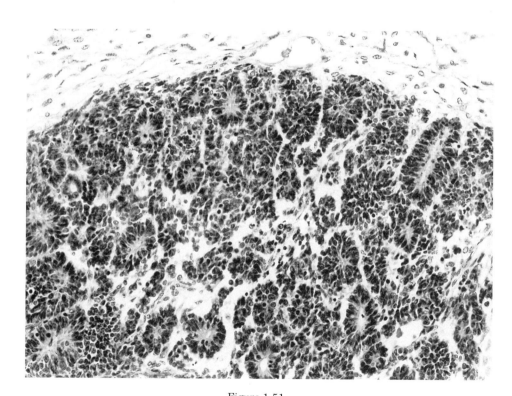

Figure 1-51
NEUROEPITHELIAL ROSETTES VERSUS TUBULOGENESIS IN NEPHROBLASTOMA
Rosettes in a primitive neuroepithelial tumor of the kidney (top) often lack the nuclear concentration around the center of the rosette that is usual in early tubular formations of nephroblastomas (bottom).

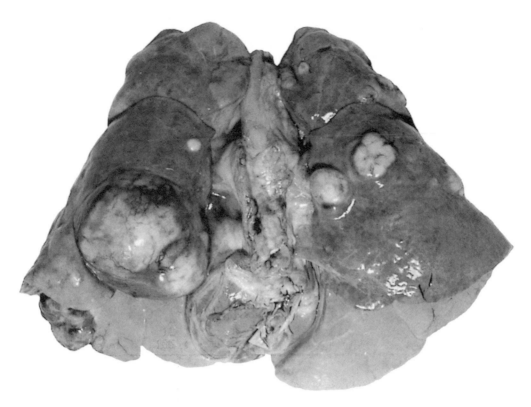

Figure 1-52
NEPHROBLASTOMA
Lung metastases. (Fig. 67 from Fascicle 12, 2nd Series.)

Table 1-5

STAGING OF PEDIATRIC RENAL TUMORS (NATIONAL WILMS TUMOR STUDY)

Stage	Definition
I	*Limited to kidney and completely resected.* Renal capsule intact. Renal sinus may be infiltrated but not beyond hilar plane.
II	*Tumor infiltrates beyond kidney, but completely resected.* Includes cases with tumor penetration of renal capsule or infiltration of renal vessels beyond the hilar plane, biopsied tumors, and those with local spillage confined to flank. Simple protrusion of the tumor beyond capsule or hilar plane acceptable for state I designation.
III	*Residual nonhematogenous tumor confined to abdomen.* Includes cases with one of the following: a) Tumor in abdominal lymph nodes; b) Diffuse peritoneal contamination by direct tumor growth, tumor implants, or spillage into peritoneum before or during surgery; c) Involvement of specimen margins grossly or microscopically; d) Residual tumor in abdomen.
IV	*Hematogenous metastases.*
V	*Bilateral renal involvement at diagnosis.* The tumors in each kidney should be separately substaged in these cases.

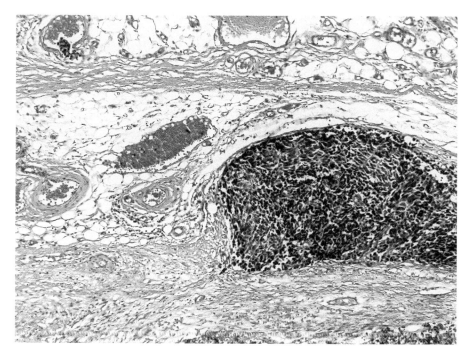

Figure 1-53
"HORIZONTAL ANALYSIS" OF RENAL TUMOR CAPSULE
The outermost tumor cells are in the same layer as perirenal fat, despite being overlain by a fibrous capsule. This appearance is consistent with a stage II designation by the NWTS definition.

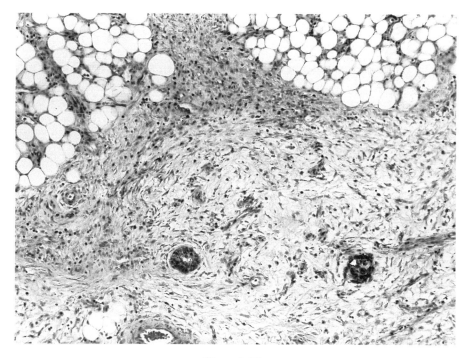

Figure 1-54
INFLAMMATORY PSEUDOCAPSULE
Reactive granulation tissue surrounds the kidney and tumor. In this field, two small islands of tumor are present within the pseudocapsule.

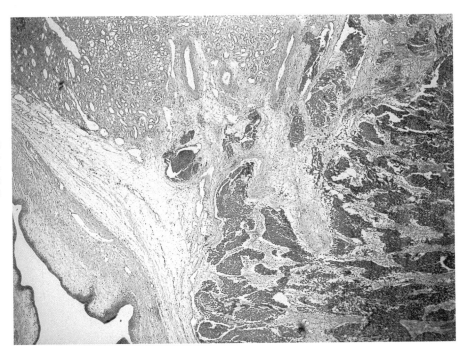

Figure 1-55
NEPHROBLASTOMA
Tumor cells are present within the vessels and soft tissue of the renal sinus. Note the adjacent pelvicaliceal structure and lack of encapsulation of the cortex in the sinus.

necrosis of the peripheral regions of the neoplasm. The presence of an inflammatory pseudocapsule does not necessarily disqualify a lesion from being stage I, although relapse rates are somewhat higher in such cases, requiring that the inflammatory nature of the capsule be noted in histologic descriptions (81).

The renal sinus is a major source of confusion in differentiating stage I from stage II lesions (fig. 1-55). The renal sinus is the most common site of extension of tumors beyond the renal parenchyma and it is essential that this region be generously sampled for histologic analysis. The NWTS definition for stage I accepts minor degrees of infiltration of the soft tissues and vessels of the renal sinus as long as the infiltration remains within the hilar plane. This criterion is difficult to apply in practice since the hilar plane of neoplastic kidneys is usually distorted by the tumor. If extensive infiltration of the renal sinus is present, a stage II designation is generally preferred. Simple protrusion of encapsulated tumor into or beyond the hilar plane is of no significance and such lesions can be classified as stage I.

In a study of stage I cases performed by the NWTS, four features were associated with an increased rate of relapse: the presence of an inflammatory pseudocapsule; invasion of the renal sinus; extensive infiltration of the renal capsule without complete penetration; and tumor infiltration of intrarenal vessels (81). When all four of these features were absent, no relapses were observed. These cases are currently being considered by the NWTS for a therapeutic trial using nephrectomy alone. It is important, therefore, that pathologists sample the renal sinus, tumor-kidney junction, tumor capsule, and uninvolved renal parenchyma generously in order to evaluate these features.

The distinction of stage II from stage III nephroblastoma is based in part upon evaluation of the specimen margin. This analysis is complicated by the extreme friability of most nephroblastomas, creating a situation where tumor cells are usually displaced during sectioning of the gross specimen. This problem is compounded by retraction of the specimen capsule as it is incised. Problems with margin evaluation can be largely avoided if specimen surfaces are carefully inked prior to sectioning or selectively inked at foci suspicious for capsular involvement. The common practice of incising nephrectomy specimens in the operating room, while edifying for the surgical staff, often renders the specimen surface unevaluable and should be avoided.

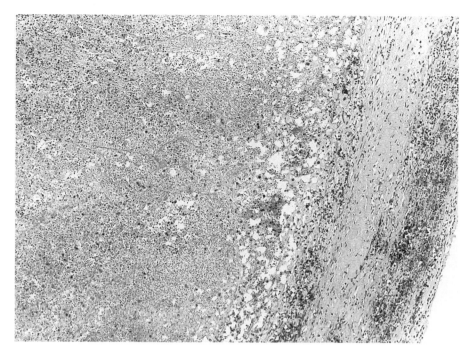

Figure 1-56
NEPHROBLASTOMA
Total tumor necrosis due to
chemotherapy.

Tumor thrombi in renal veins are another potential source for staging confusion, since the resected vein margin usually retracts when severed and tumor protruding from the lumen may seem to represent marginal involvement. The surgeon is best able to determine whether or not the tumor thrombus extends to the resection margin.

Bilateral nephroblastomas occur in approximately 5 percent of cases and are designated stage V by the NWTS. This designation has several disadvantages. Since the staging scheme represents a numerical progression that relates to increasing likelihood for tumor relapse and death, the stage V designation can falsely suggest that the prognosis is even worse than that for stage IV. However, the prognosis in bilateral cases is determined by the stage of the most advanced tumor as well as by the presence or absence of other prognostic determinants, such as anaplasia. A stage V tumor that has stage I nephroblastomas of favorable histology in both kidneys generally has a very favorable outcome (26). Such cases can be assigned a substage designation using the stage of the most advanced lesion as the substage determinate (e.g., stage V, substage I). It has been suggested that the stage V designation be replaced by a prefix, such as the letter "B" (20).

Treatment. Therapy for nephroblastoma is one of the great success stories in modern oncology (37,86). Dactinomycin and vincristine are the most effective drugs for most of cases with favorable histology and are now in standard use around the world. These chemicals are used in conjunction with surgery, without radiotherapy, for all stage I and II lesions with favorable histology. Tumors with unfavorable histology are treated similarly, as long as they are stage I. Radiotherapy and more toxic chemotherapeutic agents are used for patients with stage I to V disease. Most patients with nephroblastomas are treated with the relatively nontoxic regimens since almost 70 percent have low-stage lesions with favorable histology.

The effects of therapy on the histology of nephroblastoma has been studied by the NWTS (86). Actively proliferating embryonal cell types rich in blastemal cell populations usually undergo a dramatic response while mature tubular and skeletal muscle cells tend to remain unaltered (figs. 1-56, 1-57). Anaplastic cells are unaffected. Infiltrating populations of histologically viable-appearing embryonal elements with easily identifiable mitoses appearing after recent therapy are a sign of treatment failure.

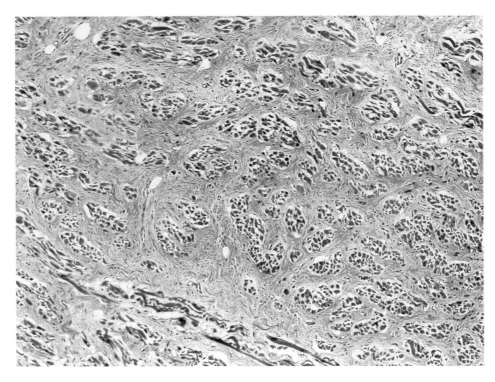

Figure 1-57
NEPHROBLASTOMA
Persistence of mature skeletal muscle following chemotherapy. Mature, nonreplicating cell types are often unaffected by therapy, but do not necessarily imply a poor therapeutic result.

Prognosis. As indicated by the histologic classification and staging schemes, the majority of nephroblastomas are low stage, have a favorable histology, and are associated with an excellent prognosis. A favorable outcome can be expected even among neoplasms with small foci of cellular anaplasia and small, focal areas of capsular penetration. Prognosis is apparently not effected primarily by tumor size or weight. The most significant unfavorable factors are age at detection, high stage, and unfavorable histology.

NEPHROBLASTOMATOSIS AND NEPHROGENIC RESTS

Precursors of nephroblastoma are encountered in 25 to 40 percent of cases (19,22,27,58,70). Similar lesions have been observed in approximately 1 percent of routine postmortem examinations in infants (24). Recent studies have helped to clarify the formerly complex and confusing concepts and terminology concerning these lesions (19,22).

The term nephrogenic rest has been proposed for abnormally persistent foci of embryonal cells that are capable of developing into nephroblastomas (22). The term supplants the designation persistent nodular blastema, since the lesions are not always nodular and often contain no blastemal cells. Nephrogenic rests are further classified into perilobar (PLNR) and intralobar (ILNR) types. These categories have a number of distinguishing structural features (figs. 1-58, 1-59) (Table 1-6). The major subtypes can be further categorized on the basis of their apparent function into incipient, dormant, involuting (sclerosing), hyperplastic, and neoplastic.

The term *nephroblastomatosis* is more specifically defined as designating the presence of diffuse or multifocal nephrogenic rests (or their neoplastic derivatives). Nephroblastomatosis can be further categorized according to the type of rests present. When only PLNR or ILNR are present, the designations *perilobar* or *intralobar nephroblastomatosis* is used; *combined nephroblastomatosis* refers

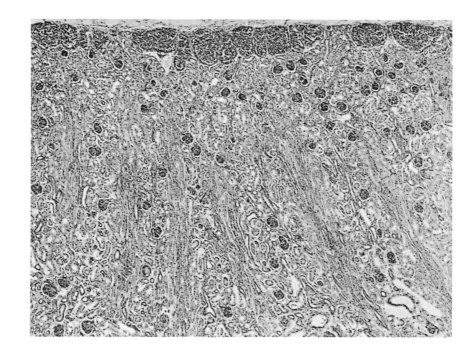

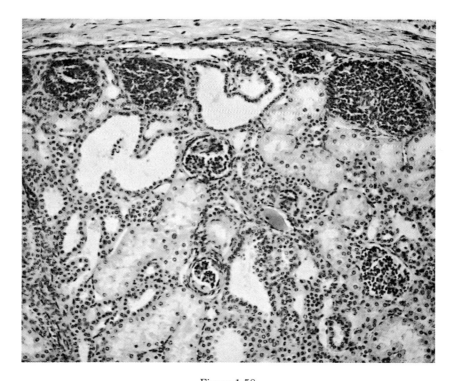

Figure 1-58
PERILOBAR NEPHROGENIC RESTS

Top: These rests are of microscopic size and composed of blastemal cells. Such rests are termed "incipient" in a neonate and "dormant" in an older infant or child. (Fig. 21 from Fascicle 12, 2nd Series.)

Bottom: Higher magnification of incipient or dormant rests, showing size relationship to adjacent glomeruli. (Fig. 25B from Fascicle 12, 2nd Series.)

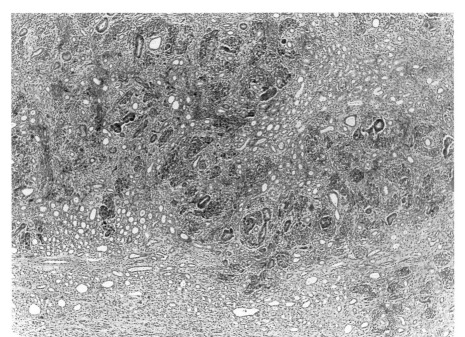

Figure 1-59
INTRALOBAR
NEPHROGENIC REST
This relatively small, blastemal lesion could be termed incipient or dormant, depending upon the age of the patient. Note the characteristic interstitial location, intermixed with normal nephronic elements.

Table 1-6

FEATURES DISTINGUISHING PERILOBAR FROM INTRALOBAR RESTS

	Perilobar Rests	Intralobar Rests
Position in lobe	Peripheral	Random
Margins	Sharp, demarcated	Irregular, interspersed
Composition	Blastema, tubules	Stroma, blastema, tubule
	Stroma scanty or sclerotic	Stroma often predominates
Distribution	Often unifocal	Usually multifocal

to the presence of both PLNR and ILNR. The extremely rare variant originally described by Hou and Holman (49), in which the entire renal parenchyma is composed of actively proliferating embryonal elements, is designated *universal nephroblastomatosis* (fig. 1-60, 1-61).

Both PLNR and ILNR can be subdivided into categories that reflect their development and morphology (19,22). *Incipient rests* are microscopic lesions with no evidence of proliferation, maturation, or involution which occur in newborns or young infants. *Dormant rests* describe the same lesions in an older patient (fig. 1-58). *Involuting (sclerosing) rests* are the most fre-

quently encountered lesions, especially in PLNR. These rests usually contain well-formed tubular structures lined by a single layer of low cuboidal basophilic epithelium containing few or no mitotic figures and encased in a dense collagenous stroma (fig. 1-62). The end stage of a sclerosing rest is termed an *obsolescent rest*. These lesions are composed entirely of collagenous stroma and are difficult to identify with certainty in the absence of other rests (fig. 1-63). *Hyperplastic rests* have undergone diffuse or focal proliferative overgrowth (fig. 1-64). Their most distinctive feature is a tendency to preserve the original shape of the rest. For example, if the original perilobar rest

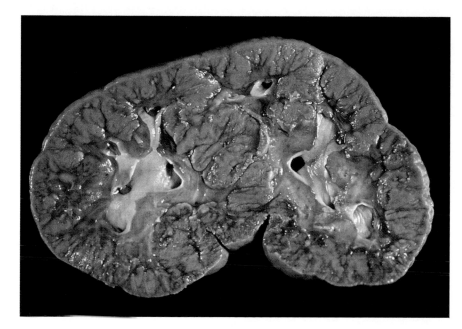

Figure 1-60
UNIVERSAL OR PANLOBAR
NEPHROBLASTOMATOSIS
The kidneys of this prematurely born neonatal male weighed 220 g combined, approximately ten times normal. Note extreme distortion of lobar architecture throughout. (Courtesy of Dr. Maria M. Rodriguez, Miami, FL.)

Figure 1-61
UNIVERSAL
NEPHROBLASTOMATOSIS
Mature and immature elements are intermingled throughout the renal parenchyma.

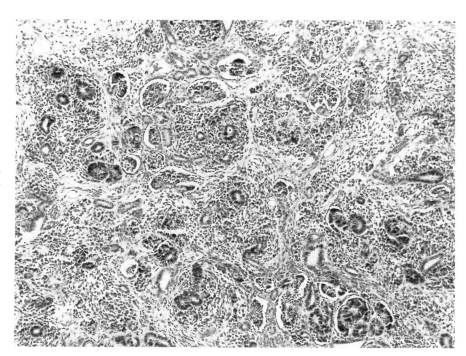

formed a more or less continuous band around the surface of the kidney (diffuse perilobar nephroblastomatosis), the hyperplastic overgrowth would produce the lesions seen in figures 1-65 and 1-66. The term *hyperplastic diffuse perilobar nephroblastomatosis* is appropriate for this abnormality. Diffusely hyperplastic overgrowth of discrete nephrogenic rests preserves

the original shape of the rest (fig. 1-67). The shape of the lesion is the most reliable clue to its nature. A small biopsy taken from the lesions shown in figures 1-65 to 1-67 could not be distinguished histologically or cytologically from nephroblastoma. Some rests have histologic features suggesting a hyperplastic growth superimposed upon a previous involutional phase, such

45

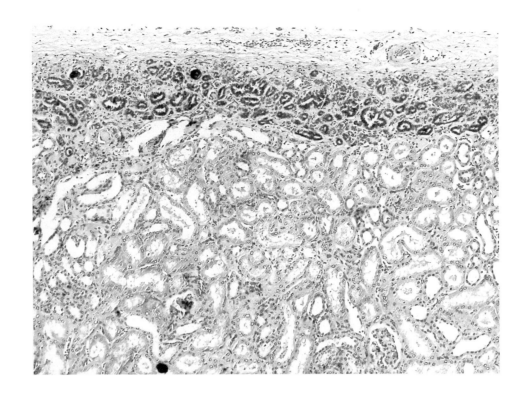

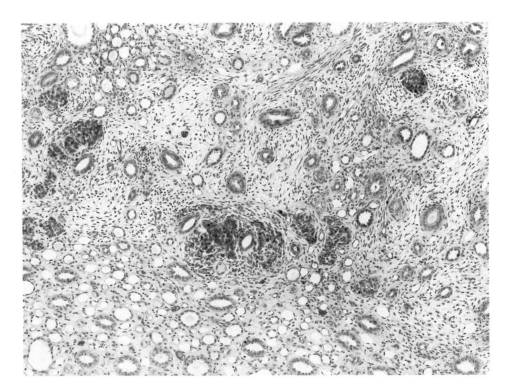

Figure 1-62
NEPHROGENIC RESTS

Top: Sclerosing perilobar nephrogenic rest.
Bottom: Sclerosing intralobar nephrogenic rest. This lesion is composed primarily of mature spindle cell stroma, though a few blastemal islands remain. When the latter elements are not present, sclerosing intralobar rests can resemble focal renal dysplasia.

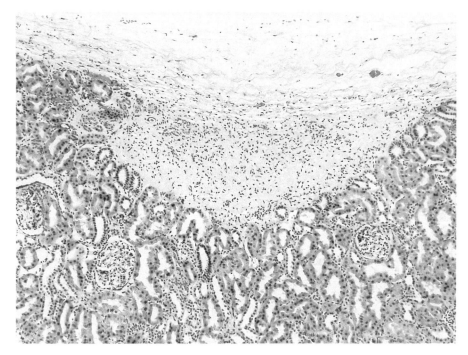

Figure 1-63
OBSOLESCENT PERILOBAR NEPHROGENIC REST
This lesion could be distinguished from other causes of focal scarring only by the presence of other perilobar rests in the adjacent cortical surface.

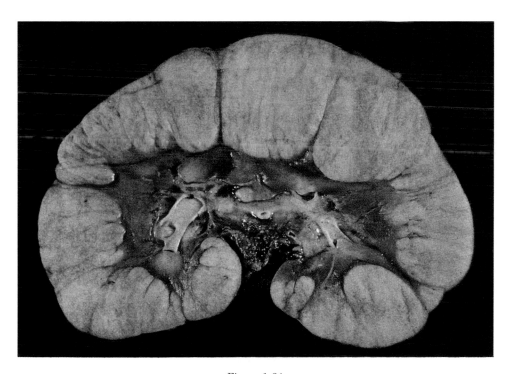

Figure 1-64
HYPERPLASTIC PERILOBAR NEPHROBLASTOMATOSIS
The kidney is enlarged but preserves its reniform shape due to relatively uniform overgrowth of a peripheral rim of nephroblastic tissue. (Courtesy of Dr. Frederic B. Askin, St. Louis, MO.)

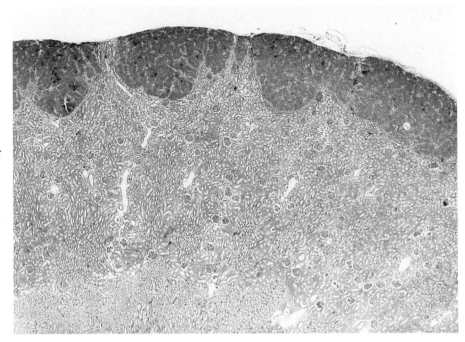

Figure 1-65
DIFFUSELY
HYPERPLASTIC
PERILOBAR
NEPHROBLASTOMATOSIS
A nearly confluent rind of perilobar rest tissue has undergone uniform overgrowth. Compare the size of this lesion to that of glomeruli. A more advanced stage of this process is shown in figure 1-64.

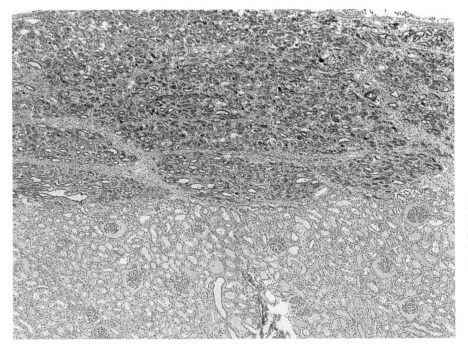

Figure 1-66
DIFFUSELY
HYPERPLASTIC
PERILOBAR
NEPHROBLASTOMATOSIS
IN THE
SCLEROSING STAGE
The thickness of the abnormal rind in this specimen implies a previously hyperplastic state that has subsequently become quiescent and assumed the appearance of a sclerosing perilobar rest.

as would occur with focal hyperplasia within a rest (figs. 1-68, 1-69). *Neoplastic rests,* within which one or more clonal neoplasms have developed, are recognized by their propensity for spherical expansile growth (figs. 1-70–1-72). As the knowledge of hyperplastic and neoplastic rests increases, it is apparent that many of the individual tumors in children diagnosed as multicentric nephroblastomas were actually hyperplastic rests. A developmental scheme illustrating the relationship between various phases of nephrogenic rest pathobiology is illustrated in figure 1-73.

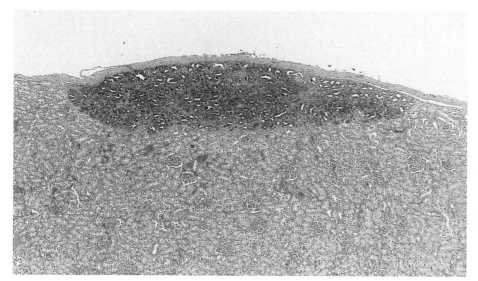

Figure 1-68
MULTIFOCAL
HYPERPLASIA
IN PERILOBAR
NEPHROGENIC REST
Proliferating embryonal foci of various shapes and sizes are separated by structures similar to those in sclerosing perilobar rests.

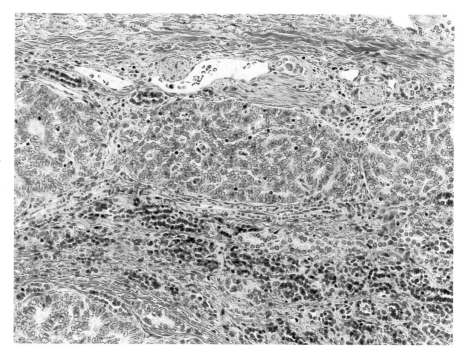

PLNR and ILNR have distinctive epidemiologic features. PLNR was found in approximately 1 percent of infant autopsies whereas ILNR was found in only 0.1 percent (24). Not surprisingly, the prevalence of both types of rests is substantially higher in association with nephroblastoma than in the general infant population (Table 1-7). The association with metachronous bilateral nephroblastoma is especially relevant. Patients with any type of nephrogenic rest in a kidney removed for nephroblastoma should be considered at increased risk for tumor formation in the remaining kidney; the risk is the greatest with intralobar rests (22). In contrast, when nephrogenic rests are not found in a generous sampling of renal parenchyma, the risk for contralateral nephroblastoma is negligible. Both types of nephrogenic rests are associated with certain syndromes carrying a high risk for nephroblastoma (see Table 1-2).

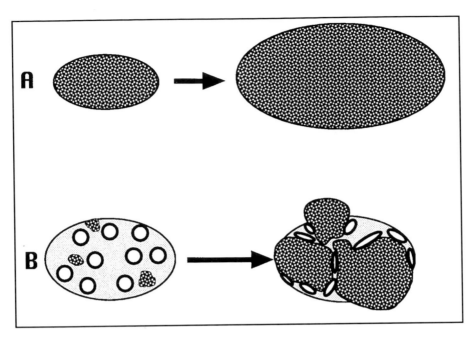

Figure 1-69
DIAGRAM OF MULTIFOCAL HYPERPLASIA IN PERILOBAR NEPHROGENIC REST

A: A uniform hyperplasia involving all cells of a rest.

B: A nodular or focal hyperplasia involving only susceptible cells in a sclerosing rest. The latter appearance suggests renewed proliferative activity in a rest that was in the process of regression. (Fig. 8 from Beckwith JB. Precursor lesions of Wilms' tumor: clinical and biological implications. Med Pediatr Oncol 1993;21:158–68.)

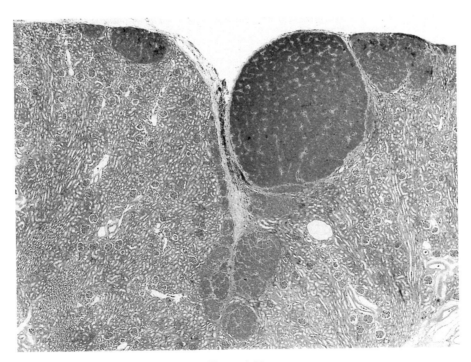

Figure 1-70
NEOPLASTIC PERILOBAR NEPHROGENIC REST

The larger rounded nodule seen near the center is an early nephroblastoma compressing adjacent rest elements at its periphery. The other structurally similar lesions in this field are dormant in hyperplastic rests and have a more irregular shape.

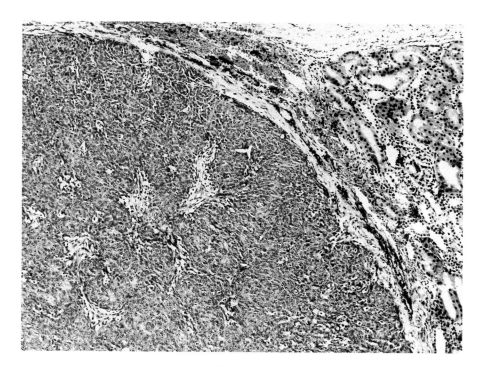

Figure 1-71
NEOPLASTIC PERILOBAR REST
Note the compressed rest remnants at the periphery of the expanding tumor.

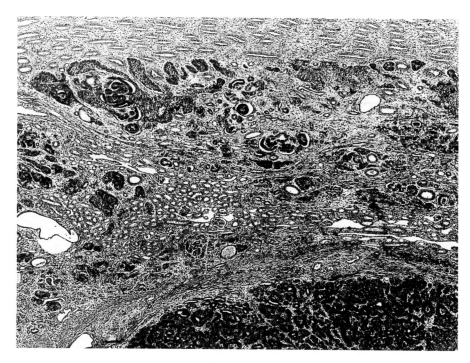

Figure 1-72
NEOPLASTIC INTRALOBAR REST
The edge of the nephroblastoma at the bottom of the field has a sharply defined border and dense cellularity. Most of the remainder of the field is occupied by intralobar nephrogenic rest tissue mingled with normal cortical and medullary structures. This appearance can easily be mistaken for tumor infiltration of the renal parenchyma.

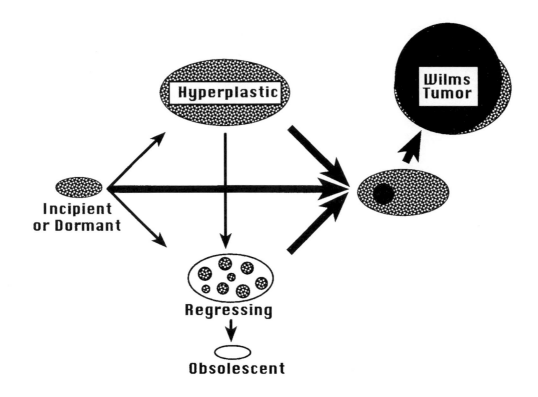

Figure 1-73
DIAGRAMMATIC REPRESENTATION OF THE POTENTIAL FATES OF NEPHROGENIC RESTS
(Fig. 4 from Beckwith JB. Precursor lesions of Wilms' tumor: clinical and biological implications. Med Pediatr Oncol 1993;21:158–68.)

Table 1-7

APPROXIMATE PREVALENCE OF NEPHROGENIC RESTS
IN SELECTED PATIENT POPULATIONS

Patient Category	Perilobar Rests (%)	Intralobar Rests (%)
Infant autopsies	0.01	0.001
Dysplastic kidneys	0.04	Unknown
Nephroblastoma cases		
Unilateral	0.25	0.15
Synchronous bilateral	0.80	0.40
Metachronous bilateral	0.40	0.75

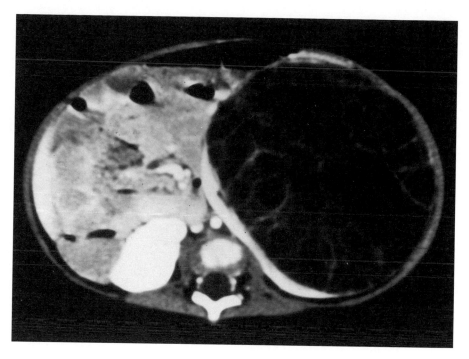

Figure 1-74
CYSTIC NEPHROMA
Computed tomographic image. (Courtesy of Dr. J. Fergall Magee, Vancouver, Canada.)

CYSTIC NEPHROMA AND CYSTIC, PARTIALLY DIFFERENTIATED NEPHROBLASTOMA

Definition. Cystic nephroma (CN) and cystic, partially differentiated nephroblastoma (CPDN) are benign neoplasms currently considered by many experts to be part of the spectrum of nephroblastoma (87–89). This concept is difficult to contest when the lesions contain foci of blastemal cells (CPDN) but is questionable when tumors comprise only cysts and nondescript fibrous stroma. Current evidence supports a spectrum of changes from pure multicystic tumors to obvious nephroblastomas with cysts; the separation of one end of the spectrum into a distinct category of multilocular cyst is not preferred.

General and Clinical Features. CN and CPDN can be solitary and unilateral, multilocular, have no communication among locules or with the renal pelvis, be true cysts lined by epithelium, lack fully developed nephrons in septa, or be sharply demarcated from an otherwise normal remaining kidney (87–89). Tumors occur in both adults and children; affected adults are most often female. Children are usually less than 2 years of age. Most tumors are asymptomatic and present as palpable masses, though hematuria is occasionally a presenting symptom. The cystic nature of the lesion is easily recognized by ultrasonography or CT (fig. 1-74). It is important to note that nephroblastomas, clear cell sarcomas, and mesoblastic nephromas may also be predominantly cystic.

Pathologic Findings. Grossly, CN and CPDN are multicystic lesions that usually measure 5 to 10 cm in greatest dimension. By definition, they are sharply circumscribed from the adjacent kidney and appear as bulging masses, often with a bosselated surface. Cysts range from a few millimeters to 4 cm in diameter and are filled with colorless fluid. The intervening septa must conform to the contours of the cyst and do not contain nodular masses (fig. 1-75). Hemorrhage, necrosis, and calcification are not features of either CN or CPDN. Extension of the lesion beyond the renal capsule may occur and does not negate the diagnosis. Regions of expansile solid tumor indicate a diagnosis of cystic nephroblastoma rather than CPDN (figs. 1-19, 1-76).

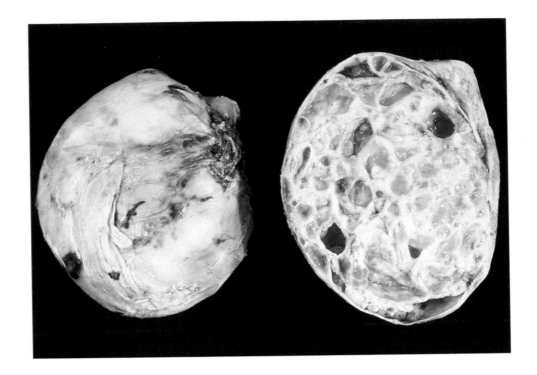

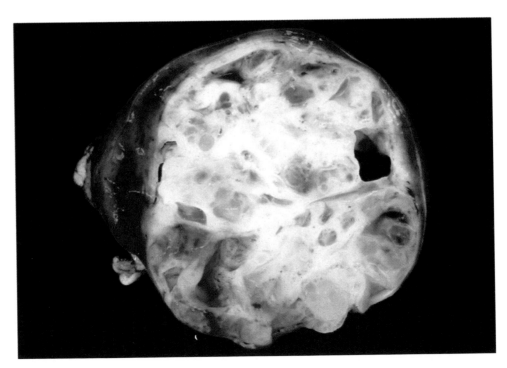

Figure 1-75
CYSTIC, PARTIALLY DIFFERENTIATED NEPHROBLASTOMA
Top: Gross appearance of external and sectioned surfaces. (Courtesy of Dr. Beverly B. Dahms, Cleveland, OH.)
Bottom: This illustration shows the sharp, smooth border between lesion and kidney. (Courtesy of Dr. Esperanza M. Tiamson, Baltimore, MD.)

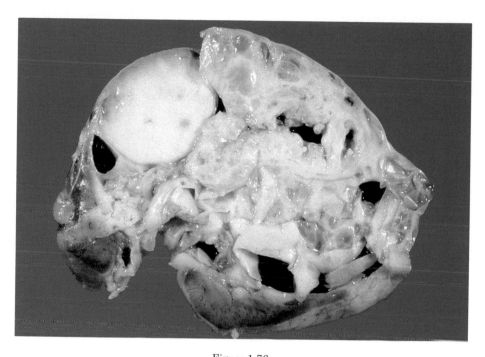

Figure 1-76
CYSTIC NEPHROBLASTOMA WITH A DISTINCT SOLID REGION
The latter finding excludes the diagnosis of cystic, partially differentiated nephroblastoma or cystic nephroma. (Courtesy of Dr. Craig W. Zuppan, Loma Linda, CA.)

The microscopic features confirm the gross appearance (figs. 1-77, 1-78). Lesions are sharply circumscribed from the adjacent renal parenchyma and do not contain entrapped renal elements. The septa are predominantly fibrous and molded to the cystic spaces. They may contain small foci of blastema or abortive tubules lacking proliferative activity. The cysts are lined by cuboidal, often "hobnailed" cells. Long cilia have been identified on these cells using scanning electron microscopy (90). This suggests differentiation toward collecting duct epithelium.

Differential Diagnosis. Since these lesions represent a part of the spectrum of nephroblastomatous disease, some difficulty in differentiating certain cases of CPDN from nephroblastoma is expected. The distinction is not difficult to make, however, and any case of nephroblastoma that is predominantly cystic and contains such scant cellularity that it might be considered CPDN is probably adequately treated by nephrectomy alone. The presence of expansile solid regions of nephroblastomatous tissue not molded by the cystic spaces is the primary feature distinguishing nephroblastoma from CPDN (fig. 1-76).

CN must be distinguished from polycystic kidneys. The most important criterion is a lack of mature renal parenchymal elements in the fibrous septa. Cartilage may occur in both CN and CPDN and this feature is not helpful in separating these lesions from dysplastic kidneys.

Prognosis. As defined here, CN and CPDN are benign neoplasms adequately treated by total resection. Some potential for recurrence exists if CPDN is incompletely excised, but metastases have not been documented. Some cystic carcinomas and sarcomas of adult kidneys have been reported to arise in CN, but it has not been conclusively proven that these lesions arose in preexistent cystic lesions rather than representing cystic change in a malignant neoplasm.

MESOBLASTIC NEPHROMA

Definition. This is a monomorphous renal neoplasm usually recognized in early infancy and uncommon among patients older than 1 year of age. These tumors have been described under other names, most notably *leiomyomatous hamartoma*, but the term initially suggested by

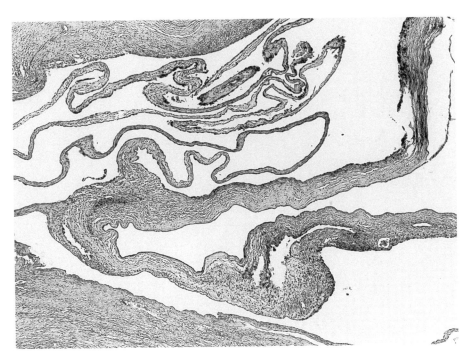

Figure 1-77
CYSTIC NEPHROMA
Only mature elements are present in the septa.

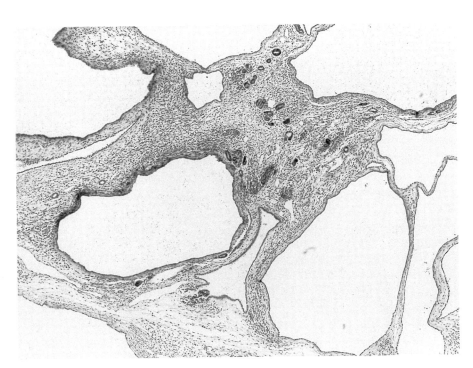

Figure 1-78
CYSTIC, PARTIALLY DIFFERENTIATED NEPHROBLASTOMA
Embryonal elements are present, but conform to the septa between cysts.

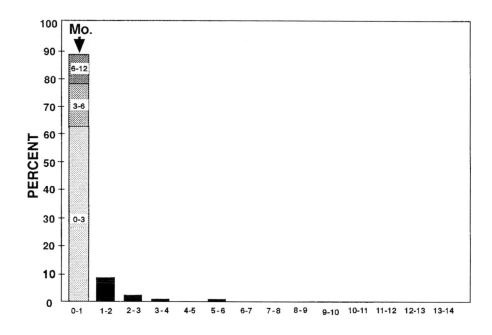

Figure 1-79
MESOBLASTIC NEPHROMA
Age distribution curve based on 238 pediatric cases in National Wilms Tumor Study pathology center.

Bolande is preferred (95,96,118). They could be considered part of the spectrum of monomorphous nephroblastomas but their distinctive clinicopathologic features warrant a separate designation.

General and Clinical Features. Mesoblastic nephroma is a congenital neoplasm most commonly recognized during the first 3 months of life (fig. 1-79). With the widespread application of ultrasound imaging, many cases are recognized prior to birth. The histogenesis is controversial (95,111,118). Most experts believe the tumor is a neoplasm rather than a hamartoma. The predominant view is that mesoblastic nephroma is a proliferative lesion of early nephrogenic mesenchyme. The tumor has been reported occasionally in children with Beckwith-Wiedemann syndrome but has not been reported in other syndromes associated with nephroblastoma (119).

The median age at diagnosis is 2 months and at least 90 percent of cases appear within the first year of life. Rare cases have been reported in older children and adults, although it remains uncertain whether the adult lesions are histolog-ically identical to infantile mesoblastic nephroma (104). There is no sex predilection. Most cases are detected because of an abdominal mass, although polyhydramnios and premature delivery often occur in affected fetuses and nonimmunological hydrops has been reported (91,99,103). Some patients with mesoblastic nephromas have hypercalcemia, attributed to excessive production of prostaglandin E by the tumor (113,116). Hyperreninism is not uncommon (98,107,120). In such cases, the hormone is produced by entrapped renal elements rather than tumor cells.

Pathologic Findings. Grossly, mesoblastic nephromas vary from 0.8 to 14 cm in greatest dimension (mean, 6.2 cm). They appear as solitary, unilateral masses with soft or firm, bulging cut surfaces indistinguishable from nephroblastomas (figs. 1-79, 1-80). Cysts, hemorrhage, and necrosis are common features (fig. 1-81). Cysts are occasionally the predominant gross feature (100). Most mesoblastic nephromas are centered near the hilus of the kidney and nearly all involve the renal sinus. Recognizing this, both surgeon and pathologist should take particular

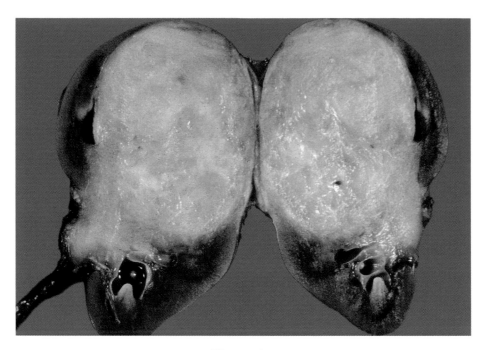

Figure 1-80
MESOBLASTIC NEPHROMA
Gross appearance of the classic pattern. Note the whorled, myomatous appearance of the sectioned surface, the extensive involvement of the medial aspect of the kidney, and lack of a sharply demarcated tumor-kidney junction. (Courtesy of Dr. Jane Chatten, Philadelphia, PA.)

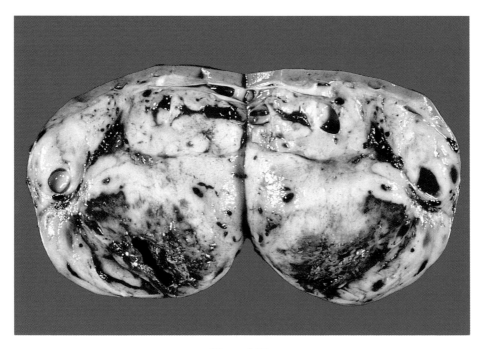

Figure 1-81
MESOBLASTIC NEPHROMA
Gross appearance often associated with the cellular pattern, with foci of hemorrhage, necrosis, and scattered cysts. (Courtesy of Dr. Ona Marie Faye-Petersen, New York, NY.)

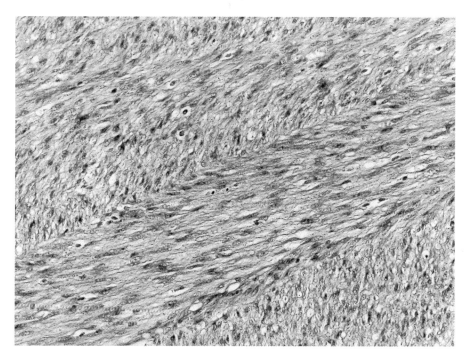

Figure 1-82
MESOBLASTIC NEPHROMA
The spindle cells forming the lesion are not densely aggregated and a prominent interlacing bundle pattern is characteristic of the classic pattern.

care to establish that the medial aspect of the nephrectomy specimen is free of tumor. Mesoblastic nephromas are well demarcated but commonly extend beyond the renal capsule.

Microscopically, mesoblastic nephromas are predominantly monomorphic neoplasms composed of spindled mesenchymal cells of fibroblastic or myofibroblastic lineage. They can be divided into two major types: classic and cellular. The classic subtype is that originally described by Bolande (96) although fewer than one third of mesoblastic nephromas have this histology. The cellular pattern is most common.

In the classic pattern, the tumor resembles infantile fibromatosis. It is characterized by intersecting fascicles of spindle cells resembling fibroblasts or myofibroblasts interspersed with scanty collagen fibers (figs. 1-82, 1-83). Dilated, thin-walled vascular spaces are often prominent. Mitotic activity is variable but generally less conspicuous than in the cellular pattern. The tumor margins are irregular with radiating bands of cells extending into the renal parenchyma and the perirenal soft tissue (figs. 1-84–

1-86). There is usually little compression of adjacent renal structures, suggesting that the tumor and fetal kidney were growing as an integrated unit. Entrapped renal elements can be misinterpreted as components of the neoplasm, especially since they are often not completely mature in these infants. Extensions of tumor tissue characteristically consist of long, narrow "tongues" of spindle cells that may continue for some distance beyond the gross margins of the tumor, especially at the hilus of the kidney. It is for this reason that wide surgical margins and careful pathologic documentation are important. Abnormal metaplastic changes in tubules or glomeruli adjacent to or entrapped by the lesion are present in many specimens (figs. 1-87, 1-88). These metaplastic cells have an embryonal appearance and may exhibit papillary hyperplasia, a feature that can be mistaken for evidence of mixed stromal and epithelial nephroblastoma. Small nodules of hyaline cartilage are often encountered. Extramedullary hematopoiesis is common. We have not observed skeletal muscle in mesoblastic nephromas.

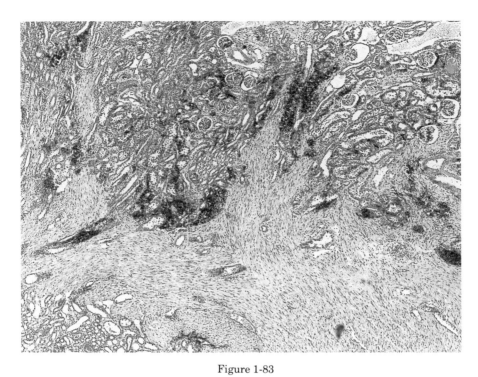

Figure 1-83
MESOBLASTIC NEPHROMA
In this classic pattern, the tumor interdigitates with renal parenchyma without compression or distortion of renal structures.

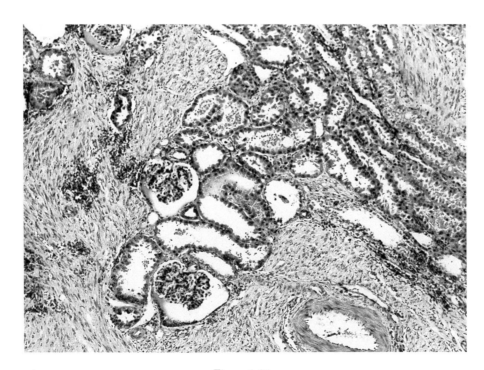

Figure 1-84
MESOBLASTIC NEPHROMA
Classic pattern showing interdigitating tumor-kidney junction with minimal distortion of adjacent structures.

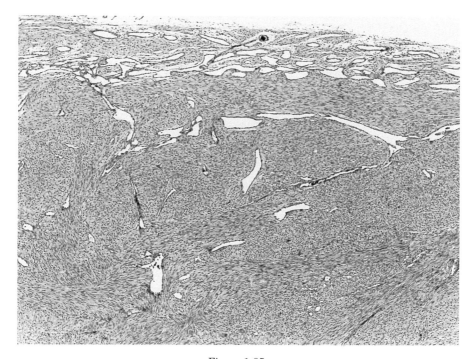

Figure 1-85
MESOBLASTIC NEPHROMA
Perirenal invasion, with characteristic angiomatous vascular proliferation at the advancing edge.

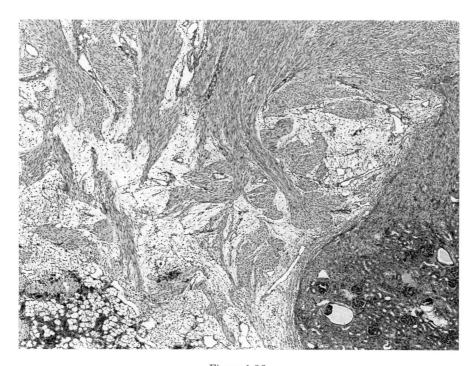

Figure 1-86
MESOBLASTIC NEPHROMA
Extension into the renal sinus and along structures medial to the kidney is an important feature of most lesions.

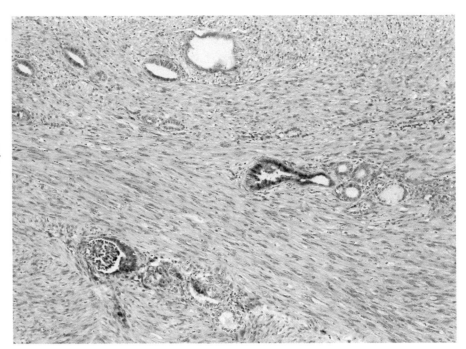

Figure 1-87
MESOBLASTIC NEPHROMA
Embryonal metaplasia of Bowman capsule and entrapped tubules.

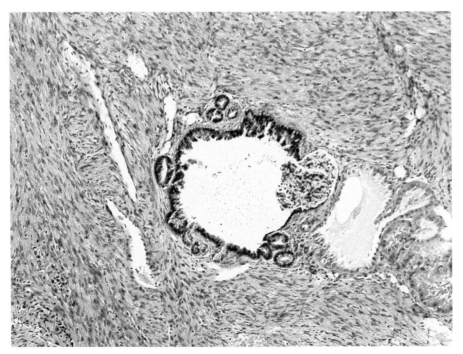

Figure 1-88
MESOBLASTIC NEPHROMA
Embryonal metaplasia of Bowman capsule and entrapped nephrons is sometimes accompanied by epithelial hyperplasia.

The cellular pattern is characterized by increased cellular density and a high proliferative rate, imparting a sarcomatous appearance to the tumor. Cellular and classic patterns may coexist (fig. 1-89). These mixed lesions suggest that at least some cellular mesoblastic nephromas arise within regions of classic morphology. Recognition of the classic pattern, often found at the periphery of cellular lesions, can be helpful in microscopic evaluation. Cellular mesoblastic nephromas most commonly consist of plump cells with large, vesicular nuclei and abundant

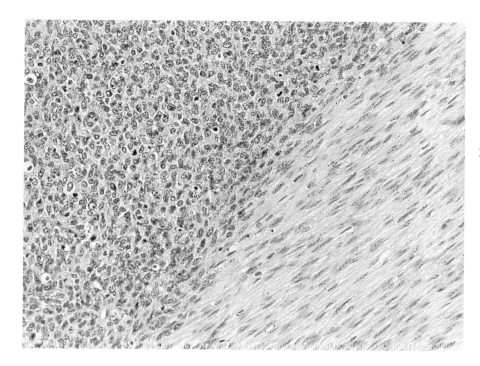

Figure 1-89
MESOBLASTIC NEPHROMA
Cellular and classic appearance.

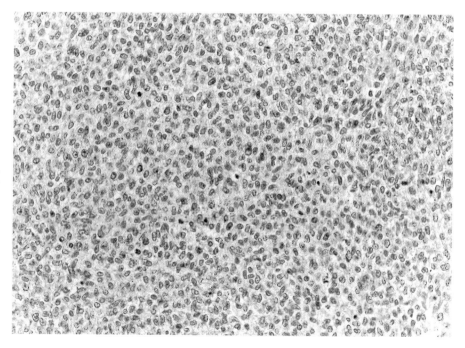

Figure 1-90
MESOBLASTIC
NEPHROMA

The most common variant is cellular, composed of plump spindle cells growing in a diffuse pattern.

cytoplasm (figs. 1-89, 1-90). Lesions are usually sharply circumscribed without the interdigitating margins of classic lesions. Mild to moderate nuclear pleomorphism may be present and the cells often grow in sheets reminiscent of fibroblast cell cultures. Some specimens resemble adult-type fibrosarcomas while others are com-

posed of smaller, more densely packed, less pleomorphic spindle cells reminiscent of the so-called infantile fibrosarcoma (fig. 1-91).

Immunohistochemical reactions in both types of mesoblastic nephroma have been consistently positive using antibodies directed toward fibrocytes, myofibroblasts, and smooth muscle cells

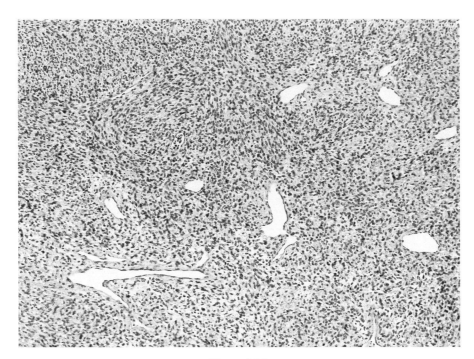

Figure 1-91
MESOBLASTIC NEPHROMA
Cellular variant composed of monomorphous sheets of closely packed spindle cells imparting a small blue-cell appearance.
Note the prominent irregular vascular spaces, which are a feature of many cellular mesoblastic nephromas.

(110,117). Epithelial markers have been positive only for entrapped epithelium. In addition to vimentin, desmin, and actin, reactions for fibronectin have been positive. Negative reactions have occurred using antibodies to laminin (106).

Ultrastructural studies have revealed elongated mesenchymal cells with prominent arrays of anastomosing rough endoplasmic reticulum (fig. 1-92) (109,110). Thin cytoplasmic filaments are often present. Basal lamina is absent and only sparse tight junctions of the macula adherens type have been observed.

Special Techniques. The DNA content of mesoblastic nephromas has been reported by several groups (93,112). We have observed slight increases in DNA content, especially in cellular specimens. Others have found mesoblastic nephromas to be predominantly diploid.

Karyotypic studies have revealed a variety of abnormalities but trisomy 11 has been the most frequent finding (114,115). The significance of this finding remains unclear but it may be a useful marker in cases where the diagnosis is

difficult. Interestingly, a similar genetic abnormality has been reported in congenital fibrosarcoma of the leg (92).

Differential Diagnosis. Mesoblastic nephroma must be differentiated from other pediatric renal neoplasms (Tables 1-8–1-10). Previously treated nephroblastomas may be especially rich in well-differentiated spindled stroma and one should be wary of the diagnosis of a mesoblastic nephroma in such cases. The most commonly encountered and challenging problem is the differentiation of mesoblastic nephroma from clear cell sarcoma. Both tumors occur in early life and both are exclusively mesenchymal. Entrapped renal elements and embryonal metaplastic changes are often present. Helpful features in differential diagnosis are listed in Table 1-9 but no single criterion can be relied upon. Rhabdoid tumor is more easily distinguished from mesoblastic nephroma but the occasional spindled appearance of a rhabdoid tumor or a mesoblastic nephroma with unusually prominent nucleoli can lead to diagnostic difficulties.

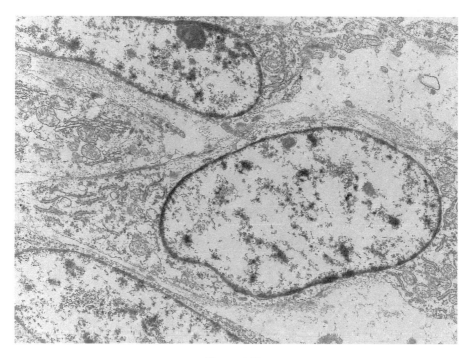

Figure 1-92
MESOBLASTIC NEPHROMA
Electron micrograph. (Courtesy of Dr. Gary W. Mirabeau, Denver, CO.)

Table 1-8

DIFFERENTIAL DIAGNOSIS OF NEPHROBLASTOMA AND MESOBLASTIC NEPHROMA

FEATURES DIAGNOSTIC FOR NEPHROBLASTOMA

Skeletal muscle, other heterologous cell types. (Note: cartilage and squamous epithelium are present in kidneys with mesoblastic nephromas, but these represent renal dysplasia and are not intrinsic to the tumor.)

Blastema

FEATURES SUPPORTIVE FOR NEPHROBLASTOMA

Age over 1 year

Nephrogenic rests

Bilateral renal tumors

Mode of Dissemination. Almost all mesoblastic nephromas are predominantly localized to the kidney at the time of treatment, although they may infiltrate the adjacent perirenal fat. Recurrences and metastases are uncommon. The case material in the NWTS pathology center currently includes 24 of 330 (7 percent) patients with known recurrences. This figure almost certainly exaggerates the true incidence of adverse events since material from every recurrent or metastatic case reported in the American literature has been specifically requested and unusual cases have naturally accumulated in this reference center (Table 1-11) (94). Local recurrence, usually to the flank, is the major problem and underscores the need for wide surgical resection. Metastases reported to date have involved only lung and brain. With a single exception, we are

Table 1-9

DIFFERENTIAL DIAGNOSIS OF CLEAR CELL SARCOMA OF KIDNEY AND MESOBLASTIC NEPHROMA

FEATURES SUPPORTIVE, BUT NOT DIAGNOSTIC, OF MESOBLASTIC NEPHROMA

    Diagnosis in first 6 months of life

    Tongues of spindle cells extending radially from tumor surface

    Diffuse or interlacing bundle growth pattern

    Lack of classic clear cell carcinoma cord pattern

    Randomly distributed dilated "staghorn" vessels, coexistent renal dysplasia

    Coarse nuclear chromatin

    High cell density with overlapping nuclei

    High mitotic rate, muscle-specific actin or desmin positivity

    DNA index over 1.0

    Trisomy 11

    Prominent branching, anastomosing endoplasmic reticulum on electron microscopy

FEATURES SUPPORTIVE, BUT NOT DIAGNOSTIC, OF CLEAR CELL SARCOMA

    Age over 1 year at diagnosis

    Classic clear cell carcinoma cord pattern

    Delicate chromatin pattern or empty-appearing nuclei

    Prominent collagenous sclerosis, hyalinization

    Abundant mucosubstances in lesion

    Metastases to bone or other extrapulmonary sites

Table 1-10

DIFFERENTIAL DIAGNOSIS OF MESOBLASTIC NEPHROMA AND RHABDOID TUMOR OF KIDNEY

FEATURES SUPPORTIVE OF RHABDOID TUMOR

Associated tumor in midline posterior cranial fossa

Metastatic disease

Cytoplasmic inclusions

Large nucleoli

Large polygonal cells with prominent acidophilic cytoplasm

Angioinvasive tumor

Table 1-11

SITES OF RECURRENCE OR METASTASIS OF MESOBLASTIC NEPHROMA

Sites	Cases
Abdominal recurrence only	18
Abdomen and lung	1
Lung metastasis only	4
Brain metastasis only	1

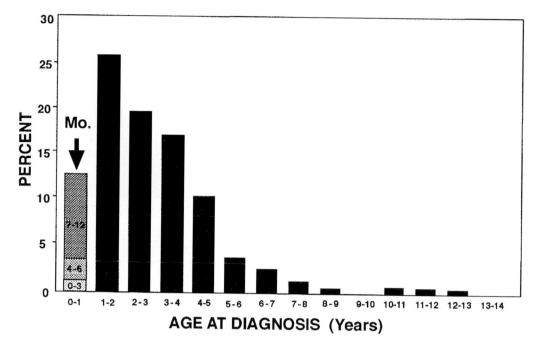

Figure 1-93
CLEAR CELL SARCOMA OF KIDNEY
Age distribution of 156 cases in National Wilms Tumor Study pathology center.

aware of no recurrences appearing more than 1 year after nephrectomy. Despite a tendency to local infiltration, the prognosis of mesoblastic nephroma is excellent. Surgical resection is the preferred treatment and local recurrence the most often observed complication.

Prognosis. We have not been able to document a consistent relationship between histologic pattern and prognosis, independent of patient age and tumor stage (94,97,101,102,105, 108,110). Patients older than 6 months of age at diagnosis tend to have highly cellular lesions and higher relapse rates than younger infants.

CLEAR CELL SARCOMA

Definition. This rare pediatric neoplasm is distinguished from nephroblastoma primarily by a histologic pattern having a significant component of clear cells, a predilection for metastases to bone, and a poor prognosis (122,128,130). Recognizing the inordinate frequency of bone involvement, some authors have suggested the term *bone-metastasizing renal tumor of child-*

hood for clear cell sarcoma of kidney. Although neither term is entirely satisfactory, clear cell sarcoma of kidney (CCSK) is currently preferred. This neoplasm is so rare that pathologists unconnected with referral centers cannot be expected to be familiar with the spectrum of histologic patterns (127,130,133–136). This section attempts to compensate for the lack of adequate published descriptions of CCSK by providing more photographs and descriptive detail than might seem appropriate for a rare entity.

General and Clinical Features. CCSK is a neoplasm of unknown etiology. The cells are histologically undifferentiated and most investigators have assumed a differentiation toward primitive nephrogenic mesenchyme. These neoplasms comprise 5 percent of primary pediatric renal tumors. CCSK is rare during the first 6 months of life and in young adults; the incidence peaks during the second year of life and progressively falls thereafter (fig. 1-93). We are aware of no well-documented case occurring beyond the third decade. In the NWTS series, males were

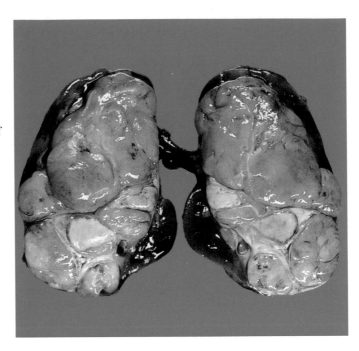

Figure 1-94
CLEAR CELL SARCOMA OF KIDNEY
Gross appearance. (Courtesy of the Department of
Pathology, The Children's Hospital, Denver, CO.)

affected more frequently than females (sex ratio, 1.6 to 1). An even higher male predominance has been observed by others (127). No racial or geographic predisposition has been observed and the disease is neither familial nor associated with specific malformations, chromosomal defects, genetic abnormalities, or unusual syndromes.

Pathologic Findings. Grossly, the tumors vary in weight from 126 to nearly 3000 g (median weight, 520 g). All lesions have been unilateral and unicentric. The botryoid-like intrapelvic extensions sometimes seen in nephroblastomas have not been observed and involvement of the renal vein is uncommon. The tumor-kidney junction is sharply defined and the tumor is usually confined within the renal capsule. Most often, CCSK seems to arise from the medullary or central regions of the kidney. On section, the surface is usually homogeneous and light brown or gray, and often seems mucoid. Most lesions have a tough, dense texture but some may be soft. Lesions are more often irregular than spherical but lack the multinodular appearance characteristic of nephroblastoma (fig. 1-94). Cysts are often present and may be the predominant feature in some specimens.

The light microscopic features are distinctive and represent the only secure foundation for the diagnosis. In many cases, the diagnosis can be

suspected by visual inspection of a glass slide stained with hematoxylin and eosin (fig. 1-95). CCSKs tend to have a homogeneous, pale blue appearance with gradual rather than demarcated transitions in density. This is in contrast to nephroblastoma, which is usually a uniform dark blue or variegated with sharply demarcated blue and pink regions. General visual appearance notwithstanding, a large number of histologic patterns can exist in CCSKs.

Most CCSKs have the *classic pattern* (figs. 1-96–1-98). At low magnification, the tumor appears monomorphous with a uniform pattern comprising cell cords or nests of 6 to 10 cells in width separated by evenly dispersed small vascular channels. The channels are usually of capillary size and accompanied by a component of spindle cells. These vascular septa appear as long parallel arrays connected by numerous short arcades. The plane of section with respect to these arrays determines whether the pattern is cordlike or alveolar. The prominence of the vascular septa depends upon the number of stromal cells accompanying the vessels. In well-fixed material, the cells comprising the cords are uniform in size and distribution but with indistinct borders. These are rarely as densely packed as those of nephroblastomatous blastema and nuclei are more commonly separated than overlapping. The

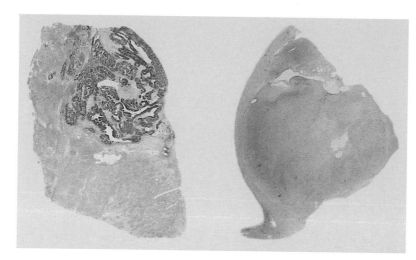

Figure 1-95
NEPHROBLASTOMA VERSUS
CLEAR CELL SARCOMA
OF KIDNEY
Comparison of unmagnified H&E stained slide of nephroblastoma (left) with CCSK. Note the more uniform appearance and paler blue color of CCSK.

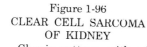

Figure 1-96
CLEAR CELL SARCOMA
OF KIDNEY
Classic pattern, with cell cords demarcated by delicate fibrovascular arcades.

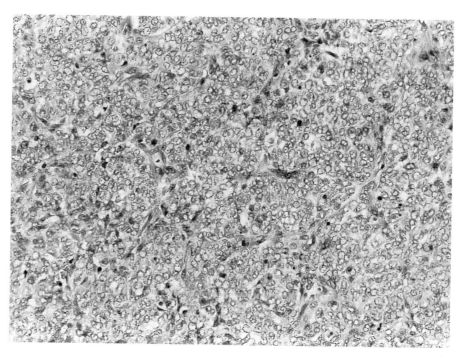

mitotic rate is variable but deceptively lower than that in other malignant pediatric renal neoplasms. Most specimens contain numerous vesicles (fig. 1-97). Although these structures often appear to be intracytoplasmic in usual preparations, thin sections and electron micrographs reveal most to be intercellular. Depending upon the fixative used, these vacuoles appear empty or filled with pale-staining or granular mucopolysaccharides. This material is a conspicuous feature of most specimens, including the variant patterns. It contributes to the pale, ve-

sicular appearance of most specimens and is the basis for the term "clear cell" sarcoma. However, most CCSKs are not composed entirely of clear cells but have at least some fields in which the cytoplasm is more condensed and acidophilic (fig. 1-98). When cells with acidophilic cytoplasm predominate, the lesion may resemble a rhabdoid tumor. The nuclei are usually uniform with such finely granular and evenly dispersed chromatin that they may appear almost empty. Nucleoli tend to be small and sparse. Fine nuclear grooves may be seen but are insufficiently

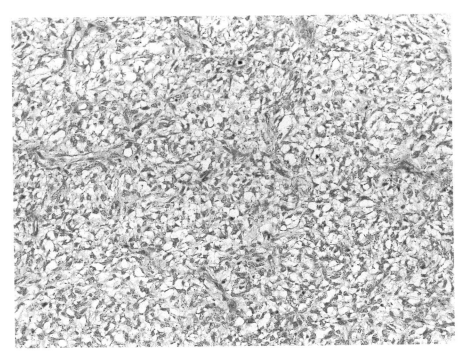

Figure 1-97
CLEAR CELL SARCOMA OF KIDNEY
Classic pattern, showing numerous cytoplasmic vesicles.

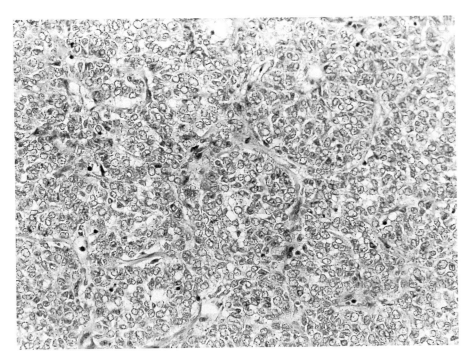

Figure 1-98
CLEAR CELL SARCOMA OF KIDNEY
In this field, the tumor cell cytoplasm is more compact and less vesicular. Note the pale, frequently empty-appearing nuclei.

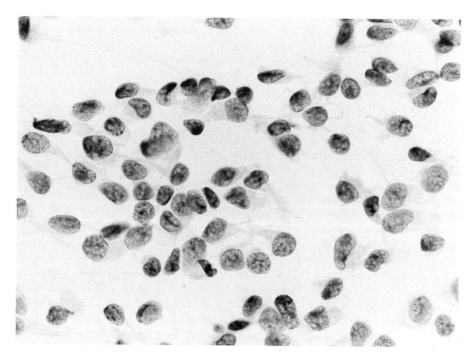

Figure 1-99
CLEAR CELL SARCOMA OF KIDNEY
Fine needle aspiration cytology.

prominent in usual tissue sections to be helpful in the diagnosis. These nuclear grooves are more prominent in aspirated specimens (fig. 1-99), but the diagnostic usefulness of this finding has not yet been established (123).

The tumor-kidney junction is distinctive. Although the tumor margin seems sharp under low magnification, higher magnification reveals tumor cells percolating for short distances into the adjacent renal parenchyma (figs. 1-100, 1-101). This is in contrast to nephroblastomas, which usually have either a sharply defined pushing border or an aggressively invasive, widely infiltrating margin. Invasion of blood vessels by the tumor is not a prominent feature of CCSK but may be seen in the form of cohesive tumor thrombi near the advancing margin of some specimens.

The infiltrative nature of CCSK characteristically results in entrapment and separation of individual nephrons or collecting ducts at the periphery of the tumor (figs. 1-100, 1-101). The cells of these entrapped tubules often assume an embryonal appearance which can be readily mistaken for the tubules of nephroblastoma, espe-

cially when they undergo hyperplastic overgrowth. Similar areas of "embryonal metaplasia" may be seen in the entrapped nephronic elements of mesoblastic nephromas and rhabdoid tumors, but larger groups of nephrons tend to be entrapped by these neoplasms.

While the classic pattern of CCSK is usually distinctive, some specimens contain regions that differ dramatically in histology and it is these variant patterns which most often lead to diagnostic difficulty. In most cases, more than one variant pattern appears in the same lesion. Fortunately, at least some foci of the classic pattern are usually also present. The *variant pattern* usually reflects morphologic transformations of the classic pattern. Some of these primarily involve the cell cords and nests while others involve the septa. For descriptive purposes, we refer to "cord cells" and "septal cells" without necessarily implying that these cell categories are biologically distinct.

The *epithelioid pattern* is most likely to be confused with nephroblastoma. This pattern occurs focally within the tumor and may form discrete, expansile nodules of higher cell density

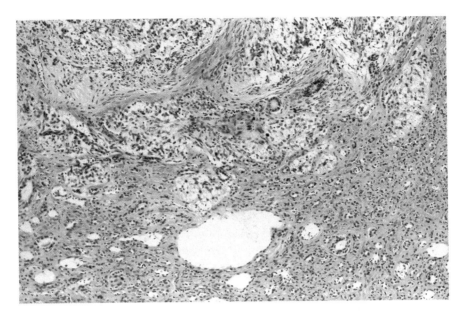

Figure 1-100
CLEAR CELL SARCOMA OF KIDNEY
Tumor-kidney junction, showing the entrapment of individual nephrons by tumor cells extending a short distance into the adjacent renal parenchyma.

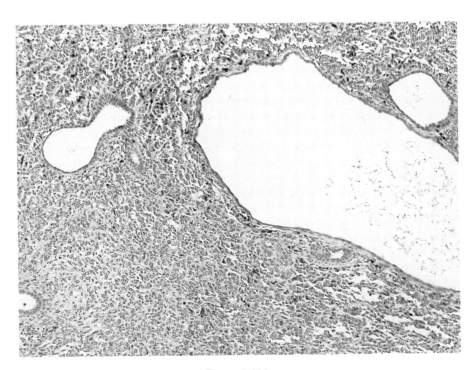

Figure 1-101
CLEAR CELL SARCOMA OF KIDNEY
Entrapped single renal tubules, with cystic dilatation of one tubule. Note the rather embryonal, metaplastic appearance of tubular epithelium, which can lead to an erroneous diagnosis of nephroblastoma.

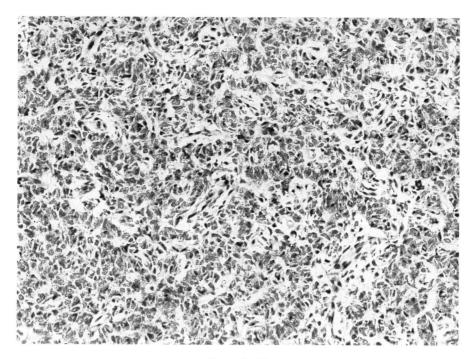

Figure 1-102
CLEAR CELL SARCOMA OF KIDNEY
Cord cells have become condensed, creating cohesive epithelioid ribbons that can be confused with nephroblastoma.

than the surrounding pale, uniform cells, suggesting that epithelioid foci may grow more rapidly than the rest of the tumor. These epithelioid structures seem to result from condensation of cell cords into cohesive ribbons and rarely form rosettes or tubular structures (figs. 1-102, 1-103) (135). The intervening vascular septa are usually retained between the condensed cell cords but are not always conspicuous.

Early condensation of cord cells usually occurs centrally but may develop along the vascular septa, forming perivascular rosettes on cross section. Increasing condensation forms progressively distinct "ribbon" formations that vary from one to several cells in width and usually follow the pattern of the original cell cords. A characteristic variation is the formation of undulating, elongated ribbons of single cell thickness, producing a sharply defined "filigree" pattern (fig. 1-104). Within the broader cords of the ribbon pattern, coalescent aggregates of interstitial mucin, similar to those forming the cytoplasmic vacuoles, can create a tubular appearance (fig. 1-105). These lumina can become dilated to form grossly apparent cysts. Well-developed tubular

formations are rare but when present can lead to an erroneous diagnosis of nephroblastoma (130, 135). Despite the strong resemblance of these changes to tubular differentiation, they do not react with antibodies to cytokeratins. In contrast, entrapped renal tubules are strongly reactive.

A *spindled pattern* can sometimes be prominent in CCSK. The pattern is formed by some combination of spindle cell expansion of the septa of the classic pattern and elongation of the cord cells (figs. 1-106, 1-107). When the spindle cell expansion is extreme, cord cells may be obliterated, resulting in a complex pattern of intersecting spindle cell bundles reminiscent of a mesoblastic nephroma or other spindle cell neoplasm. When cord cells are elongated, their nature usually remains evident but the distinction between cord cells and septal cells may be entirely lost, producing broad sheets of spindle cells mimicking a variety of sarcomatous lesions.

In the *sclerosing pattern*, abundant collagenous sclerosis is usually present, at least focally. The presence of collagenous sclerosis can actually assist in the recognition of CCSK, since collagen is rarely conspicuous in untreated

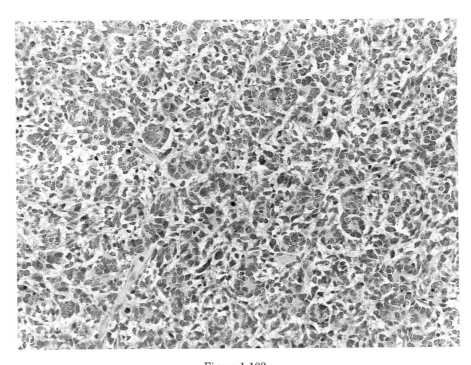

Figure 1-103
CLEAR CELL SARCOMA OF KIDNEY
Rosette formation is a rare finding in some specimens. In a few specimens, true tubular lumina are encountered.

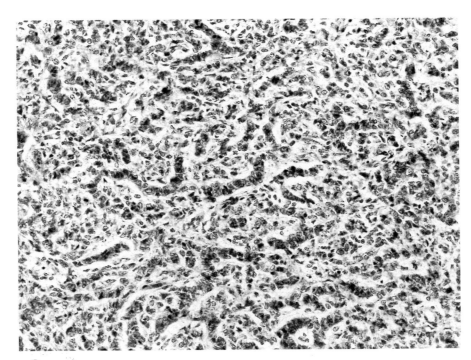

Figure 1-104
CLEAR CELL SARCOMA OF KIDNEY
Filigree pattern.

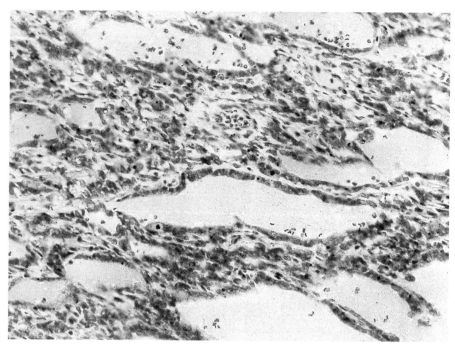

Figure 1-105
CLEAR CELL SARCOMA OF KIDNEY
Tumor tubules filled with mucin produce a striking epithelioid pattern. The cells lining the spaces in this specimen were negative with cytokeratins and epithelial membrane antigen immunostains, in contrast to entrapped renal tubules, which can stain positively.

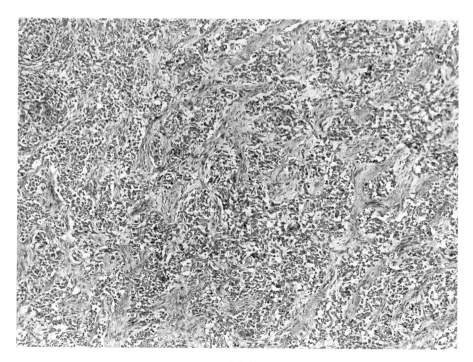

Figure 1-106
CLEAR CELL SARCOMA OF KIDNEY
Proliferation of septal cells imparts a prominent spindled pattern to some lesions.

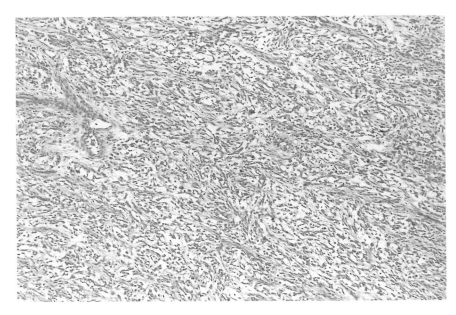

Figure 1-107
CLEAR CELL SARCOMA OF KIDNEY
Cord cells have acquired a spindled configuration. Vascular septa are still recognizable.

nephroblastomas except in areas of infarction. The sclerosis is often limited to cord cells and the process usually preserves the original dimensions of the cell cord as well as the original vascular septa (fig. 1-108). This produces a distinctive pattern of "chicken wire" vessels set in a poorly cellular sclerotic background. Collagen bundles from the sclerotic septa can extend diffusely in a pericellular pattern, isolating single cells or small groups of cells in a dense matrix that may become hyalinized. This can produce an osteosarcomatoid appearance similar to that of a rhabdoid tumor (fig. 1-109).

Mucopolysaccharide is a fundamental component of CCSK and may be present in amounts that obscure the original classic pattern. When this material accumulates diffusely between cord and septal cells, it imparts a *myxoid pattern* (fig. 1-110). Coalescent pools of mucopolysaccharide may give a cystic appearance.

The *cystic pattern* may arise by several mechanisms, most of which have been described and illustrated above: unlined cysts may result from intercellular accumulations of interstitial mucins (fig. 1-110); cysts lined by renal tubular epithelium result from dilatation of entrapped nephrons or collecting ducts; and cysts lined by

pseudoepithelial structures result from the accumulation of mucosubstances within ribbons of the epithelioid pattern (fig. 1-105). The cells lining pseudoepithelial structures do not manifest cytokeratin antigenic determinants.

The *palisading pattern* is one of the more distinctive variants of CCSK, and is observed in approximately 15 percent of specimens (fig. 1-111). This pattern is characterized by the focal presence of arrays of parallel spindle cell nuclei alternating in tigroid fashion with nuclear free zones. The resemblance to the nuclear palisades of neurilemomas is striking, but in our limited experience, these areas have not manifested S-100 protein or ultrastructural features suggesting neurilemomas.

In the *sinusoidal (pericytomatous) pattern*, blood vessels comprising a part of the classic CCSK pattern become distended, so that the tumor resembles a hemangiopericytoma (fig. 1-112). Evidence supporting angiopericytomatous differentiation in CCSK has not yet emerged.

A *pleomorphic (anaplastic) pattern*, characterized by the presence of monstrous, polypoid nuclei with multipolar mitotic figures (fig. 1-113), is occasionally seen. It has been encountered in metastatic foci following therapy but also in primary

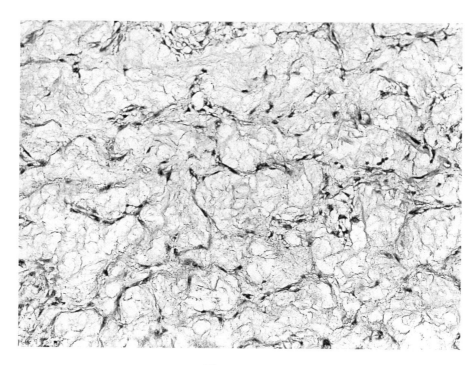

Figure 1-108
CLEAR CELL SARCOMA OF KIDNEY
In this example of the sclerosing pattern, a distinctive pattern is created by the persistence of vascular septa with complete collagenous sclerosis of cell cords.

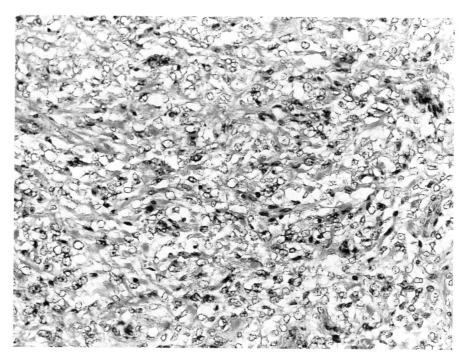

Figure 1-109
CLEAR CELL SARCOMA OF KIDNEY
Hyalinizing pattern.

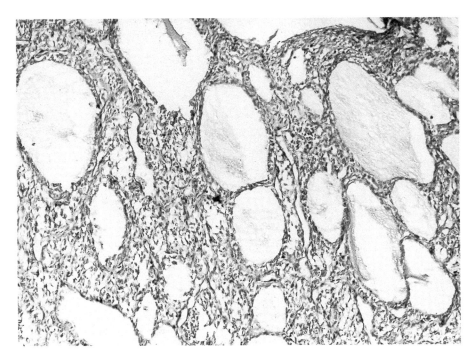

Figure 1-110
CLEAR CELL SARCOMA OF KIDNEY
Myxoid and cystic pattern.

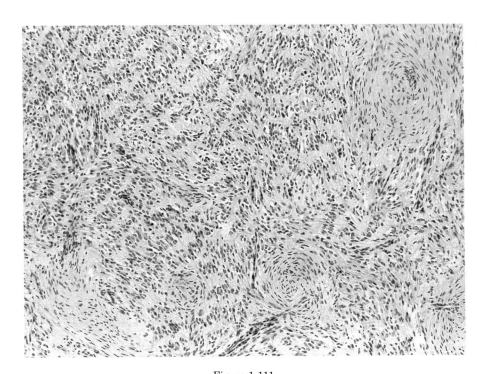

Figure 1-111
CLEAR CELL SARCOMA OF KIDNEY
The palisading pattern is reminiscent of nerve sheath tumors. Negative staining for S-100 protein is helpful in distinguishing these lesions.

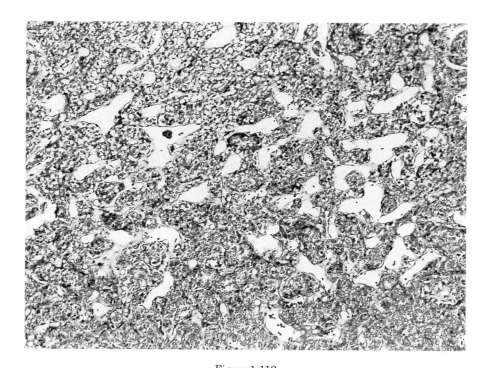

Figure 1-112
CLEAR CELL SARCOMA OF KIDNEY
A pericytomatous pattern is created by vascular dilatation, clearly delineating the fundamental pattern of clear cell sarcoma of kidney.

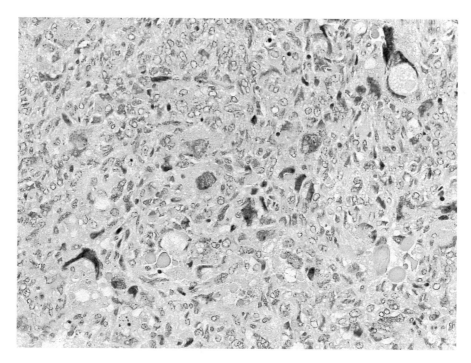

Figure 1-113
CLEAR CELL SARCOMA OF KIDNEY
Pleomorphic tumor giant cells are seen in some specimens.

Table 1-12

FEATURES DISCRIMINATING NEPHROBLASTOMA FROM CLEAR CELL SARCOMA*

Nephroblastoma	Clear Cell Sarcoma
Clinical	
Nephroblastoma syndromes	Metastases to bone, brain, or other sites (except lung, lymph nodes, liver)
Bilateral/multicentric tumors	
Gross and Light Microscopy	
Heterologous cell types (skeletal muscle, etc.)	**Classic or variant CCSK patterns form entire tumor**
Classic blastemal patterns (serpentine, etc.)	Homogeneous, pale H&E appearance
Nodular growth pattern	Tumor surrounds, isolates nephrons
Botryoid intrapelvic growth	Prominent collagen (except in treated or infarcted tumor)
Tumor in renal veins	
Nephrogenic rests	
Electron Microscopy	
Numerous desmosomes	Prominent collagen
Abundant flocculent material on cell surfaces	Prominent processes
Many organelles	
Confronting cisternae	
Many intermediate filaments	
Numerous cilia	

* Features in boldface are diagnostic, others are supportive.

lesions. In metastases, such changes are likely to be misinterpreted as a new type of tumor.

Immunohistochemical and ultrastructural studies are of limited value in the diagnosis of CCSK (121,124–127,129,131,134,136,137). Their primary contribution is in the exclusion of other pediatric renal neoplasms. The lectin pattern of CCSK resembles that of the blastemal and primitive regions of nephroblastomas (125). Vimentin has been demonstrated in many cases (121,137). By electron microscopy, the cells of CCSK generally contain a paucity of intermediate filaments, with incompletely formed cell junctions, and few distinguishing features.

Special Techniques. Only a few cases of CCSK have been examined by techniques other than light and electron microscopy. Almost all have had diploid DNA with relatively low proliferation indices (134). We are aware of several specimens in which no cytogenetic abnormality was detected, but translocation of 10;17 was identified in one published report (132).

Differential Diagnosis. CCSK must be distinguished primarily from nephroblastoma and mesoblastic nephroma (Tables 1-12, 1-13). Diagnosis is best achieved on specimens from the primary tumor since the histologic appearance of metastatic lesions can be extremely variable. In general, a mass at any site in the body from a child with a previous history of CCSK should be considered a metastasis until proven otherwise.

Differentiation of CCSK from nephroblastoma is the most frequent consideration and is difficult in some cases. We discourage the use of intraoperative frozen sections for diagnosis of pediatric neoplasms, since accurate discrimination of various entities in a small biopsy specimen is often impossible. It is important to remember that CCSK

Table 1-13

**FEATURES DISCRIMINATING MESOBLASTIC NEPHROMA
FROM CLEAR CELL SARCOMA OF KIDNEY***

Mesoblastic Nephroma	Clear Cell Sarcoma
Clinical	
Age less than 6 months	Age more than 1 year
Increased renin, calcium	Metastases (except lung)
Light Microscopy	
Classic mesoblastic pattern	**Classic CCSK pattern**
Renal dysplasia (e.g., cartilage)	**Most variant CCSK patterns**
Coarse chromatin	Fine chromatin
High mitotic rate	Low mitotic rate
Extensively infiltrating margins	Extensive sclerosis
Staghorn vessels in tumor	? Nuclear grooves
Tumor surrounds groups of nephrons	Tumor entraps isolated nephrons
Electron Microscopy	
Branching, anastomosing RER**	Prominent collagen, cytoplasmic processes
Nuclear grooves and pockets	Electron lucent cells

* Features in boldface are diagnostic, others are supportive.
**RER: Rough endoplasmic reticulum.

is a distinctive tumor so that any region of unequivocal nephroblastoma excludes the diagnosis of CCSK.

Rhabdoid tumor is not a frequent source of diagnostic confusion but occasional CCSKs may contain focal areas suggestive of rhabdoid tumor. The inconspicuous nucleoli, more lucent cytoplasm, and less aggressive infiltrative marginal pattern of CCSK are the most helpful diagnostic considerations.

Mode of Dissemination. One of the most distinctive features of CCSK is its propensity for widespread metastases. Early reports focused particularly on bony metastases but the 40 to 70 percent incidence reported in early series is misleading since metastasis was one of the criteria used in selection of cases. The incidence of bony metastases in the NWTS experience is 17 percent (124). Even this frequency has dropped substantially in recent years, apparently due to the consistent use of doxorubicin in therapeutic regimens. Other commonly observed metastatic sites are regional lymph nodes, brain, lungs, liver, and soft tissue, including periorbital fat. We have observed metastases in skeletal muscle, including distal extremities and paraspinous muscle. Other unusual sites include testis and salivary gland.

In contrast to nephroblastoma, the late onset of first relapse among cases of CCSK is a distinctive feature. Relapses after intervals as long as 5 years have been documented. Late relapses are especially prevalent among children treated with doxorubicin. The high relapse rates in patients with stage I tumors who were treated with protocols that did not include doxorubicin suggests that these late metastases actually represent retarded or inhibited growth of micrometastases that occurred early in the course of the disease. These findings tend to reduce the value of staging for CCSK of the kidney in children.

Prognosis. The inclusion of doxorubicin in therapeutic protocols for CCSK has reduced the death rate from nearly 70 percent to 30 to 40 percent. Nevertheless, late recurrences and deaths leave the ultimate outcome for these patients in doubt.

Table 1-14

RENAL NEOPLASMS MIMICKING RHABDOID TUMOR OF KIDNEY

Nephroblastoma with cytoplasmic inclusions
Renal cell carcinoma with inclusions
Collecting duct carcinoma
Transitional cell carcinoma
Mesoblastic nephroma
Rhabdomyosarcoma
Leiomyosarcoma
Neuroepithelial tumors
Metastases from extrarenal "pseudo-rhabdoid" tumor

Table 1-15

EXTRARENAL NEOPLASMS MIMICKING RHABDOID TUMOR

Rhabdomyosarcoma
Leiomyosarcoma
Ganglioneuroblastoma
Carcinoid, other neuroendocrine tumors
Epithelioid schwannoma
Melanoma
Glioma
Epithelioid sarcoma
Synovial sarcoma
Histiocytic sarcoma
Large cell lymphoma
Yolk sac tumor
Hepatocellular carcinoma
Angiosarcoma

RHABDOID TUMOR

Definition. Rhabdoid tumor is a rare malignant neoplasm characterized by a monomorphous population of large, relatively noncohesive cells with vesicular nuclei and large nucleoli. This neoplasm was initially recognized as a clinicopathologic entity during review of material from the NWTS (139,148). The name was suggested by a tendency for the tumor cells to resemble those in histologic sections of skeletal muscle tumors. Neither ultrastructural nor other features supporting a myogenic origin have been evaluated. Most rhabdoid tumors occur in the kidneys of infants. Many lesions reported as rhabdoid tumor at extrarenal sites do not conform to our definition but lack of consensus on uniform criteria for diagnosis makes the proper classification of these lesions difficult. In the following discussion, the term rhabdoid tumor of kidney is reserved for unequivocal cases. Renal neoplasms with features resembling rhabdoid tumor but having clinical, histologic, immunohistochemical, or ultrastructural features that differ from the classic form will be designated as *malignant undifferentiated neoplasm with rhabdoid features* (145).

General and Clinical Features. Rhabdoid tumor is a neoplasm of unknown etiology. An association with separate primary tumors of primitive neuroepithelial origin occurring in the midline of the posterior or middle cranial fossa has been observed in approximately 15 percent of cases (140). The histogenesis is uncertain and many cases with cytologic and even ultrastructural features resembling those of rhabdoid tumor have

been reported from extrarenal sites (142,145, 153,159,161). We have found many lesions with light microscopic features reminiscent of rhabdoid tumor of the kidney and encourage a skeptical approach to this diagnosis when the age of the patient, site of the tumor, natural history, or phenotypic features of the lesions do not correspond closely to the classic pattern (Tables 1-14, 1-15).

Rhabdoid tumors constitute only 2.5 percent of cases in the NWTS (161). The median age at diagnosis in our series was 11 months; more than 90 percent of patients were under 3 years of age, and the oldest was 8.5 years (fig. 1-114). Males predominate over females by a ratio of 1.5 to 1. Extrarenal tumors with rhabdoid features have been reported in one pair of siblings but we are aware of no familial recurrences of renal rhabdoid tumors (149). There is no association with syndromes predisposing to nephroblastoma nor have consistent genetic abnormalities been observed (143). A few rhabdoid tumors have been associated with hypercalcemia and elevated levels of parathormone (150,151). It is unlikely that parathormone is secreted by the tumor cells themselves since tests for transcription of parathormone mRNA have been negative.

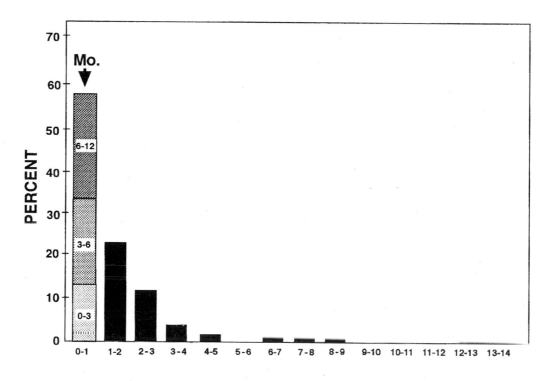

Figure 1-114
RHABDOID TUMOR
Age distribution of 120 cases in the files of the National Wilms Tumor Study pathology center.

Pathologic Findings. Grossly, rhabdoid tumors are soft, pale, bulging, relatively uniform, moderately well demarcated from the adjacent kidney, and usually lack a capsule (fig. 1-115). Although large, most weigh less than 500 g. Small tumors tend to arise in the renal medulla. These neoplasms are unicentric and unilateral but multiple renal nodules representing secondary implants may occur.

Microscopically, rhabdoid tumors have a monomorphous pattern composed of sheets of large, loosely cohesive cells with acidophilic cytoplasm and distinct cell borders. Cells with characteristic cytoplasmic inclusions tend to be clustered rather than uniformly distributed and not all cells of any given neoplasm contain these structures (figs. 1-116–1-119). The growth pattern is infiltrative with invasion of local blood vessels (fig. 1-117). Cross-striations have not been observed in the cytoplasm of rhabdoid tumors. Rarely, tumor cells may be organized into fairly distinctive cords or tubule-like structures

reminiscent of a nephroblastoma (fig. 1-120). The nuclei of rhabdoid tumor cells are large and vesicular with very large nucleoli.

Necrosis, with preservation of cells around blood vessels, may create a superficial resemblance to the serpentine blastemal patterns of nephroblastoma, but the cells of rhabdoid tumor are much larger and the fibromyxoid stroma associated with blastemal nephroblastoma is not a feature. The stroma of rhabdoid tumors tends to be densely collagenous and may become hyalinized (fig. 1-121). Basophilic ground substance may accumulate to such a degree as to suggest chondroid differentiation (fig. 1-122). Scattered infiltrates of eosinophils or multinucleated histiocytes may be prominent in some tumors. Variant patterns of rhabdoid tumor have been observed; they are listed in Table 1-16 and reviewed in detail elsewhere (160).

Immunohistochemical studies of rhabdoid tumors have resulted in a conflicting and frustrating degree of variability (147,151,153–158,160,162).

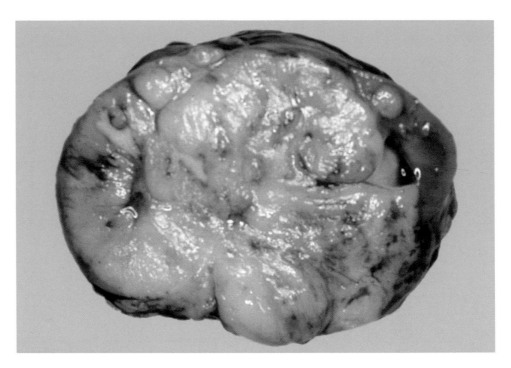

Figure 1-115
RHABDOID TUMOR
Gross appearance.

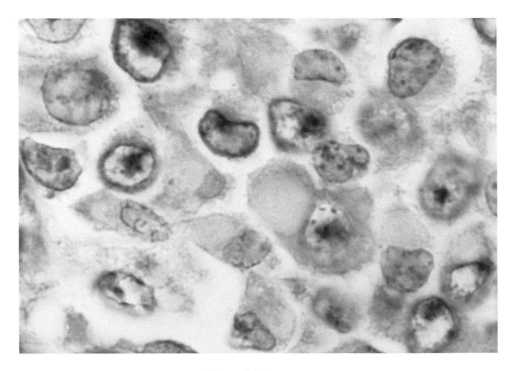

Figure 1-116
RHABDOID TUMOR
Characteristic appearance in well-fixed, routinely processed sections.

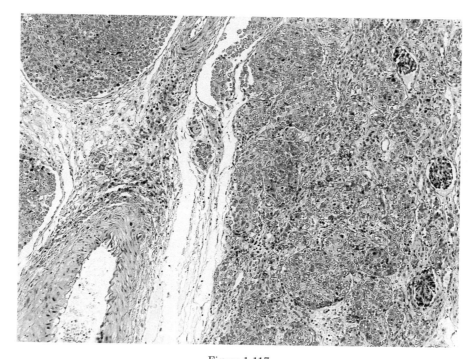

Figure 1-117
RHABDOID TUMOR
Aggressive infiltration of vessels in the renal parenchyma and sinus is characteristic of this neoplasm.

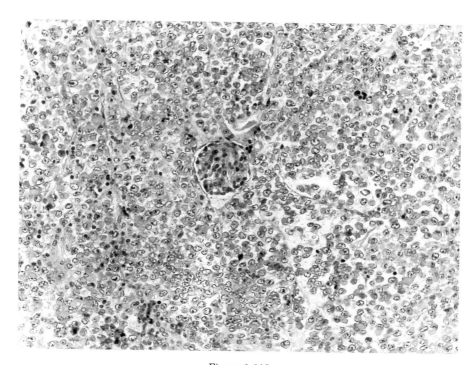

Figure 1-118
RHABDOID TUMOR
Sheets of tumor cells surround a centrally placed glomerulus, a result of the aggressive invasive growth pattern of this lesion.

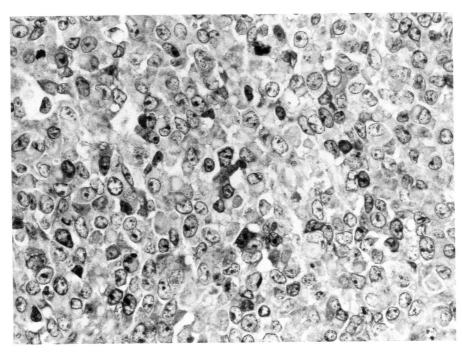

Figure 1-119
RHABDOID TUMOR
Note the characteristic vesicular nuclei, prominent nucleoli, and occasional pale cytoplasmic inclusions in this diffuse growth pattern.

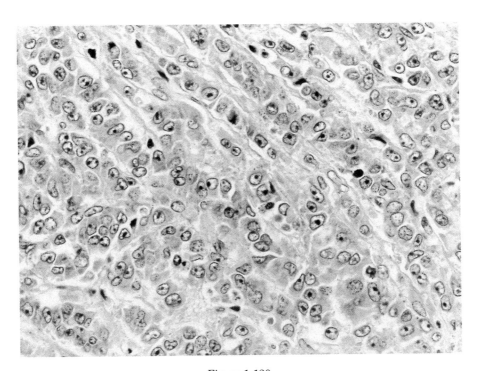

Figure 1-120
RHABDOID TUMOR
Epithelioid pattern, possibly resulting from replacement of preexistent tubular structures in the renal medulla.

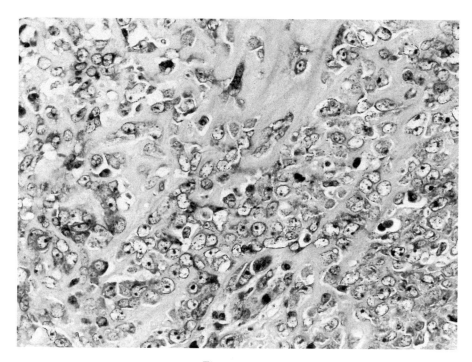

Figure 1-121
RHABDOID TUMOR
Hyalinizing pattern.

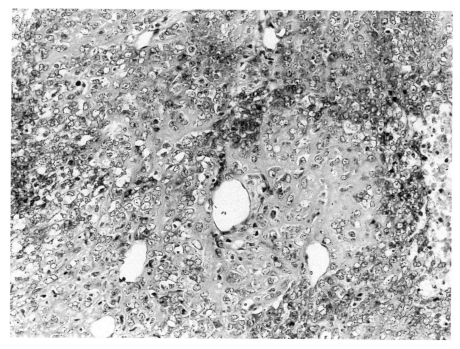

Figure 1-122
RHABDOID TUMOR
Chondroid pattern is focally present in many specimens.

Table 1-16

VARIANT PATTERNS OF RHABDOID TUMOR

Sclerosing patterns
    Fibrotic
    Osteosarcomatoid
    Chondroid
Epithelioid patterns
    Trabecular
    Mucoid
    Alveolar
    Pseudoglandular
Spindled patterns
    Broad fascicular
    Myxoid
    Pericytomatous
    Storiform
    Palisading
Lymphomatoid patterns
    Solid
    Histiocytoid

This variability is caused in part by the inclusion of questionable examples and may be compounded by nonspecific binding of antibodies to the filamentous cytoplasmic inclusions of these lesions (160). Contamination of tumor by other cell types may account for positive immunohistochemical reactions in some cases (147). The most consistently positive reactions for renal rhabdoid tumors are with antibodies to vimentin and cytokeratins. Epithelial membrane antigen is present in most cases. Positive results for neural markers as well as desmin and actin have been observed (157). The immunohistochemical profile of rhabdoid tumor of the kidney remains a controversial and confusing topic awaiting more accurate definition of the tumor itself.

In contrast to immunohistochemistry, ultrastructural studies have produced relatively consistent results (147,148,151,153–157,160). Prominent aggregates of filaments range in thickness from 6 to 10 nm. These filaments characteristically form tightly whorled structures adjacent to the nucleus (fig. 1-123). Other filamentous bundles resembling tonofilaments are usually also present. Primitive cell junctions are commonly observed. Cytoplasmic organelles and glycogen are present but usually not abundant. Dense core granules, alternating thick and thin filaments, and cell-associated basal laminae have been conspicuously absent, suggesting that these lesions are not differentiating toward neuroendocrine, skeletal muscle, or smooth muscle cells. It should be emphasized that whorled aggregates of filaments are not diagnostic of rhabdoid tumor and can be seen in a number of other neoplastic entities (161), and otherwise classic rhabdoid tumors of kidney may contain few if any cells with filamentous inclusions.

The distinctive cells of rhabdoid tumor lend themselves to cytologic diagnosis, especially in cases of infantile renal tumors with disseminated disease. Successful application of this approach has been reported by several groups (138, 144). The distinctive large and vesicular nuclei, prominent central nucleoli, and cytoplasmic inclusions can be diagnostic in an appropriate clinical setting.

Special Techniques. Although monosomy of chromosome 22 has been reported, no consistent karyotypic abnormalities have been described in the few cases of rhabdoid tumor studied to date (141,143). Flow cytometry has revealed diploid DNA (153).

Differential Diagnosis. Differentiating rhabdoid tumor from other renal neoplasms of infancy and childhood is usually straightforward. The problem is more complicated for renal tumors occurring in older individuals and for extrarenal lesions resembling rhabdoid tumor. The entities listed in Tables 1-14 and 1-15 are far more likely than rhabdoid tumor when diagnostic difficulties arise.

A recently described abdominal neoplasm, desmoplastic small round cell tumor, has histologic features similar to those of rhabdoid tumor in some cases (146,152). This lesion is seen in older children and young adults rather than in infants. The distinctive pattern of nesting, neuroendocrine type cells set in a desmoplastic stroma differs from the usual appearance of rhabdoid tumor.

Portions of nephroblastoma, mesoblastic nephroma, and clear cell sarcoma may resemble rhabdoid tumor but other areas contain more

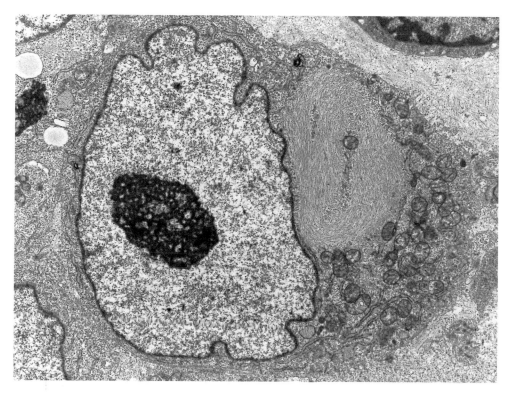

Figure 1-123
RHABDOID TUMOR
The characteristic electron microscopic appearance of a whorled aggregate of intermediate filaments can occur in many other neoplasms. (Courtesy of Dr. Gary W. Mierau, Denver, CO.)

characteristic histologic patterns and the differential diagnosis should only be a problem when small amounts of tissue are available for histologic examination. The distinguishing features of these lesions are detailed in their respective sections of this atlas. Occasional renal cell and transitional cell carcinomas may have features resembling those of rhabdoid tumor (153,161). Ultrastructural studies usually reveal the correct diagnosis when well-developed cell junctions, intracytoplasmic lumina with microvilli, or other features of renal cell or transitional cell carcinoma are observed.

Mode of Dissemination. Rhabdoid tumor is a very aggressive neoplasm which disseminates early and metastasizes widely. Metastases are both hematogenous and lymphatic.

Prognosis. Rhabdoid tumor of kidney is one of the most lethal neoplasms of childhood: 80 percent of patients in the NWTS died of their cancers. Most deaths occur within 1 year of diagnosis (161).

OTHER RENAL TUMORS

A small number of renal tumors have been documented in individual case reports. Typical renal cell carcinoma may occur in children. This entity is described in detail under renal tumors of adult kidneys (169). Other examples are briefly described.

Ossifying Renal Tumor of Kidney

This is a rare neoplasm characteristically presenting as a calcified mass in the renal pelvis, where it mimics a renal calculus both clinically and radiologically (163,168). The majority of known cases are in boys less than 1 year of age. Hematuria is the usual presenting symptom.

The lesion is relatively small and attached to the renal parenchyma at or near the papilla so that most of the mass lies free in the pelvic cavity. Grossly, tumors resemble renal calculi except for the firm attachment to the parenchyma. Microscopically, ossifying renal tumors are composed of

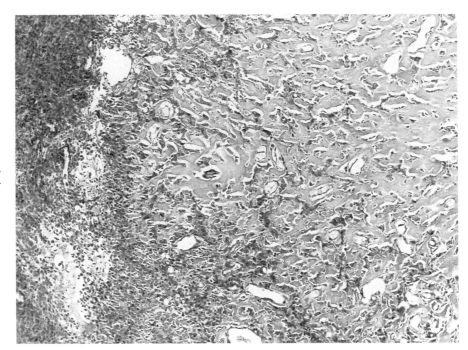

Figure 1-124
OSSIFYING RENAL
TUMOR OF INFANCY
Spindle cells with focal osteoid matrix characterize this lesion.

proliferating spindle cells admixed with partially calcified osteoid matrix (fig. 1-124). Prognosis is excellent: there are no known cases with recurrences or metastases.

Renal Lymphangioma

A rare cause of unilateral or bilateral nephromegaly, this lesion can resemble infantile polycystic disease, nephroblastomatosis, or renal vein thrombosis (170). The lesion is predominantly cortical but usually involves the medulla as well. Despite the name, the nature of this lesion is uncertain and it may represent diffuse lymphangiectasia rather than a neoplasm. Dilatation of lymphatics in the perirenal soft tissues of one case, along with marked ascites, tends to favor the non-neoplastic hypothesis.

Nephrogenic Adenofibroma

This is a solitary, benign tumor of the kidney in children and young adults (167). It has a distinctive composite appearance, with unencapsulated regions of renal cell proliferation resembling nephroblastic nephroma surrounding discrete nodules of embryonal epithelium having a tubular or tubulopapillary configuration. The epithelial

elements may contain psammoma bodies and often have a low mitotic rate (fig. 1-125). Tubular elements resembling collecting duct carcinomas may be seen in some specimens (fig. 1-126).

Hydropic Cell Variant of Nephroblastoma

This is a unique tumor composed of markedly enlarged, hydropic cells forming a thick rind around the kidney (165,166). Of the reported cases, at least one contained regions clearly recognizable as nephroblastoma and this lesion appears to represent a rare and distinctive alteration of tubular epithelial cells in nephroblastoma. It should not be confused with other renal tumors composed of clear cells.

Intrarenal Teratomas

These are rare primary renal neoplasms in children (164). We consider many reported cases to be examples of teratoid nephroblastoma. The files of the NWTS pathology center contain only two examples of renal teratoma; one of these was limited to the renal sinus and did not involve the renal parenchyma. True renal teratoma differs from teratoid nephroblastoma by the formation of recognizable nonrenal organs such as brain, gastrointestinal tract, or skin.

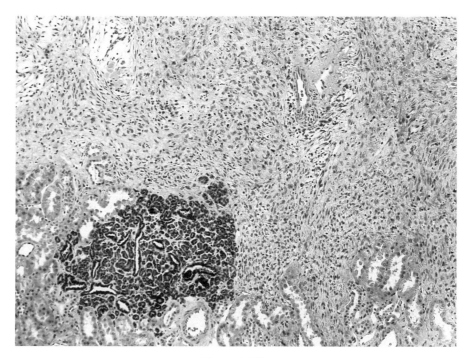

Figure 1-125
NEPHROGENIC ADENOFIBROMA
Spindle and myxoid stroma with adenomatous foci are characteristic.

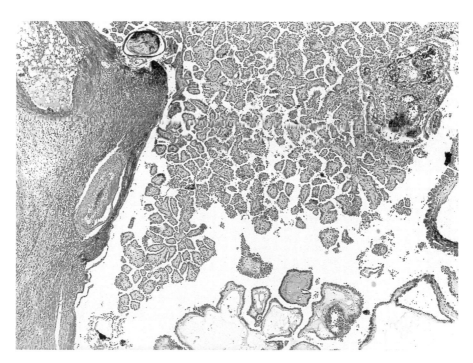

Figure 1-126
NEPHROGENIC ADENOFIBROMA
Foci resembling collecting duct carcinoma are seen in some lesions.

Table 1-17

RENAL TUMORS OF ADULTS

Renal cell carcinoma

    Clear cell (hypernephroid) type

    Papillary type

    Granular cell type

    Chromophobe cell type

    Sarcomatoid type

    Collecting duct type

Renal cortical adenoma

Oncocytoma

Rare tumors with epithelial or renal parenchymal differentiation

Mesenchymal tumors

Non-neoplastic tumorous conditions

TUMORS OF ADULTS

CLASSIFICATION

The broad separation of renal tumors according to patient age rather than histology is an arbitrary but widely accepted practice whose usefulness has been validated by many years of experience. Exceptions to this method of classification are well known, however, and the reader should be aware that renal neoplasms characteristically arising in infants and children may occur in adults and lesions usually arising in the kidneys of older individuals are observed in children. Renal tumors included in this section are categorized in Table 1-17.

RENAL CELL CARCINOMAS

Definition. This group of malignant neoplasms differentiate in whole or in part toward mature renal tubular structures. In the broadest sense, these neoplasms could be simply designated adenocarcinomas, but current usage prefers the term "renal cell" to distinguish them.

General Features. Renal neoplasms, primarily renal cell carcinomas (RCC), account for 3 percent of adult malignancies; approximately 27,000 cases result in more than 10,000 deaths per year in the United States (182). Tumors are found among all ethnic groups and geographic areas: there is no race predilection. Men are affected more than women (ratio, 1.6 to 1). The disease arises mainly in adult kidneys but tumors have been observed in infants as young as 6 months of age (229). The incidence increases with advancing age, with a peak in the sixth decade of life among patients with a median age of 55 years.

Renal cell neoplasms have been studied for more than 100 years but the etiology and histogenesis remain obscure. The term "hypernephroma," for example, was introduced by Grawitz to describe the clear cell type of renal cell carcinoma in the belief that the tumor arose from heterotopic adrenal (hypernephroid) rests in the kidney (193,211). Modern studies strongly indicate differentiation toward mature renal tubular structures, but in most cases, the exact portion of the nephron involved has been difficult to confirm (178,209,232,264). A variety of agents, including viruses, estrogens, lead compounds, X rays, and over 100 chemicals including aromatic hydrocarbons can induce RCC in experimental animals (173). None of these agents has been proven to be an important etiologic factor for renal cancers in humans, however. A slightly increased frequency of kidney cancer has been documented in men exposed to cadmium and rare cases have been observed after exposure to thorotrast (225,261). The most important known etiologic factor for RCC in men involves constituents of tobacco, whether smoked or chewed (178).

Cytogenetic studies of RCC have shown that most tumors exhibit consistent chromosomal abnormalities. Most commonly observed is a terminal deletion of the short arm of one of the two homologous chromosomes 3, beginning at 3p13 (227,247,263). Using restriction fragment length polymorphism (RFLP) analysis, DNA sequence deletions have been found consistently on chromosome 3 in RCC, mainly of the clear and granular cell types (265). These findings suggest that there is a recessive suppressor gene of chromosome 3 that may predispose to development of RCC when deleted. Genetic abnormalities are not constant for all subtypes, however. The papillary type, for example, most commonly exhibits trisomy of chromosome 17 and trisomy or tetrasomy of chromosome 7 (226,227).

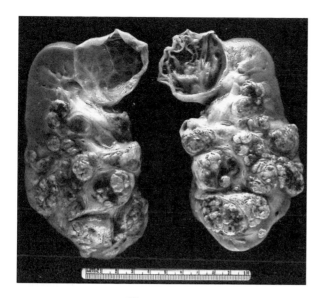

Figure 1-127
RENAL CELL CARCINOMA, CLEAR CELL TYPE
There is a multinodular tumor and a cortical retention cyst in this kidney. (Fig. 8-41 from Farrow GM. Diseases of the kidney. In: Murphy WM, ed. Urological pathology. Philadelphia: WB Saunders, 1989:409–82.)

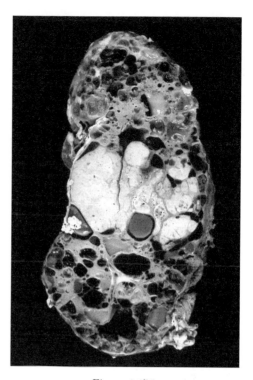

Figure 1-128
RENAL CELL CARCINOMA
This tumor arose in a kidney with adult-type polycystic renal disease.

RCCs are commonly associated with other renal diseases, malformations, and paraneoplastic syndromes. Authentic examples of RCC have been documented in supernumerary kidneys as well as teratomas (186,187). It must be noted, however, that if rigid diagnostic criteria are applied, most cases of extrarenal RCC are poorly documented tumors attributed to a renal cell origin primarily because of their clear cell histology (235).

RCCs are often associated with cysts (fig. 1-127). In most cases, the cyst is of the common variety generally considered a cortical retention cyst but associations with both acquired and hereditary polycystic disease have been well documented (figs. 1-128, 1-129) (185,190,207,212,219, 228). The renal neoplasms associated with acquired polycystic disease in patients on chronic hemodialysis generally occur after dialysis for several years (mean, 3.5 years) and the frequency of RCC varies directly with both the duration of dialysis and the incidence of cysts (198,210). The clinical significance of this association is not clear. Although renal tumors have been found in 25 percent of patients with acquired cystic disease, not all lesions have been malignant and

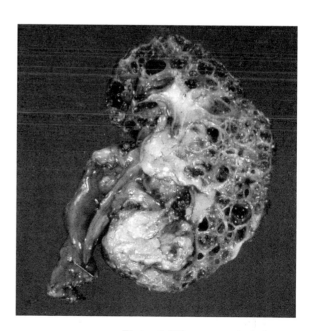

Figure 1-129
RENAL CELL CARCINOMA
This tumor is in the lower pole of a kidney with acquired polycystic disease associated with chronic hemodialysis. (Courtesy of Dr. Myron R. Melamed, New York, NY.)

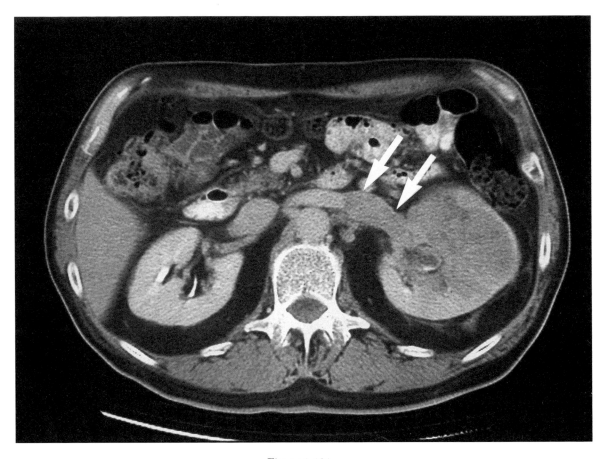

Figure 1-131
RENAL CELL CARCINOMA
As seen with computerized tomography, a large renal cell carcinoma in the kidney extends into the major renal vein (arrows). (Fig. 8-39 from Farrow GM. Diseases of the kidney. In: Murphy WM, ed. Urological pathology. Philadelphia: WB Saunders, 1989:409–82.)

renal capsule or traction on perinephric structures from the tumor itself. Flank masses are palpated in 6 to 48 percent of cases. They are usually nontender and indicative of a large tumor. An acquired scrotal mass due to varicocele secondary to obstruction of the spermatic vein has been observed in a few patients. Nonspecific symptoms such as fever (10 to 20 percent), weight loss (15 to 30 percent), fatigue (30 to 40 percent), nausea and vomiting (8 to 14 percent), and neuropathy or muscle tenderness (4 percent) are more commonly observed than the classic triad. Approximately 30 percent of patients with RCC present with signs and symptoms of metastatic disease.

Polycythemia, mostly in the form erythrocytosis, is seen in up to 6 percent of patients with RCC. Conversely, 2 to 4 percent of individuals

with polycythemia have RCC. In most cases, erythropoietin production by the tumor can be documented. Normochromic normocytic anemia unrelated to blood loss is seen in approximately 75 percent of cases. An increase in the erythrocyte sedimentation rate occurs in nearly 70 percent of patients. Hypercalcemia, attributed to production of parathormone-like substances by the tumor, may also occur.

Renal tumors are most accurately and consistently detected with some type of radiographic procedure (figs. 1-131, 1-132) (197). Calcification occurs in 10 to 15 percent of lesions and is usually localized to nonperipheral portions of the mass. Excretory urography may provide important information about the location and function of the contralateral kidney but is not particularly sensitive or specific in localizing small renal tumors.

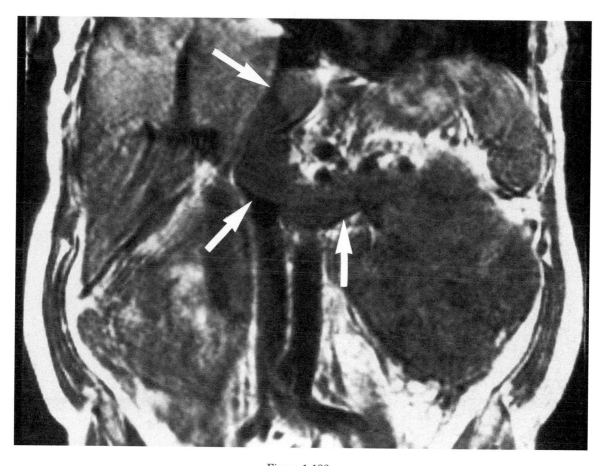

Figure 1-132
RENAL CELL CARCINOMA
As seen with magnetic resonance imaging, there is massive extension of renal cell carcinoma into the inferior vena cava (arrows).

CT is much more useful in this regard. Important staging information regarding extension to perirenal tissues, including the renal vein, vena cava, and lymph nodes, is best obtained using this technique (231). Ultrasonography is particularly useful in the evaluation of cystic lesions detected by other modalities, as well as for localizing needles in percutaneous procedures (205). The composition of the cyst and its fluid can be helpful in determining the nature of cystic tumors. In general, benign cysts appear radiologically as homogeneous spheres with regular smooth internal borders whereas neoplasms may contain nodules protruding into the cysts. Benign cysts are typically filled with clear, straw-colored fluid which is low in fat, protein, and lactic dehydrogenase while cystic carcinomas may be bloody, contain necrotic tissue, and

have an elevated fat, protein, or lactic dehydrogenase content. Renal arteriography is no longer the procedure of choice in the evaluation of renal masses and is generally reserved for special situations. In RCC, the arteriogram often shows neovascularity in the tumor, arteriovenous fistulas, and pooling of the contrast medium accentuating the capsular vessels (236). MRI may provide accurate staging information as well as a three-dimensional representation of the tumor to help plan a surgical approach (221).

Significant advances in the appropriate classification of RCCs have resulted from the application of immunohistochemistry, electron microscopy, cytogenetics, and molecular genetics. It now seems clear that a number of distinctive entities exist and that a classification is warranted. Categorizing neoplasms into subgroups

Table 1-19

CLASSIFICATION OF RENAL CELL CARCINOMA

Clear cell (hypernephroid)
Papillary
Granular cell
Chromophobe cell
Sarcomatoid
Collecting duct

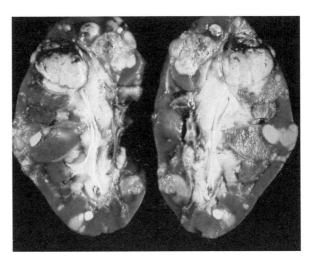

Figure 1-133
RENAL CELL CARCINOMA
The tumors are multiple and bilateral. (Fig. 8-40 from Farrow GM. Diseases of the kidney. In: Murphy WM, ed. Urological pathology. Philadelphia: WB Saunders, 1989:409–82.)

with similar pathologic features may be helpful in designing appropriate therapeutic strategies and predicting the likelihood of progression, however, considerable heterogeneity often exists within a single neoplasm and the likelihood of heterogeneity tends to increase with tumor size. At best, any classification scheme can only serve as a short-term structure upon which to build future knowledge. In the case of the RCCs listed in Table 1-19, the scheme is most valuable for small tumors since these neoplasms are most likely to be histologically uniform.

Pathologic Findings. *RCC, Clear Cell (Hypernephroid) Type.* This is the most common histologic variant, accounting for approximately 70 percent of RCCs. This tumor has been the subject of intense interest and its histogenesis remains controversial. Most lesions are solitary and randomly distributed in the renal cortex. They occur with equal frequency in either kidney. Multiple neoplasms may occur and in such cases, coexistence of a carcinoma with an adenoma is the rule. Multicentricity in the same kidney occurs in approximately 4 percent of cases whereas bilaterality occurs in 0.5 to 3.0 percent (fig. 1-133) (217). The pathologic criteria for the distinction of multicentricity from intrarenal or contrarenal metastases have not been established but a significant difference in the morphology of various tumors in the same or opposite kidneys favors a metastatic origin. Among multifocal cases, 75 percent have synchronous lesions; the remainder are asynchronous (266). Multicentricity and bilaterality are often associated with familial cases and associated conditions such as von Hippel-Lindau syndrome (fig. 1-130) (249). In one such case, as many as 15 discrete carcinomas were found (189).

RCC, clear cell type is characteristically a well-differentiated tumor which protrudes from the renal cortex as a rounded, bosselated mass. The interface of the tumor and the adjacent kidney is usually well demarcated, with a "pushing margin" (fig. 1-134). Rarely, RCC may be diffusely infiltrative (fig. 1-135). These neoplasms may be over 15 cm in greatest dimension (fig. 1-136) but the frequency of small lesions is rapidly increasing in countries where radiologic imaging techniques are widely applied. Size itself is not a determinant of behavior and all RCCs of the clear cell type are malignant tumors. Associated cysts are usually spatially separated from the neoplasm (fig. 1-127). On section, areas of necrosis, cystic degeneration, hemorrhage, and calcification are commonly present (figs. 1-137, 1-138). Calcification, and even ossification, typically occurs within necrotic zones and has been demonstrated in 10 to 15 percent of RCC cases (177). Variations in consistency tend to accompany tumor size, with small tumors being much more homogeneous than large lesions.

Although cystic changes occur in up to 26 percent of cases, only 5 percent of RCC, clear cell type are so predominantly cystic as to suggest a benign tumor (figs. 1-139, 1-140) (241). These *multilocular cystic renal cell carcinomas* have been considered a subtype of the clear cell variety.

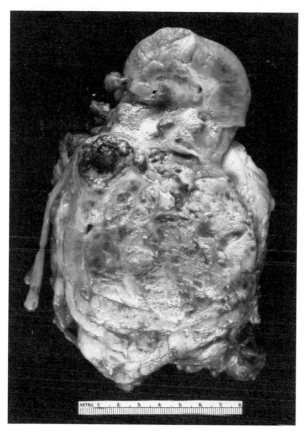

Figure 1-134
RENAL CELL CARCINOMA
The tumor grows with a "pushing" margin. (Fig. 8-45 from Farrow GM. Diseases of the kidney. In: Murphy WM, ed. Urological pathology. Philadelphia: WB Saunders, 1989:409–82.)

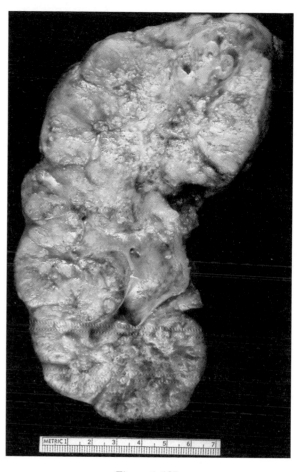

Figure 1-135
RENAL CELL CARCINOMA
This unusual tumor is diffusely infiltrative.

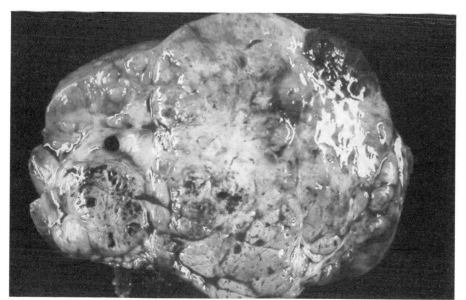

Figure 1-136
RENAL CELL
CARCINOMA,
CLEAR CELL TYPE
This large, golden yellow tumor has a variegated surface.

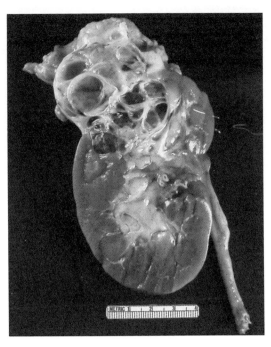

Figure 1-137
RENAL CELL CARCINOMA, CLEAR CELL TYPE
There are widespread zones of hemorrhage and necrosis.

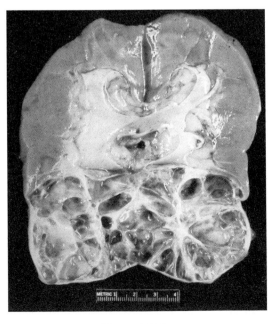

Figure 1-139
RENAL CELL CARCINOMA
This is a multilocular cystic renal cell carcinoma. (Fig. 8-47 from Farrow GM. Diseases of the kidney. In: Murphy WM, ed. Urological pathology. Philadelphia: WB Saunders, 1989:409–82.)

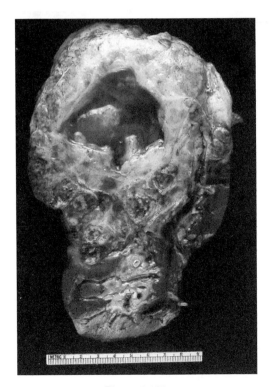

Figure 1-138
RENAL CELL CARCINOMA
This tumor exhibits central cystic degeneration. (Fig. 8-46 from Farrow GM. Diseases of the kidney. In: Murphy WM, ed. Urological pathology. Philadelphia: WB Saunders, 1989:409–82.)

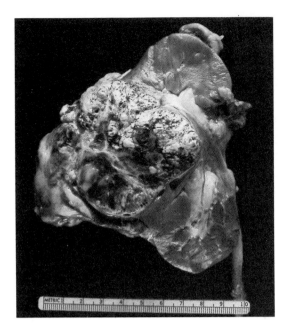

Figure 1-140
RENAL CELL CARCINOMA
This multilocular renal cell carcinoma must be distinguished from multilocular cyst.

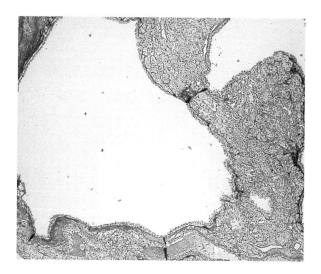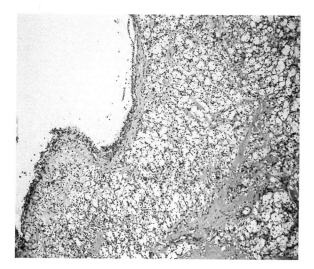

Figure 1-141
MULTILOCULAR RENAL CELL CARCINOMA
Left: Cystic spaces are lined by clear cells which form sheet-like aggregates.
Right. This sheet of clear cells is renal cell carcinoma.

They are distinguished from cystic nephroma (multilocular cyst) by the presence of nodular aggregates of clear cells in at least some portions of the cyst wall (fig. 1-141). These nodular aggregates are invariably of clear cell type and nuclear grade I. Not surprisingly, few if any have recurred or metastasized following nephrectomy. Among cases associated with polycystic kidney, the tumor appears as a solid mass against a backdrop of variable-sized cysts (see figs. 1-128, 1-129).

The clear cell type of RCC is typically golden due to the rich lipid content of its cells (figs. 1-142, 1-143A): cholesterol, neutral lipids, and phospholipids are abundant. These accumulate as droplets in the cytoplasm of tumor cells due to deficient glycogenolysis and lipolysis associated with unresponsiveness of the tumor cell adenylate cyclase to glucagon and beta-catecholamines (224). The lipid content is markedly similar to that of proximal convoluted tubules (232).

Microscopically, the clear cell type of RCC is characterized by cells interspersed with abundant, thin-walled blood vessels (fig. 1-144). The cells are filled with lipids and cholesterol which are ordinarily dissolved in usual histologic preparations, creating a clear cytoplasm surrounded by a distinct cell membrane (fig. 1-143B). These neutral lipids can be identified in unfixed material using oil red O and Sudan IV reactions. The phospholipid components are the most resistant

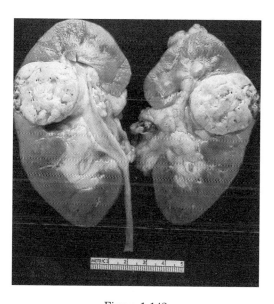

Figure 1-142
RENAL CELL CARCINOMA, CLEAR CELL TYPE
This tumor is circumscribed and golden yellow. (Fig. 8-43 from Farrow GM. Diseases of the kidney. In: Murphy WM, ed. Urological pathology. Philadelphia: WB Saunders, 1989:409–82.)

to solvents and may be identified with Sudan black B reactions. Glycogen can be identified by the periodic acid-Schiff reaction. Both types of cytoplasmic substance are readily observed in electron microscopic preparations. Other cytoplasmic components include hyaline intracytoplasmic

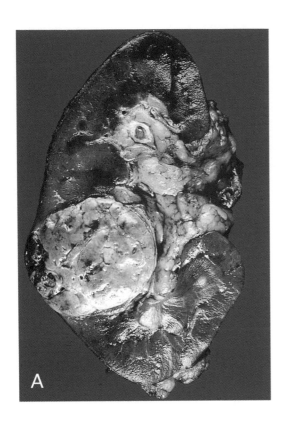

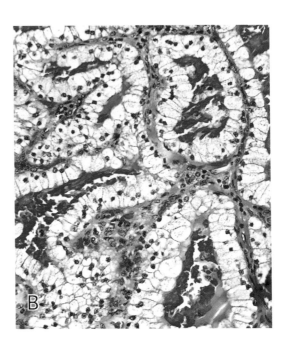

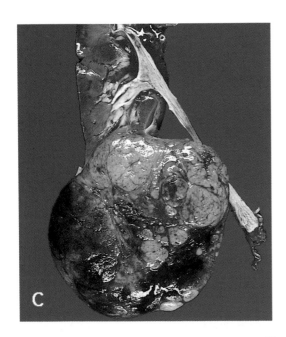

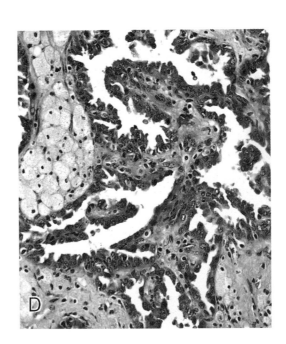

Figure 1-143
RENAL CELL CARCINOMA, CLEAR CELL AND PAPILLARY TYPES

A: Renal cell carcinoma, clear cell type: The golden color results from cytoplasmic lipids.
B: Renal cell carcinoma, clear cell type: The cells are in an acinar arrangement and feature optically clear cytoplasm.
C: Papillary renal cell carcinoma: The golden yellow color is due to lipid-laden stromal macrophages (xanthoma cells).
D: Papillary renal cell carcinoma: Neoplastic cells cover papillary structures with numerous stromal xanthoma cells.

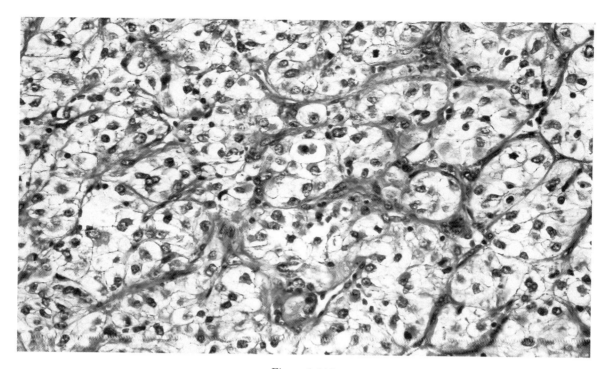

Figure 1-144
RENAL CELL CARCINOMA, CLEAR CELL TYPE
Alveolar architecture is created by thin-walled vascular septa.

globules and structures resembling Mallory bodies (195,218). The hyaline globules are 5 to 7 μm in greatest dimension and stain brightly acidophilic in usual preparations (fig. 1-145) but also react positively with periodic acid-Schiff, phosphotungstic acid, and Luxol fast blue reagents.

RCC, clear cell type exhibits various architectural patterns. Well-differentiated tumors usually have a uniform pattern, predominantly of the alveolar (fig. 1-146) or acinar variety (fig. 1-147). In these patterns, rounded collections of cells are peripherally demarcated by a network of delicate interconnecting capillary or sinusoidal structures and supported by a network of thin reticulin fibers. No luminal differentiation is apparent in the alveolar pattern but a central, rounded luminal space filled with lightly acidophilic serous fluid or erythrocytes occurs in the acinar pattern. Solid sheets of neoplastic cells punctuated by zones of hemorrhage, necrosis, and fibrosis are characteristic of poorly differentiated neoplasms.

In well-preserved preparations, nuclei tend to be round and uniform with finely granular, evenly distributed chromatin. Depending upon the degree of differentiation, nucleoli may be

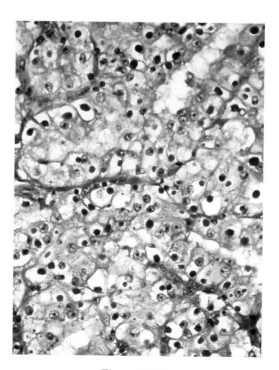

Figure 1-145
RENAL CELL CARCINOMA, CLEAR CELL TYPE
In addition to nuclei, many cells contain hyaline cytoplasmic globules 5 to 7 μm in diameter.

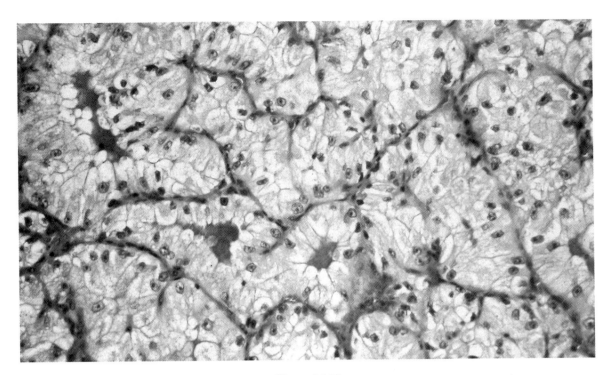

Figure 1-146
RENAL CELL CARCINOMA, CLEAR CELL TYPE
Alveolar and acinar architecture are mixed.

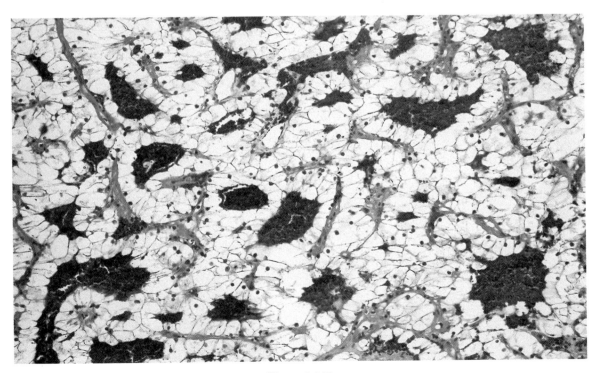

Figure 1-147
RENAL CELL CARCINOMA, CLEAR CELL TYPE
Acinar architecture is exhibited in this example. Pseudoglandular spaces are filled with erythrocytes.

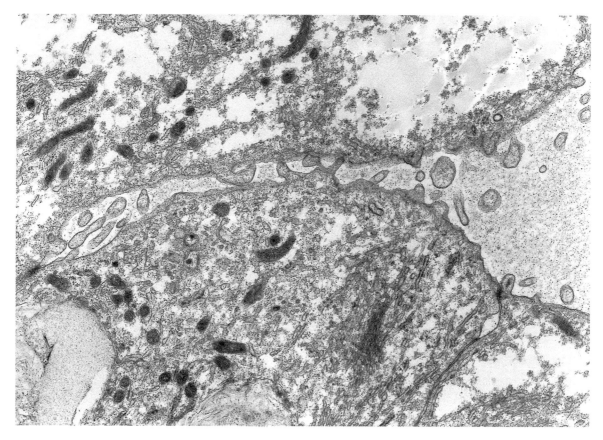

Figure 1-148
RENAL CELL CARCINOMA, CLEAR CELL TYPE
There are microvilli on the luminal aspect of the cell membrane (X3500). (Fig. 8-31 from Farrow GM. Diseases of the kidney. In: Murphy WM, ed. Urological pathology. Philadelphia: WB Saunders, 1989:409–82.)

absent, sparse, or large and prominent. Very large nuclei lacking nucleoli or bizarre nuclei may occasionally occur.

Ultrastructurally, cells tend to have a tubular differentiation characterized by arrangement around microlumina, varying amounts of brush border (fig. 1-148), and demarcation of groups of cells by basal lamina. Abundant lipid vacuoles and glycogen are characteristically present (fig. 1-149). Other organelles, such as Golgi and rough endoplasmic reticulum, are either absent or sparse.

Immunohistochemical studies indicate that the antigenic composition of RCCs is variable. These neoplasms manifest determinants common to renal tubules but evidence suggests that they develop from an uncommitted or primitive cell rather than any particular portion of the nephron (192). Cells comprising the clear cell type of RCC tend to react with antibodies to brush border antigens, low molecular weight cytokeratins, and vimentin (262,264). A significant number of cases are reactive to placental alkaline phosphatase. Rare cases reactive for carcinoembryonic antigens, alpha-fetoprotein and S-100 protein antigen, have been observed. These neoplasms do not react with antibodies to Tamm-Horsfall protein (199). Antibodies to lectins demonstrate variable antigenic composition (260). These studies indicate that even well-differentiated carcinomas may have lectin components in common with both proximal and distal tubules.

RCC, Papillary Type. This type of RCC is a histologically distinct tumor that comprises 10 to 15 percent of cases (180,230,234). Small tumors must be distinguished from true renal cortical adenomas (see section on adenoma). Papillary carcinomas are almost all larger than 3 cm in greatest dimension. In one large series, the

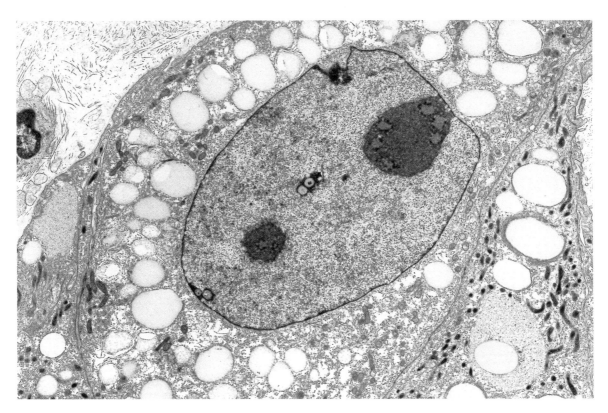

Figure 1-149
RENAL CELL CARCINOMA, CLEAR CELL TYPE

The tumor cells feature cytoplasmic glycogen and lipid droplets (X2500). (Fig. 8-30 from Farrow GM. Diseases of the kidney. In: Murphy WM, ed. Urological pathology. Philadelphia: WB Saunders, 1989:409–82.)

mean size was 8 cm and a few tumors measured up to 23 cm in greatest dimension (234).

Grossly, the papillary type of RCC is well circumscribed and eccentrically situated in the renal cortex (fig. 1-150). More than 80 percent of cases are confined to the cortex within the renal capsule at the time of nephrectomy (fig. 1-151). The cut surface of papillary RCC varies from light gray to golden yellow, depending upon the amount of lipid-laden macrophages in the stroma (fig. 1-143C). Intratumoral hemorrhage and necrosis are observed in two thirds of cases, a finding that correlates with radiographic studies showing reduced or absent tumor vascularity (174, 179,246). Tumors of this type are found in the walls of cysts (fig. 1-152) (219), are more often associated with cortical adenomas than other renal cell carcinomas, and are more often multiple.

Microscopically, RCC papillary type is characterized by a single layer of cells arranged over fibrovascular stalks (fig. 1-153). Most often, the entire tumor is papillary but tubules may exist in some cases. Accumulation of lipid-laden macrophages (xanthoma or foam cells) in the stalk is a characteristic feature (figs. 1-143D, 1-154). These xanthoma cells may greatly expand the papillary cores. Tumor necrosis may liberate large quantities of lipid and cholesterol crystals may form (fig. 1-155). Psammomatous calcifications may be abundant (fig. 1-156).

In most instances, tumor cells are small and cuboidal to low columnar with darkly acidophilic or slightly basophilic cytoplasm. Cells with clear cytoplasm are very unusual in renal carcinomas with this architectural arrangement. Large quantities of hemosiderin have been observed in the neoplastic cells of a few tumors (fig. 1-157) (204). The pigment occurs in areas distant from obvious hemorrhage and its source is unknown. Nuclei tend to be small, regular, and low grade. Nuclear enlargement, hyperchromasia, and anaplasia are distinctly unusual (fig. 1-158).

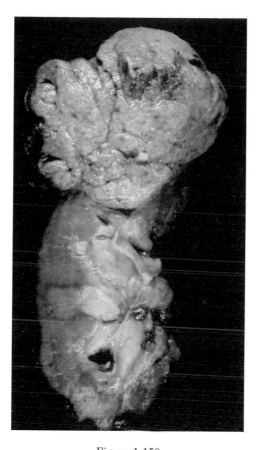

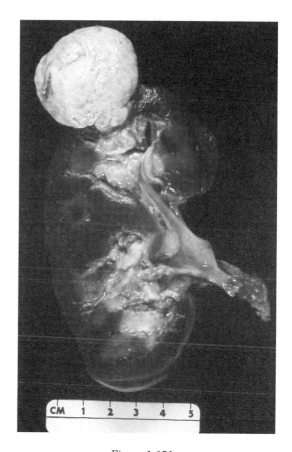

Figure 1-150
PAPILLARY RENAL CELL CARCINOMA
A golden yellow, circumscribed tumor is eccentrically
located in the upper pole of the kidney.

Figure 1-151
PAPILLARY RENAL CELL CARCINOMA
The golden color is due to numerous lipid-laden stromal
macrophages (xanthoma cells).

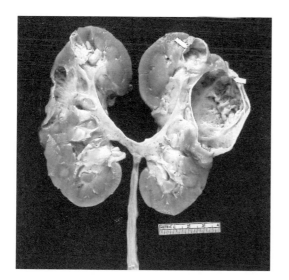

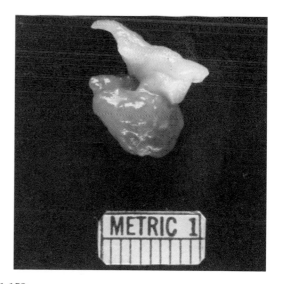

Figure 1-152
PAPILLARY RENAL CELL CARCINOMA
Left: These tumors are predominantly cysts with a localized mural nodule in each.
Right: The mural nodule projects upon a broad stalk.

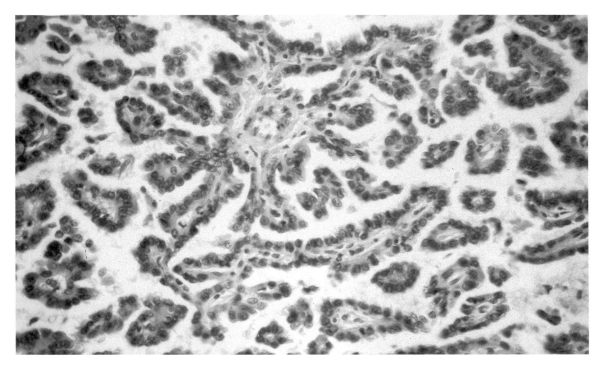

Figure 1-153
PAPILLARY RENAL CELL CARCINOMA
A single layer of cuboidal cells covers a fibrovascular papillary stalk.

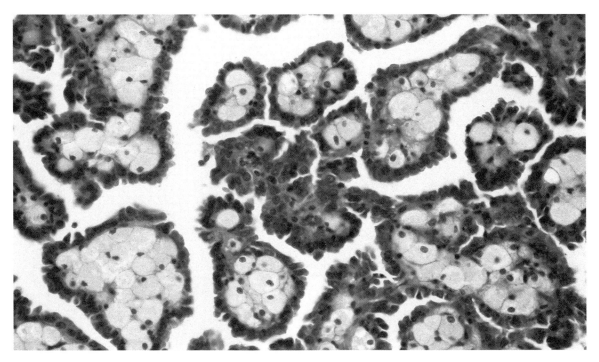

Figure 1-154
PAPILLARY RENAL CELL CARCINOMA
Stromal xanthoma cells are abundant.

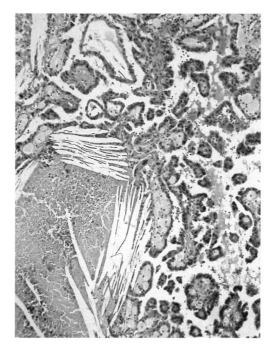

Figure 1-155
PAPILLARY RENAL CELL CARCINOMA
Tumor necrosis releases lipids which form cholesterol clefts.

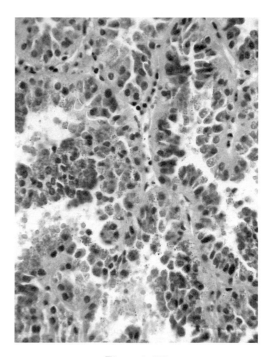

Figure 1-157
PAPILLARY RENAL CELL CARCINOMA
Hemosiderin granules are abundant in the neoplastic cells.

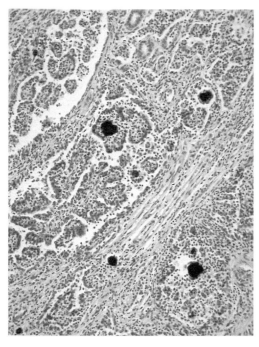

Figure 1-156
PAPILLARY RENAL CELL CARCINOMA

Psammomatous calcifications are present in the tumor. (Fig. 8-56 from Farrow GM. Diseases of the kidney. In: Murphy WM, ed. Urological pathology. Philadelphia: WB Saunders, 1989:409–82.)

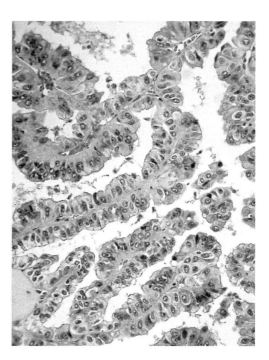

Figure 1-158
PAPILLARY RENAL CELL CARCINOMA
This higher grade tumor exhibits nuclear anaplasia.

Table 1-20

BROWN TUMORS OF THE KIDNEY: MACROSCOPIC CHARACTERISTICS

	Oncocytoma	Chromophobe Cell Renal Carcinoma	Granular Cell Renal Carcinoma
Color	Mahogany brown	Grey-brown	Variably brown
Tumor configuration	Circumscribed, rounded	Circumscribed, rounded	Irregularly invasive
Cut surface	Homogeneous, central scar	Homogeneous	Variegated
Tumor necrosis	Absent	Minimal to absent	Extensive

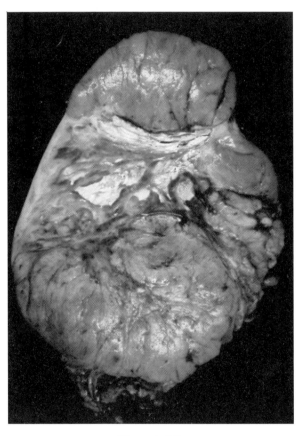

Figure 1-159
RENAL CELL CARCINOMA, GRANULAR CELL TYPE
The tumor is dark brown. Foci of necrosis are present.

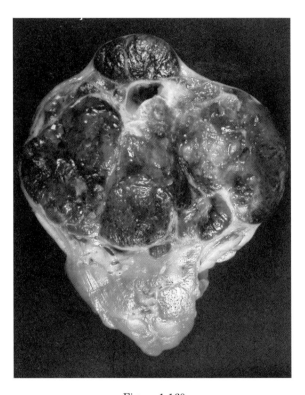

Figure 1-160
RENAL CELL CARCINOMA, GRANULAR CELL TYPE
A dark brown tumor exhibits "pushing" type invasion.

RCC, Granular Cell Type. This type accounts for approximately 7 percent of cases. As indicated, tumors comprised entirely of granular cells do occur, but many high-grade RCCs contain granular cell components (177).

Grossly, the granular cell type resembles the clear cell variant in size but hemorrhage and necrosis are more likely to be present (fig. 1-159) (Table 1-20). The tumor surface is brown, due to the phospholipid content of the numerous cytoplasmic organelles that fill its cells (figs. 1-160, 1-161). Local invasion, especially of the renal vein, is typical of this neoplasm.

Microscopically, cells may be arranged in sheets or alveoli, often interspersed with areas of necrosis (fig. 1-162) (Table 1-21). Tumor cells have abundant, acidophilic or chromophilic cytoplasm and

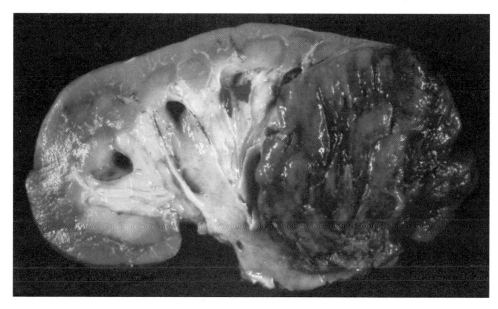

Figure 1-161
RENAL CELL CARCINOMA, GRANULAR CELL TYPE
A dark brown tumor extends into the lower pole calices.

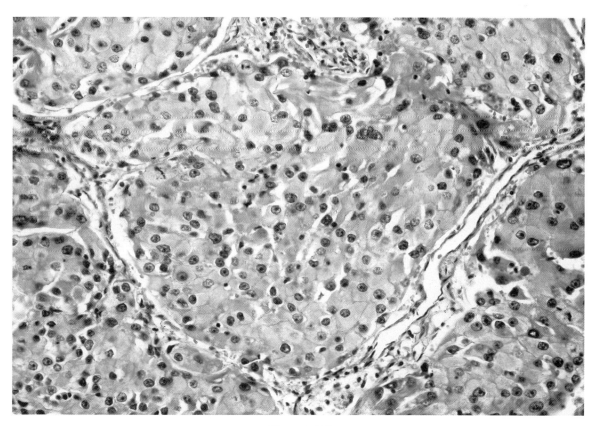

Figure 1-162
RENAL CELL CARCINOMA, GRANULAR CELL TYPE
There is an alveolar arrangement of cells with eosinophilic cytoplasm and nuclear anaplasia.

Table 1-21

**GRANULAR CELL TUMORS OF THE KIDNEY:
MICROSCOPIC CHARACTERISTICS**

	Oncocytoma	Chromophobe Cell Renal Carcinoma	Granular Cell Renal Carcinoma
Architecture	Rounded organoid cell groups	Sheets of cells divided by fine septa	Disorganized
Cellular features	Uniform small eosinophilic cells	Mixture of granular and transparent cells	Variable mixture of pleomorphic cells
Nuclear features	Round, regular, 8-10 microns	Slightly variable, slight hyperchromasia, 10-15 microns	Nuclear variability, 15-20 microns or more
	Nucleoli inconspicuous, no mitoses	Nucleoli inconspicuous few or no mitoses	Prominent nucleoli, plentiful mitoses
Ultrastructure	Mitochondria	Mitochondria and vesicles	Mitochondria, rough endoplasmic reticulum, lysosomes

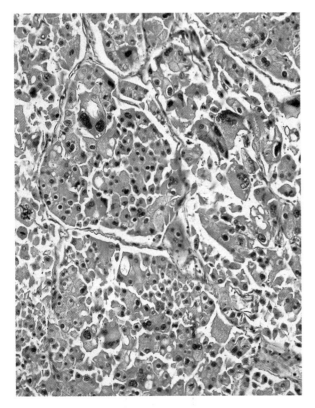

Figure 1-163
RENAL CELL CARCINOMA,
GRANULAR CELL TYPE AND ONCOCYTOMA
This high-grade carcinoma exhibits cellular pleomorphism and nuclear anaplasia.

moderately well-defined borders (fig. 1-163). Lipid and glycogen may occur in small amounts but are not important histologic features. In contrast to the clear cell type of RCC, nuclei are often of high grade. Pleomorphism, coarsely granular chromatin, and prominent nucleoli are characteristic (fig. 1-164). Mitoses are uncommon except in very anaplastic areas. Ultrastructurally, tumor cells are rich in mitochondria, rough endoplasmic reticulum, and Golgi apparatus.

RCC, Chromophobe Cell Type. This is a distinctive variant that may have been confused with oncocytoma and variants of RCC in the past (Tables 1-20, 1-21) (256). As currently defined, these tumors constitute approximately 5 percent of renal neoplasms. A similar neoplasm can be induced in rats, where it seems to differentiate toward the proximal nephron (172). In humans, however, the presence of numerous cytoplasmic vesicles containing the enzyme carbonic anhydrase C suggests differentiation toward the intercalated cells of collecting ducts (254).

Grossly, tumors range from 2 to 22 cm in greatest dimension (mean, 8 cm) (fig. 1-165). All lesions have been well-circumscribed and solitary. The cut surface is typically gray to brown and lacking in hemorrhage or necrosis (fig. 1-166A) (181).

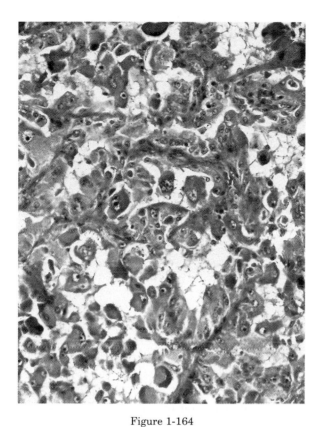

Figure 1-164
RENAL CELL CARCINOMA,
GRANULAR CELL TYPE
There is nuclear pleomorphism and nucleoli are prominent.

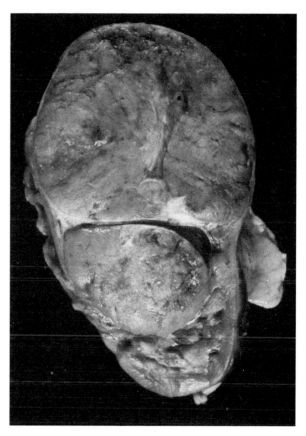

Figure 1-165
RENAL CELL CARCINOMA,
CHROMOPHOBE CELL TYPE
This large renal tumor is brown.

Microscopically, tumor cells are arranged in broad alveoli (fig. 1-167). The cells have well-defined borders and abundant cytoplasm. In most cases, the cytoplasm is distended with numerous microvesicles, giving it a "plant cell" appearance and a pale acidophilic staining in usual histologic preparations (fig. 1-166B). In some cases, the predominant cell type contains numerous mitochondria, which are granular and strongly acidophilic. Intimate admixtures of pale transparent and brightly acidophilic cells in any particular tumor are the rule (fig. 1-168). The transparent cells are often oriented along the vascular septa (figs. 1-169, 1-170). The nuclei of both cell types are similar. They are 10 to 15 mm in diameter and slightly pleomorphic, with coarsely granular chromatin and occasional prominent nucleoli conforming to a nuclear grade 2 renal neoplasm.

The microvesicles of both types of chromophobe cells can be stained by the Hale colloidal iron technique, indicating a content of mucopolysaccharides unique to RCCs (256,257). When observed using electron microscopy, the cytoplasmic vesicles are round to oval and vary in size from 150 to 300 nm (figs. 1-171, 1-172). Typically, they are complex, with vesicles occurring inside vesicles. They tend to be concentrated adjacent to and surrounding the nucleus. Mitochondria exist more peripherally. This arrangement accounts for the light microscopic appearance of a perinuclear transparent zone in many tumor cells. Immunohistochemically, tumor cells react positively with antibodies to cytokeratins, epithelial membrane antigen, soybean agglutinin, and carbonic anhydrase C. They do not react for vimentin.

RCC, Sarcomatoid Type. This is a particularly poorly differentiated, anaplastic variant comprising 1.5 percent of cases (200). The histogenesis is obscure but these tumors are classified

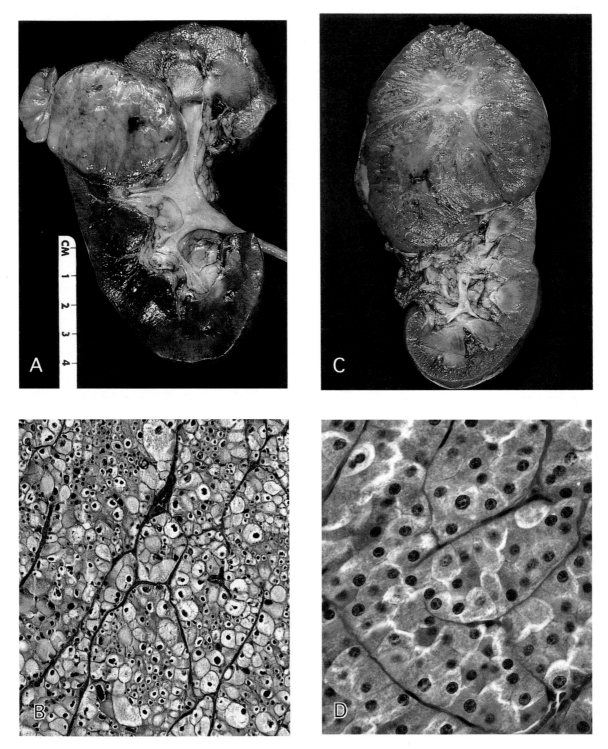

Figure 1-166
RENAL CELL CARCINOMA, CHROMOPHOBE CELL TYPE AND ONCOCYTOMA

A: Chromophobe cell carcinoma: This tumor is tan and relatively homogeneous.

B: Renal cell carcinoma, chromophobe cell type: The tumor cells vary from pale and transparent to acidophilic and granular.

C: Renal oncocytoma: This mahogany brown tumor exhibits a stellate central scar.

D: Renal oncocytoma: The cells are in tight alveolar arrangements and feature acidophilic cytoplasm. The nuclei are round and regular and exhibit no or single small nucleoli.

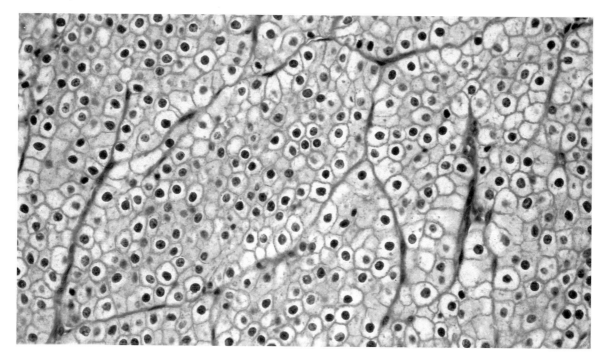

Figure 1-167
RENAL CELL CARCINOMA, CHROMOPHOBE CELL TYPE
The tumor features a mixture of acidophilic granular cells and pale transparent cells. Prominent cell borders impart a plant-like appearance.

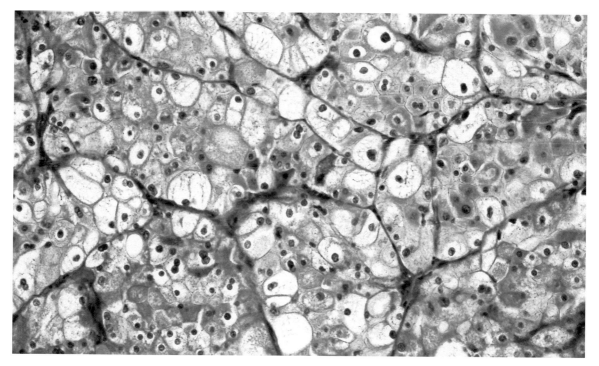

Figure 1-168
RENAL CELL CARCINOMA, CHROMOPHOBE CELL TYPE
Granular and transparent cells are intermixed in an irregular pattern.

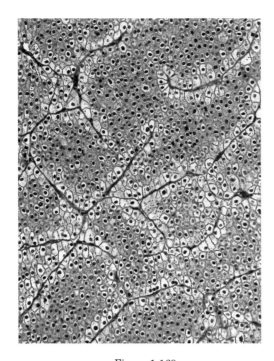

Figure 1-169
RENAL CELL CARCINOMA,
CHROMOPHOBE CELL TYPE

The transparent cells are oriented along the thin vascular septa.

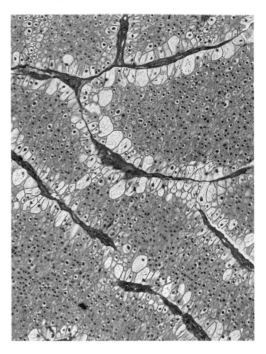

Figure 1-170
RENAL CELL CARCINOMA,
CHROMOPHOBE CELL TYPE

There is a striking orientation of transparent cells along the vascular septa.

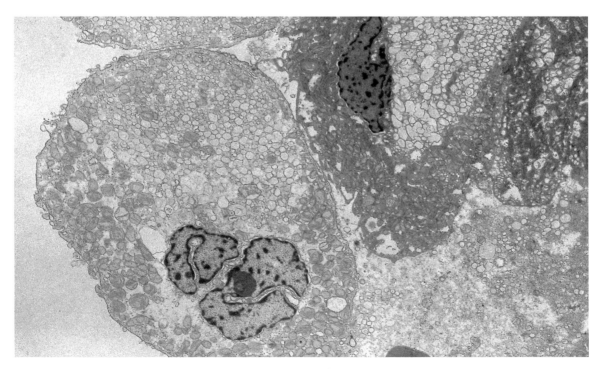

Figure 1-171
RENAL CELL CARCINOMA, CHROMOPHOBE CELL TYPE

Cytoplasmic vesicles of 150 to 300 nm are present in the cytoplasm, along with mitochondria.

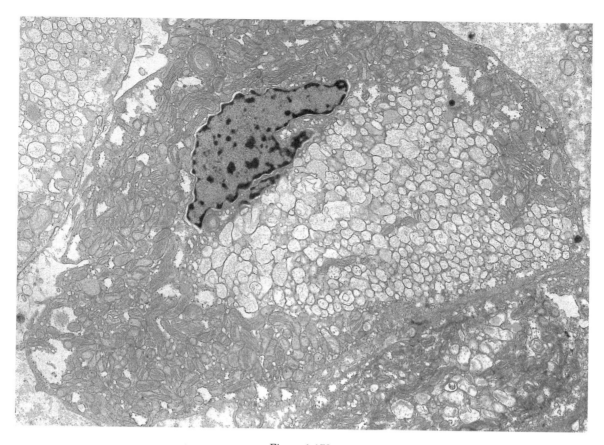

Figure 1-172
RENAL CELL CARCINOMA, CHROMOPHOBE CELL TYPE
The cytoplasmic vesicles are often paranuclear with mitochondria present in the more peripheral cytoplasm.

among the carcinomas because either light microscopic, immunohistochemical, or ultrastructural features showing evidence of epithelial differentiation are invariably present. The proportion of sarcomatous and carcinomatous differentiation in any particular tumor may be variable (250). The carcinomatous component in a sarcomatoid tumor is poorly differentiated in more than 75 percent of cases. A few reported cases had areas of chondrosarcoma and osteosarcoma; these tumors could be appropriately designated carcinosarcoma (200,233,240).

Grossly, the sarcomatoid type of RCC is usually a large, invasive tumor and many cases are widely disseminated at diagnosis (fig. 1-173). The combination of widespread metastases in association with a small primary renal tumor may occur but has been overemphasized. Depending upon the relative proportions of sarcomatous and carcinomatous elements, the sarcomatoid type

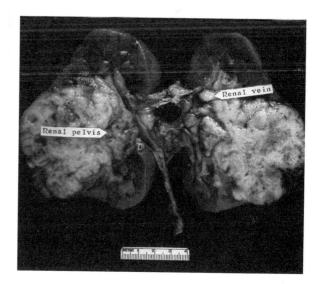

Figure 1-173
SARCOMATOID RENAL CELL CARCINOMA
The tumor is firm and fibrous and there is extensive invasion of renal structures.

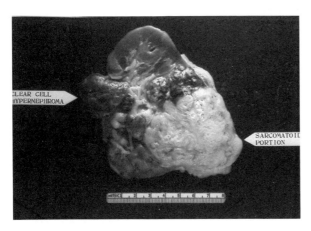

Figure 1-174
SARCOMATOID RENAL CELL CARCINOMA
This tumor exhibits a bimorphic macroscopic appearance with a firm, fibrous component and ordinary renal cell carcinoma. (Fig. 1 from Farrow GM, Harrison EG Jr, Utz DC. Sarcomas and sarcomatoid and mixed malignant tumors of the kidney in adults—Part III. Cancer 1968;22:556–63.)

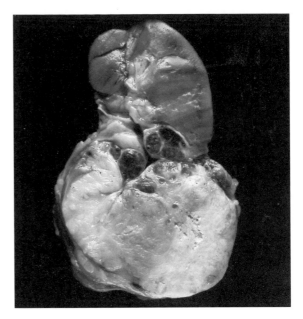

Figure 1-175
SARCOMATOID RENAL CELL CARCINOMA
Most of this bimorphic tumor is sarcomatoid, with a small component of typical carcinoma. (Fig. 2 from Farrow GM, Harrison EG Jr, Utz DC. Sarcomas and sarcomatoid and mixed malignant tumors of the kidney in adults—Part III. Cancer 1968;22:556–63.)

may present a bimorphic macroscopic appearance (figs. 1-174, 1-175) or may be heterogeneous or firm and fibrous without hemorrhage and necrosis.

Microscopically, the sarcomatoid component is characterized by interlacing or whorled bundles of spindle cells, sometimes in a storiform pattern (fig. 1-176) (258). Carcinomatous components may be distinctly separate from the spindled component and have a clear cell, granular cell, mixed, and rarely, even papillary or oncocytic morphology (fig. 1-177) (250,258). In other cases, there may be transition zones from carcinoma to sarcomatoid areas (fig. 1-178). Many tumors resemble malignant fibrous histiocytomas (figs. 1-179, 1-180). Ultrastructural studies in some cases have demonstrated desmosomal junctions among the spindle cells (196).

Not surprisingly, considerable heterogeneity has been observed using histochemical and immuno-histochemical techniques. Some tumors have reacted with antibodies to cytokeratins in both the sarcomatous and carcinomatous components (223). Immunoreactivity to desmin and smooth muscle myosin has been rarely observed among the spindle cells. Plumper elements, which may represent transition forms between carcinoma and sarcoma, have reacted positively with antibodies to epithelial membrane antigen (259).

RCC, Collecting Duct Type. This rare tumor constitutes less than 1 percent of recorded cases (194,202,213,222). Although there are some overlapping features with papillary RCC, the location in the medulla and the predominantly tubular configuration of the tumor suggest collecting duct differentiation. In the World Health Organization classification, this tumor is grouped with RCCs but designated *Bellini duct carcinoma*. An origin from the collecting ducts is further supported by atypical hyperplasia of the collecting duct epithelium adjacent to the neoplasm as well as immunohistochemical studies.

Grossly, the tumor is predominantly localized to the medulla but may invade the cortex (fig. 1-181). It produces distortion of adjacent calyces and the renal pelvis. Neither hemorrhage nor necrosis is typically present. A multicystic appearance secondary to dilated tubular structures often occurs (fig. 1-182).

Microscopically, the collecting duct type of RCC is composed of a mixture of dilated tubules and papillae (figs. 1-183, 1-184). Both tubules and papillae are lined by a single layer of cuboidal

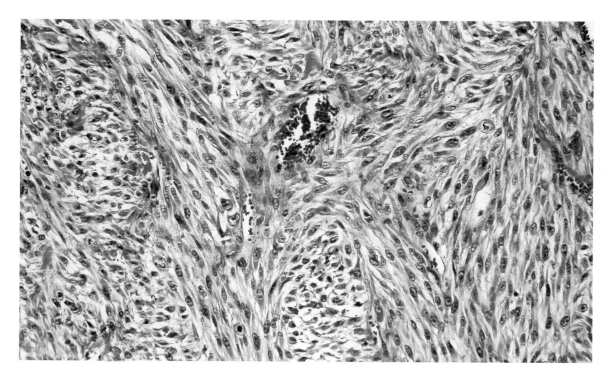

Figure 1-176
SARCOMATOID RENAL CELL CARCINOMA
There are interlacing fascicles of spindle cells.

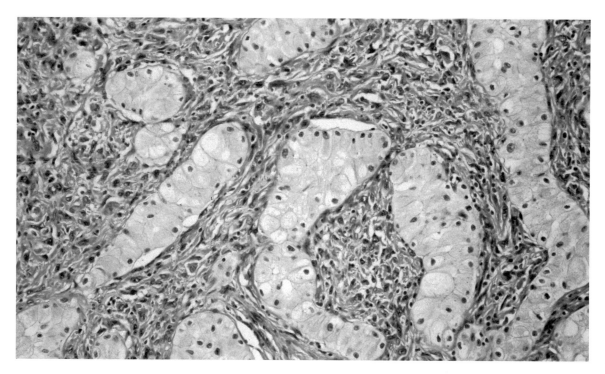

Figure 1-177
SARCOMATOID RENAL CELL CARCINOMA
This tumor features a mixture of carcinomatous and sarcomatous elements.

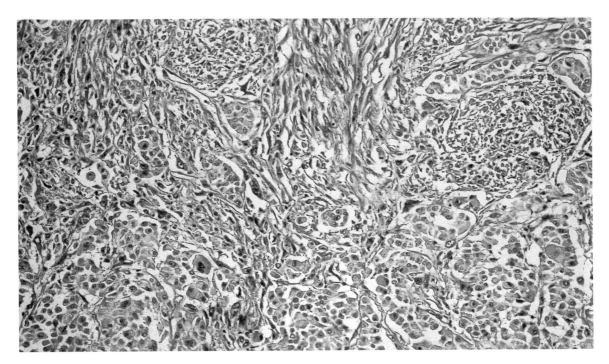

Figure 1-178
SARCOMATOID RENAL CELL CARCINOMA
In this field, a transition from typical carcinoma to sarcomatoid carcinoma may be observed.

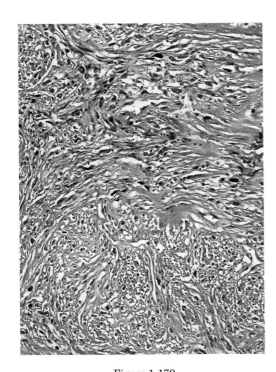

Figure 1-179
SARCOMATOID RENAL CELL CARCINOMA
This tumor is very fibrogenic and resembles malignant fibrous histiocytoma.

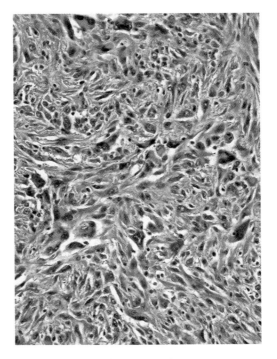

Figure 1-180
SARCOMATOID RENAL CELL CARCINOMA
This tumor exhibits giant cells and a storiform pattern resembling malignant fibrous histiocytoma.

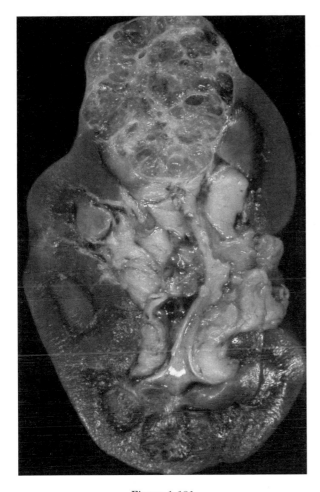

Figure 1-181
RENAL CELL CARCINOMA,
COLLECTING DUCT TYPE
This tumor is situated in both the renal cortex and medulla and is multicystic.

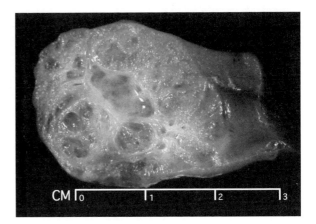

Figure 1-182
RENAL CELL CARCINOMA,
COLLECTING DUCT TYPE
This tumor, located predominantly in the renal medulla, was segmentally resected after a preoperative diagnosis of multilocular cyst.

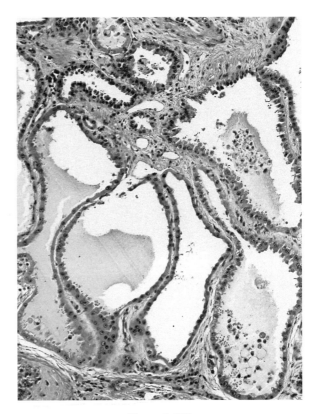

Figure 1-183
RENAL CELL CARCINOMA,
COLLECTING DUCT TYPE
This tumor is composed of dilated tubules lined by a single layer of cells.

cells with a cobblestone appearance (fig. 1-185). In most cases, the predominant pattern is tubular. These tubules may be of varying dimensions and impart a sponge-like appearance to the tumor. In well-differentiated examples, nuclear pleomorphism is minimal and mitoses infrequent (fig. 1-186). Lesions composed of anastomosing tubules with considerable nuclear hyperchromasia and pleomorphism may infiltrate the adjacent renal parenchyma and elicit a desmoplastic response (fig. 1-187). There may be atypical hyperplasia of the epithelium of the renal collecting ducts immediately adjacent to the tumor, a point of evidence for collecting duct origin (fig. 1-188). The cells of collecting duct

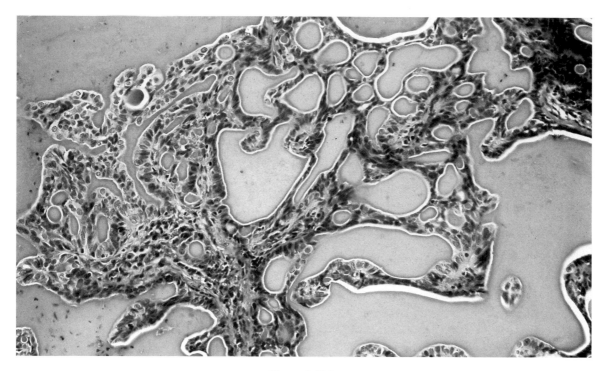

Figure 1-184
RENAL CELL CARCINOMA, COLLECTING DUCT TYPE
This tumor is composed of both dilated tubules and papillary structures.

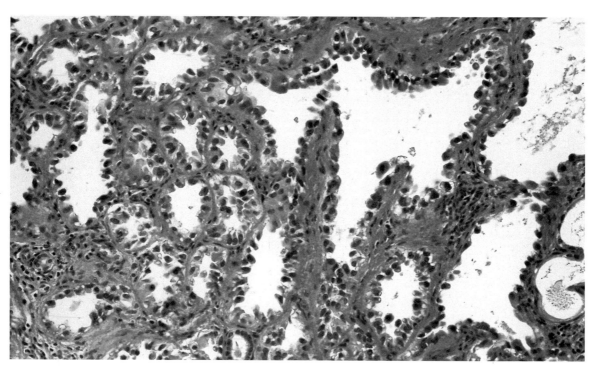

Figure 1-185
RENAL CELL CARCINOMA, COLLECTING DUCT TYPE
The tubules are lined by a single layer of cuboidal cells with a cobblestone appearance.

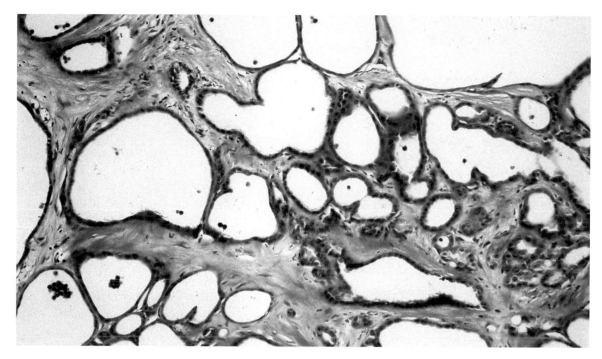

Figure 1-186
RENAL CELL CARCINOMA, COLLECTING DUCT TYPE
This specimen from an intra-abdominal metastasis demonstrates minimal morphologic features of malignancy. The kidney lesion, before metastasis, was originally interpreted as segmental polycystic renal disease.

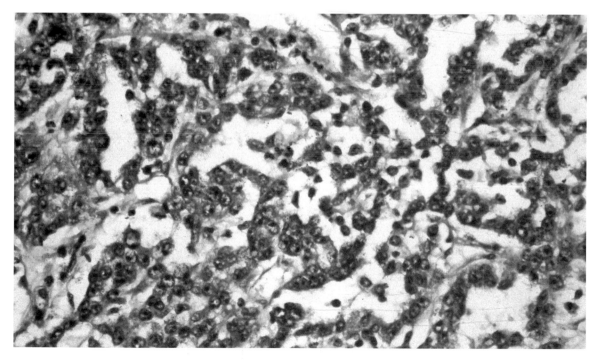

Figure 1-187
RENAL CELL CARCINOMA, COLLECTING DUCT TYPE
In this high-grade example, tubules are less well formed and there is nuclear anaplasia.

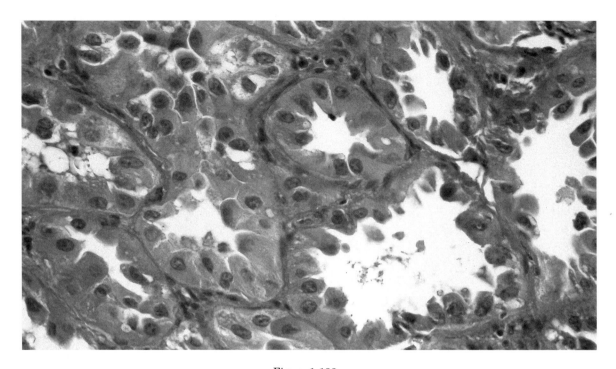

Figure 1-188
RENAL CELL CARCINOMA, COLLECTING DUCT TYPE
There is atypical hyperplasia of the collecting duct epithelium in the renal medulla immediately adjacent to the tumor.

carcinoma react positively with antibodies to both high and low molecular weight cytokeratins, peanut agglutinin, and epithelial membrane antigen (203). This immunohistochemistry is characteristic of distal tubular epithelium and differs from most other types of RCC.

Grading. Grading schemes for RCC usually rely on cytologic more than histologic criteria and emphasize the size and chromatin characteristics of the nucleus, the size and prominence of the nucleolus, and the frequency of mitoses. Nuclear grading schemes are easily correlated with quantitative morphometry and DNA ploidy as determined by flow cytometry. They are quite effective in predicting aggressive behavior following nephrectomy (Table 1-22). The preferred grading scheme is that of Fuhrman and associates (206). In this system, the entire neoplasm is classified by the highest grade of any of its component cells, regardless of their prevalence. The grading system of Fuhrman is shown in Table 1-23 (fig. 1-189).

Special Techniques. In contrast to many other epithelial neoplasms, karyotypic analysis provides clues to the etiology of some types of

RCC and is therefore mentioned in the section on general features. In summary, clear cell and granular cell types have abnormalities of chromosome 3, the most consistent change being the deletion in the short arm beginning at 3p13 (227,247,263,265). In contrast, the most common karyotypic abnormalities in papillary RCC involve chromosomes 7 and 17 and are usually manifested as trisomies (226). Consistent karyotypic aberrations have not been observed in the remaining subtypes of RCC.

Analyses of DNA ploidy using cytophotometry and flow cytometry usually correlate with determinations of nuclear grade (215,248). Quantitative measurements of DNA have not been useful as independent indicators of prognosis.

Aspiration cytology of large hypovascular renal masses, disseminated tumors, unresectable cancers, and suspected metastatic lesions involving the kidney is useful both for excluding a primary renal carcinoma and for determining the nature of mass lesions involving the kidney (fig. 1-190) (204,220,242,245). Needles of relatively large bore can be used without significant complications so that tissue fragments are available for

Table 1-22

EFFECT OF HISTOLOGIC GRADE ON SURVIVAL*

Grade	Number of Patients	Survival (%) 3-Yr	5-Yr	10-Yr
1	106	75	67	51
2	256	65	56	42
1 and 2	362	68	59	45
3	122	41	33	15
4	24	8	8	0
3 and 4	146	36	29	13
Total	508	59**	50**	36**

*Table 2 from Myers GH Jr, Fehrenbaker LG, Kelalis PP. Prognostic significance of renal vein invasion by hypernephroma. J Urol 1968;100:420–3.
**Mean survival.

Table 1-23

FUHRMAN GRADING SYSTEM

Grade	Characteristics
I	Nuclei round, uniform, approximately 10 μm; nucleoli inconspicuous or absent
II	Nuclei slightly irregular, approximately 15 μm; nucleoli evident
III	Nuclei very irregular, approximately 20 μm; nucleoli large and prominent
IV	Nuclei bizarre and multilobated, 20 μm or greater; nucleoli prominent; chromatin clumped

examination in many cases. Since needle aspirations are generally indicated only for large lesions that are expected to be either predominantly cystic or poorly differentiated, a high accuracy rate for the establishment of malignancy should be expected.

Differential Diagnosis. Differentiating RCCs from other neoplasms is usually not a problem. Difficulties arise primarily when tumors are small, papillary, oncocytic, collecting duct type, sarcomatoid type, or metastatic.

Small RCCs can be distinguished from adenomas by their pattern, cytoplasmic features, growth, and nuclear anaplasia. All clear cell, granular cell, chromophobe cell, sarcomatoid cell, and collecting duct tumors should be considered carcinomas regardless of their size at diagnosis. Papillary and tubular lesions may represent true adenomas if they lack nuclear anaplasia. Almost

all such tumors are less than 2 cm in greatest dimension and most have been incidental findings in the past.

When oncocytic cells predominate in a RCC of granular or chromophobe cell type, the tumor must be differentiated from an oncocytoma (Tables 1-20, 1-21). The distinction can be influenced by the organoid pattern of oncocytomas but is made primarily by the absence of nuclear anaplasia in these lesions. Oncocytomas may contain areas of nuclear pleomorphism and occasional foci with very large nuclei, but mitotic activity or prominent nucleoli are not characteristic, and oncocytic tumors with the latter nuclear features should be considered carcinomas.

Collecting duct carcinomas can be distinguished from the papillary type of RCC by their location, architecture, antigenic expression, and even karyotypic composition. Although rare

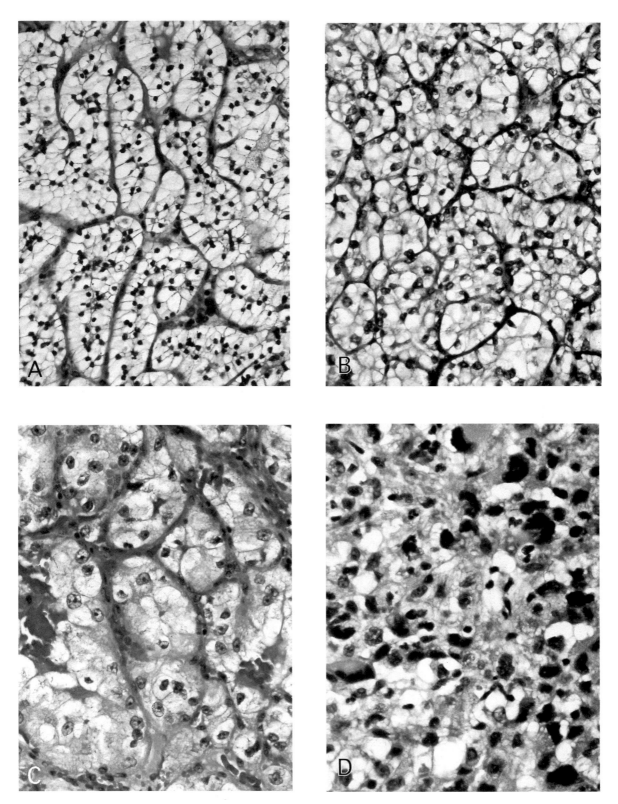

Figure 1-189
GRADING OF RENAL CELL CARCINOMA
A: Grade I; B: Grade II; C: Grade III; D: Grade IV

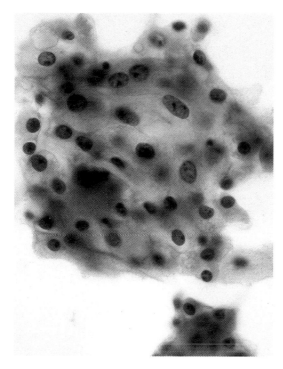

Figure 1-190
RENAL CELL CARCINOMA:
FINE NEEDLE ASPIRATION
A group of cells in an alveolar arrangement demonstrate vesiculated nuclei, prominent nucleoli, and vacuolated cytoplasm.

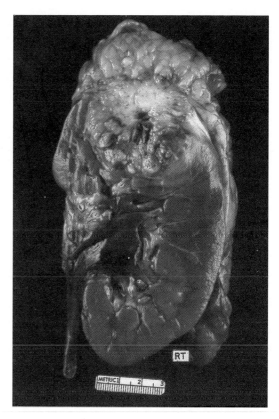

Figure 1-191
RENAL CELL CARCINOMA
This tumor extends through the renal capsule into the perirenal fat. (Fig. 8-36 from Farrow GM. Diseases of the kidney. In: Murphy WM, ed. Urological pathology. Philadelphia: WB Saunders, 1989:409–82.)

cases have exhibited some transitional cell–like foci, they differ from transitional cell carcinomas with collecting duct involvement by their architecture; immunohistochemistry; and lack of a recognizable in situ, papillary, or solid transitional cell component in the renal pelvis.

Most predominantly fibrous renal neoplasms are sarcomatoid carcinomas rather than purely mesenchymal tumors. Careful microscopic examination of generously sampled lesions almost always reveals foci of epithelial differentiation. These tumors must also be distinguished from malignant melanomas. Electron microscopy and immunohistochemistry are helpful in selected cases. Fibrous renal tumors manifesting chondrosarcomatous or osteosarcomatous elements, with or without carcinomatous foci, can be designated carcinosarcomas.

RCCs are rarely confused with metastases to the kidney. The identification of mucopolysaccharides in such cases can be diagnostic. Metastases from RCCs, in contrast, may be extremely

difficult to interpret in usual histologic preparations; radiologic co-imaging of the kidney may be necessary to clarify the situation in any particular case. Metastases from sarcomatoid RCC have been confused with primary fibrous histiocytoma of bone; metastatic papillary RCC has been misinterpreted as primary thyroid carcinoma; and metastatic clear cell RCC has been difficult to distinguish from certain primary skin and lung tumors. Demonstration of lipid and glycogen without mucopolysaccharides in the cells of such tumors is extremely helpful in confirming a renal origin. Rarely, metastatic RCC may be impossible to distinguish from cerebellar hemangioblastoma.

Mode of Dissemination. RCCs grow by direct extension, slowly compressing the adjacent kidney and attenuating the overlying capsule (fig. 1-191). Most are large at the time of detection and less than half are confined to the kidney

127

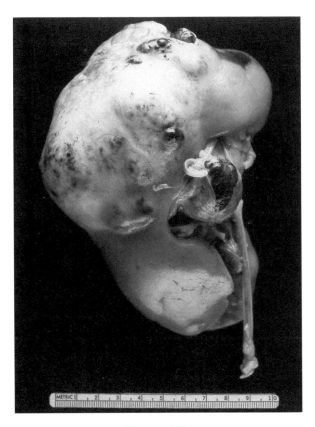

Figure 1-192
RENAL CELL CARCINOMA
This tumor extends into the main renal vein at the hilus of the kidney. (Fig. 8-37 from Farrow GM. Diseases of the kidney. In: Murphy WM, ed. Urological pathology. Philadelphia: WB Saunders, 1989:409–82.)

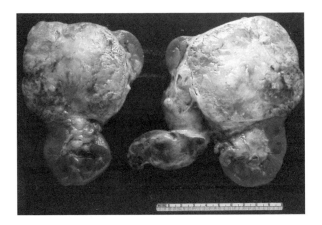

Figure 1-193
RENAL CELL CARCINOMA
Massive tumor extension into the renal vein and into the inferior vena cava.

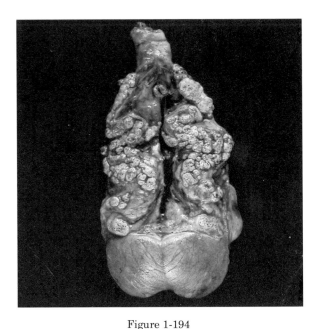

Figure 1-194
RENAL CELL CARCINOMA
Retrograde extension of tumor down the left internal spermatic vein into the spermatic cord.

(178,188). Of those tumors detected before the widespread application of modern imaging techniques, 7 percent were locally invasive, 35 percent metastatic to regional lymph nodes, and 25 percent disseminated. RCCs tend to grow into and propagate along the renal vein (figs. 1-192, 1-193) (188,208,214,237,243). In the past, this phenomenon was common and many cases of vena caval and even right atrial involvement by propagating RCC were observed. Such extensive involvement of the venous system was associated with a significant reduction in patient survival. Currently, intrarenal vein involvement is observed in approximately 16 percent of cases while involvement of the main extrarenal vein and propagation into the vena cava is noted in 8 percent and 7 percent of cases, respectively.

When metastases occur, the lung is involved in 55 percent of cases. Other organs are affected in the following descending order of frequency: lymph nodes, liver, bone, adrenal glands, kidney, brain, heart, spleen, intestine, and skin. Compared to other cancers, kidney tumors have a predilection for metastases to bone and skin (178), but metastases to unusual sites are common (figs. 1-194, 1-195).

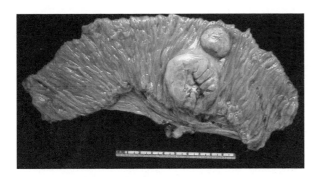

Figure 1-195
RENAL CELL CARCINOMA
Metastatic renal cell carcinoma to the small intestine.

Table 1-24

**ROBSON STAGING SCHEME
FOR RENAL CELL CARCINOMA***

Stage	Characteristics*
1	Confined to the kidney
2	Perirenal fat involvement, but confined to Gerota fascia
3	A. Gross renal vein or inferior vena cava involvement B. Lymphatic involvement C. Vascular plus lymphatic invasion
4	A. Adjacent organs other than adrenal involved B. Distant metastases

*Table 3 from Robson CJ, Churchill BM, Anderson W. The results of radical nephrectomy for renal cell carcinoma. J Urol 1969;101:297–301.

Staging. Various staging schemes have been applied to RCCs and all have demonstrated a positive correlation between the extent of tumor at the time of diagnosis and its future behavior (Tables 1-24, 1-25) (208,238,239,251). All currently used systems divide RCC into noninvasive, locally invasive, and metastatic categories. The TNM staging system of the American Joint Committee on Cancer (AJCC) and the International Union Against Cancer (UICC) is recommended (Table 1-25, fig. 1-196) although the classification of Robson and associates remains popular. Systematic lymphadenectomy would be valuable for staging RCCs, but there is little enthusiasm for this procedure in the surgical community and it is not usually performed.

Prognosis. Prognosis can be influenced by multiple factors, including tumor size, infiltrative margin, and histologic type, but tumor stage is the most important determinant of outcome. Not all factors are of equal significance and few can be considered independent variables. In general, large carcinomas are more likely to be invasive and metastatic than small lesions. An infiltrative margin is an adverse prognostic sign (171,255). Extension into the renal vein, with or without actual invasion of its wall, apparently has little effect upon short-term survival but may significantly decrease survival after 10 years (208,214). Lymph node metastases are often microscopic but have a significant impact upon survival (fig. 1-197) (Table 1-26) (251).

Prognosis can be expressed in terms of histologic subtype (171,177,180,222,255,257,258). The clear cell type is the most common and the most likely to be of low cytologic grade. These tumors spread by local invasion and tend to invade the renal vein but rarely involve lymph nodes. The overall survival rate after nephrectomy is 50 percent. The granular cell type is usually of high cytologic grade and associated with vascular invasion and distant metastases. Not surprisingly, the prognosis of patients with these tumors is much worse than for those with the clear cell type. The papillary type tends to be well differentiated; 80 percent of cases are confined to the kidney at diagnosis, although multicentricity, a propensity for late recurrence, and metastasis are features. Overall, prognosis is better than that for the clear cell type but higher grade tumors often have lymph node metastases. The chromophobe cell type tends to be localized to the kidney and most cases are of nuclear grade II. Survival following nephrectomy has been greater than 80 percent. The sarcomatoid type is lethal and few patients survive beyond 1 year following diagnosis. This tumor is particularly prone to metastasize to bones and soft tissues of the extremities, where its resemblance to a sarcoma may lead to inappropriate therapy. The collecting duct type is deceptive: more than 50 percent of reported patients have died from metastatic disease despite a tendency toward tumor localization and only moderate degrees of cellular anaplasia (222).

Table 1-25

TNM CLASSIFICATION OF RENAL CELL CARCINOMA*†

Stage	Definition
Primary tumor (T)	
TX	Primary tumor cannot be assessed
T0	No evidence of primary tumor
T1	Tumor 2.5 cm or less in greatest dimension, limited to the kidney
T2	Tumor more than 2.5 cm in greatest dimension, limited to the kidney
T3	Tumor extends into major veins or invades adrenal gland or perinephric tissue, but not beyond Gerota fascia
T3a	Tumor invades adrenal gland or perinephric tissues, but not beyond Gerota fascia
T3b	Tumor grossly extends into renal vein(s) or vena cava below diaphragm
T3c	Tumor grossly extends into vena cava above diaphragm
T4	Tumor invades beyond Gerota fascia
Lymph node (N)	
NX	Regional lymph nodes cannot be assessed
N0	No regional lymph node metastasis
N1	Metastasis in a single lymph node, 2 cm or less in greatest dimension
N2	Metastasis in a single lymph node, more than 2 cm but not more than 5 cm in greatest dimension, or multiple lymph nodes, none more than 5 cm in greatest dimension
N3	Metastasis in a lymph node more than 5 cm in greatest dimension
Distant metastasis (M)	
MX	Presence of distant metastasis cannot be assessed
M0	No distant metastasis
M1	Distant metastasis

Stage Grouping			
I	T1	N0	M0
II	T2	N0	M0
III	T1	N1	M0
	T2	N1	M0
	T3a	N0	M0
	T3a	N1	M0
	T3b	N0	M0
	T3b	N1	M0
	T3c	N0	M0
	T3c	N1	M0
IV	T4	Any N	M0
	Any T	N2	M0
	Any T	N3	M0
	Any T	Any N	M1

*American Joint Committee on Cancer (AJCC), Beahrs OH, Henson DE, Hutter RV, Kennedy BJ, eds. Manual for staging of cancer. 4th ed. Philadelphia: JB Lippincott, 1992:201–4.
†International Union Against Cancer (UICC), Hermanek P, Sobin LH, eds. TNM Classification of Malignant Tumors. 4th ed., 2nd Revision. Berlin: Springer-Verlag, 1992:148–50.

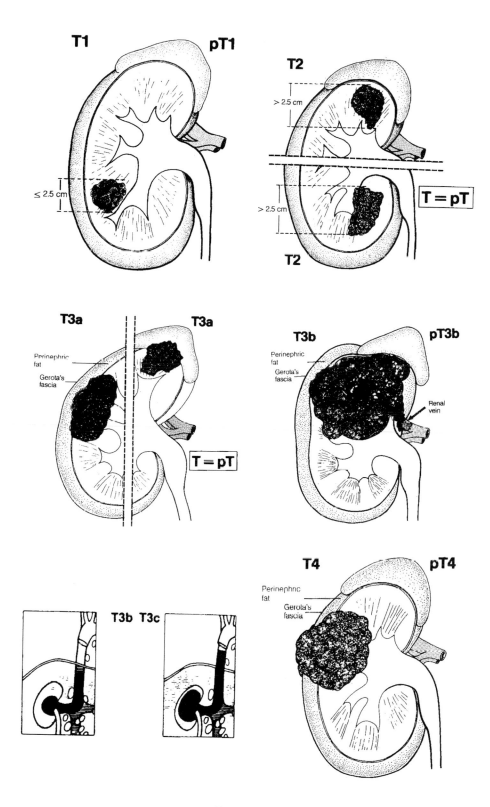

Figure 1-196

THE TNM STAGING SCHEME FOR RENAL CELL CARCINOMA

(Slightly modified from figs. 352-7,T3b,T3c from Spiessl B, ed. TNM atlas: illustrated guide to the TNM/pTNM-classification
of malignant tumours. 3rd edition. Berlin: Springer-Verlag, 1992.)

Table 1-26

LYMPHADENECTOMY IN RENAL CELL CARCINOMA*

	Total No. Patients	Patients with Metastatic Lymph Nodes (no./%)	Survival (no. patients/%/years)
Flocks and Kadesky	133	21 (16%)	3 (14%) 5
Robson et al.	76	20 (26%)	7 (35%) 3
Rafla	191	16 (8%)	4 (25%) 5
Skinner et al.	232	19 (8%)	3 (16%) 5
Middleton and Presto	66	7 (11%)	2 (29%) 5
Waters and Ritchie	67**	16 (24%)**	1 (20%) 5
Siminovitch et al.	102	9 (9%)	1 (11%) 5

*Table 2 from Siminovitch JP, Montie JE, Straffon RA. Lymphadenectomy in renal adenocarcinoma. J Urol 1982;127:1090–1.
**Includes an indeterminate number of patients with distant metastatic disease.

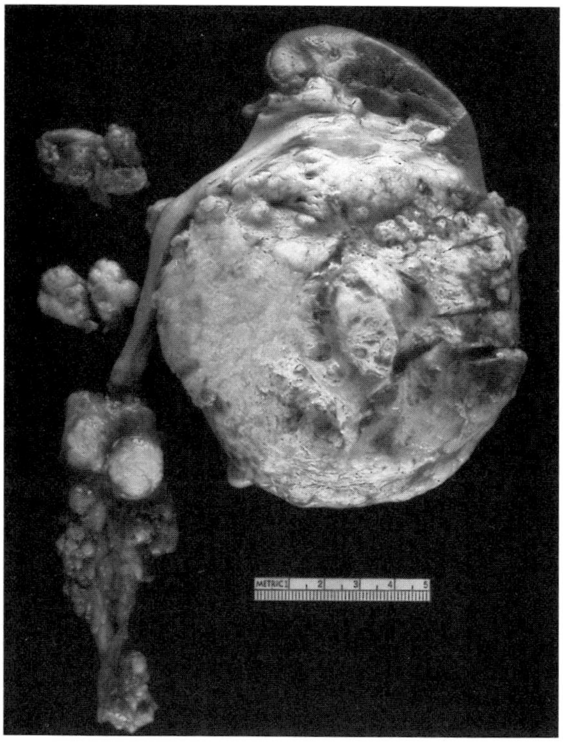

Figure 1-197
RENAL CELL CARCINOMA
Lymph node metastases in renal cell carcinoma.

RENAL CORTICAL ADENOMA

The notion that a benign epithelial neoplasm of the kidney can be defined and clearly distinguished from RCC has caused controversy and misunderstanding. All neoplasms, whether or not they have the capacity to invade and metastasize, are small at some point during their development. Many publications, including Bell's original series (175), have documented metastases from tumors measuring less than 3 cm (fig. 1-198). With the exception of oncocytoma, it has not been possible to define an unequivocally benign renal cortical neoplasm using histologic, immunohistochemical, and ultrastructural studies (176,183,201). Nevertheless, small renal cortical epithelial neoplasms are frequently found incidentally at autopsy as well as in surgically excised kidneys. These tumors occur more frequently in kidneys scarred from chronic pyelonephritis or renal vascular disease. Their frequency in autopsy studies has been as high as 22 percent. Lesions have been reported in children and are a feature of von Hippel-Lindau syndrome. They are usually well demarcated but unencapsulated, pale grey or pale yellow tumors arising in subcapsular portions of the kidney (fig. 1-199). Many have been identified in kidneys

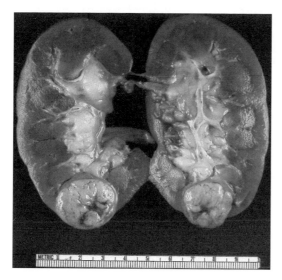

Figure 1-198
RENAL CELL CARCINOMA
This tumor is less than 3 cm in greatest dimension.

with RCC. Tumors that could be considered renal cortical adenomas are almost never larger than 2 cm in greatest dimension, although lesions measuring up to 10 cm have been described (fig. 1-200).

Microscopically, renal cortical adenomas consist of densely packed tubules lined by small, regular, cuboidal cells with rounded, uniform nuclei lacking cytologic anaplasia (fig. 1-201). Mitoses are rare. The tumors are circumscribed but not encapsulated, the interface with the normal renal parenchyma lacks significant inflammatory cells, and there is no stromal reaction. Some of these neoplasms feature a predominance of papillary structures (fig. 1-202) and some may contain psammoma bodies (fig. 1-203) or even xanthoma cells (fig. 1-204).

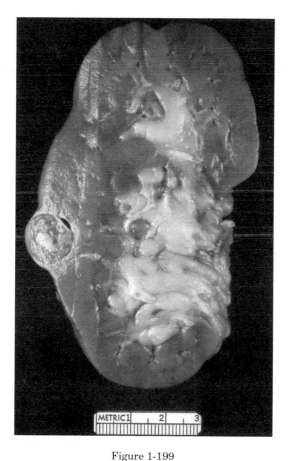

Figure 1-199
RENAL CORTICAL ADENOMA
This 1.5-cm tumor is typically situated in a subcapsular position.

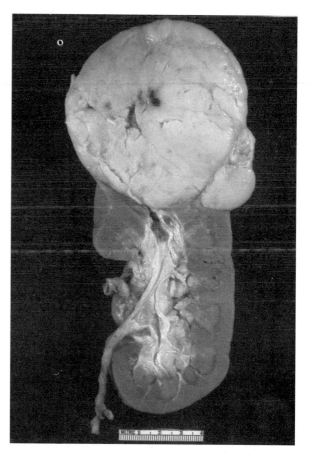

Figure 1-200
RENAL CORTICAL ADENOMA
This giant renal cortical adenoma measured over 8 cm in greatest dimension, but exhibited typical histology and no invasiveness.

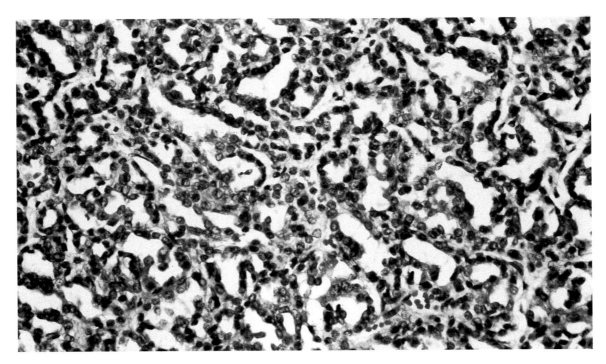

Figure 1-201
RENAL CORTICAL ADENOMA
This tumor is typically composed of tubular structures lined by cuboidal cells with nuclei less than 10 μm in diameter.

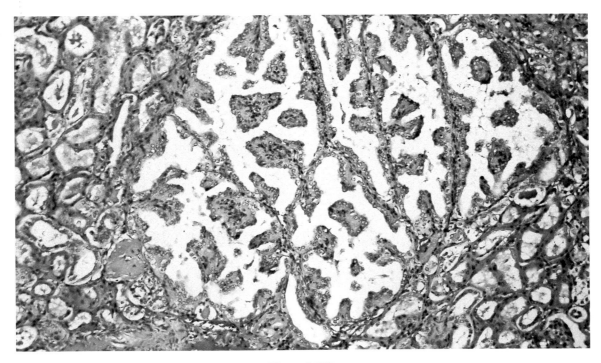

Figure 1-202
RENAL CORTICAL ADENOMA
This tiny tumor has a papillary architecture.

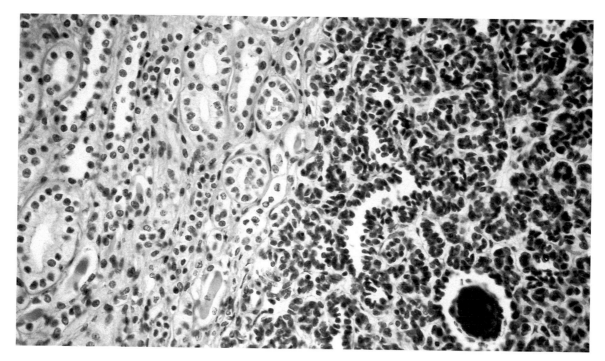

Figure 1-203
RENAL CORTICAL ADENOMA
The tumors are circumscribed but nonencapsulated. No reaction is present at the interface with the adjacent kidney. Psammomatous calcifications may be present.

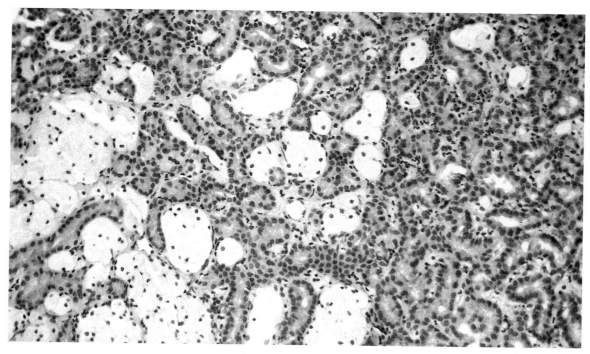

Figure 1-204
RENAL CORTICAL ADENOMA
Xanthoma cells may be present in the stroma between epithelial tubular structures.

Table 1-27

SERIES OF RENAL ONCOCYTOMAS REPORTED IN THE ENGLISH LITERATURE*

Reference	Oncocytomas	Total Tumors**	Frequency (%)
Klein and Valensi	13	198[†]	6.6
Akhtar and Kott	2	55[†]	3.9
Sarkar et al.	11	200[‡]	5.5
Yu et al.	5	107[†]	4.7
Lieber et al.	62	2797[†]	2.2
Bonavita et al.	14	1114[†]	1.3
Mitchell and Shilkin	6	42[‡]	14.3
Merino and LiVolsi	14	263[†]	5.3
Lehmann and Blessing	10	330[‡]	3.0
Barnes et al.	7	257[†]	2.7
Choi et al.	7	96[‡]	7.3
Fairchild et al.	11	219[§]	5.0
Wasserman and Ewing	4	239[‡]	1.7
Maatman et al.	11	254[†]	4.3
Giuffre and Gulliver	7	81[†]	8.6
Alanen et al.	13	562[‡]	2.3
Lawrence and Bajallan	4	130[†]	3.1
Demos et al.	1	68[†]	1.5
Thoenes et al.	20	510[†]	3.9
Total	222	7522	3.0 (mean)

* Modification of table from Lieber MM, Hosaka Y, Tsukamato T. Renal oncocytoma. World J Urol 1987;5:71–9.
**Only grade 1 tumors considered.
[†] Renal cell carcinomas and oncocytomas.
[‡] Renal adenomas and carcinomas.
[§] Radical nephrectomy specimens.

ONCOCYTOMA

Definition. Oncocytomas are neoplasms composed of cells with abundant acidophilic cytoplasm. As coined by Hamperl (277), the term oncocyte (from the Greek "onkousthai," to swell and "cyte," cell) has a general meaning; it is not surprising, therefore, that tumors of divergent histology occurring in various organs have been labeled "oncocytoma" (278,295). Widespread recognition of renal oncocytomas is credited to Klein and Valensi (279), although previous cases had been reported (295). In the kidney, oncocytoma is defined as a neoplasm composed of a uniform population of cells with abundant cytoplasm and nonanaplastic nuclei. The cytoplasm is packed with mitochondria to the virtual exclusion of other organelles, giving it a granular acidophilic appearance in preparations stained with hematoxylin and eosin (290). The lesion is assumed to differentiate toward tubular epithelium (268, 275). In an immunohistochemical study of six cases using antibodies to both proximal and distal tubular antigens, oncocytomas exhibited predominantly distal/medullary tubular antigenicity (273). The authors concluded that assignment of an exact tubular origin could not be validated but that divergent histogenesis from a common precursor stem cell was likely.

General and Clinical Features. Oncocytomas comprise an estimated 3 percent of all renal tumors requiring nephrectomy (Table 1-27) (282). For 25,000 cases of renal cancer per year in the United States, there are about 750

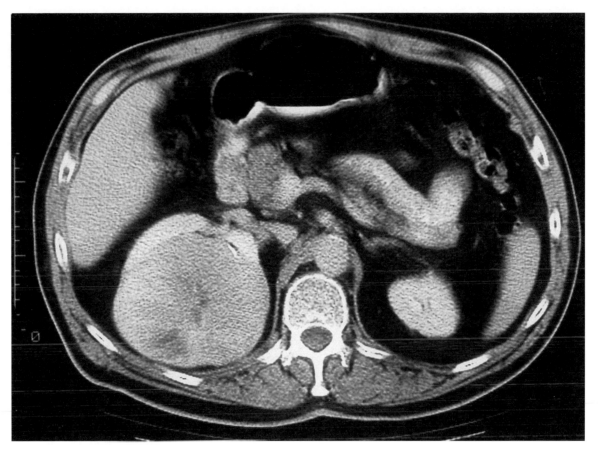

Figure 1-205
RENAL ONCOCYTOMA
Computerized tomography demonstrates a renal tumor which is circumscribed and homogeneous except for an irregular central zone which proved to be a central scar.

cases of oncocytoma. Oncocytomas affect men twice as often as women (ratio, 2.1 to 1). With a median age of 62 years (range, 10 to 94 years), patients with oncocytomas are older than those with RCC (median, 55 years). There is no association with von Hippel-Lindau disease, tuberous sclerosis, or chronic dialysis, conditions known to be related to RCC (283).

Signs and symptoms directly related to oncocytomas do not occur in most patients (282): 66 percent of patients in published cases are asymptomatic. When present, the most common manifestations are a flank or abdominal mass (19 percent), flank or abdominal pain (18 percent), microscopic hematuria (18 percent), and gross hematuria (12 percent).

Oncocytomas are ordinarily detected after an intravenous pyelogram or abdominal computed tomography for some unrelated reason. Radiographically, lesions typically have the appearance of a solid mass. Larger tumors exhibit a characteristic central stellate scar (figs. 1-205, 1-206) (272). Four typical angiographic features have been described: 1) the "lucent rim" sign; 2) a homogeneous capillary nephrogram phase; 3) absence of marked disarray in neoplastic vessels; and 4) a spoke-wheel appearance of the feeding arteries (fig. 1-207) (269,293). A relatively avascular zone may explain the central scarred foci.

Oncocytomas may also be detected in fine needle aspirations, where they appear as isolated or loosely aggregated elements with homogeneous granular cytoplasm; low nuclear-cytoplasmic ratios; and round, uniform nuclei lacking prominent nucleoli (fig. 1-208) (268). Needle aspiration is especially valuable in cases

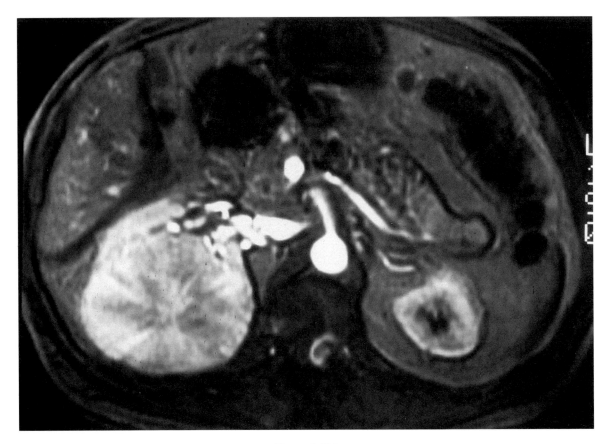

Figure 1-206
RENAL ONCOCYTOMA
This is the same tumor as illustrated in figure 1-205, examined by magnetic resonance imaging. In this image, the central scar is well visualized.

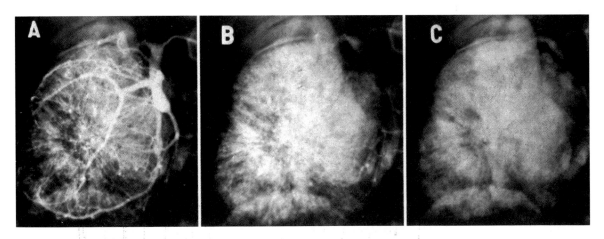

Figure 1-207
RENAL ONCOCYTOMA
A: Angiographic examination demonstrates a "spokewheel" appearance to the tumor's arterial pattern.
B: The mass is highly vascular without puddling of contrast media or A-V shunting.
C: The later phase demonstrates good encapsulation without venous-collateral circulation. (Fig. 1 from Weiner SN, Bernstein RG. Renal oncocytoma: angiographic features of two cases. Radiology 1977;125:633–5.)

in which nephrectomy should be avoided if a benign tumor can be documented (287). However, oncocytic renal tumors are often heterogeneous and might be incompletely sampled by this method.

Pathologic Findings. Oncocytomas vary considerably in size, perhaps reflecting the method of detection of these predominantly asymptomatic neoplasms (fig. 1-209). Neoplasms observed at autopsy are small (median, 2 cm) whereas clinically detected lesions are usually large (median, 6 cm). The tumors are, characteristically, well demarcated, uniformly expansile masses occurring at any renal site. Involvement of the adjacent pericapsular fat has been reported (fig. 1-210) (267,275,283). Almost all renal oncocytomas are solitary masses (282). Multicentricity, either bilateral or unilateral, has been reported in only 3 to 5 percent of cases (fig. 1-211) (282,294). Rarely, oncocytomas coexist with RCC or angiomyolipoma (283,292).

The gross appearance is so characteristic that any corroborative tests, such as electron microscopy, can be instituted at the time of macroscopic

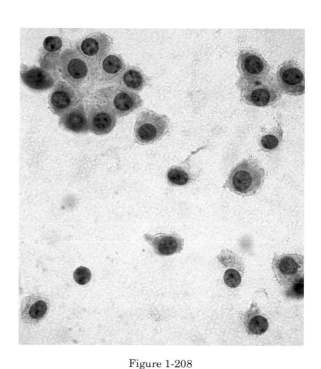

Figure 1-208
RENAL ONCOCYTOMA

In this aspiration cytology preparation, the cells exhibit small, round, and very regular nuclei with abundant granular cytoplasm.

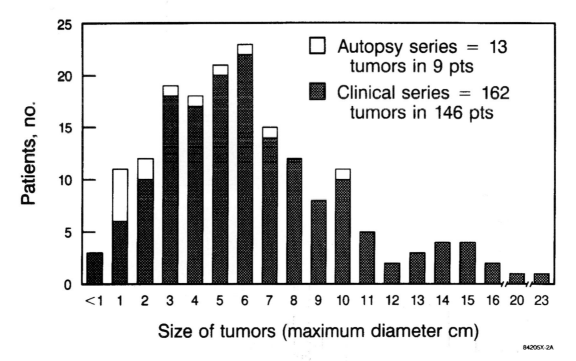

Figure 1-209
RENAL ONCOCYTOMA

Reported tumor sizes. (Fig. 8-67 from Farrow GM. Diseases of the kidney. In: Murphy WM, ed. Urological pathology. Philadelphia: WB Saunders, 1989:409–82.)

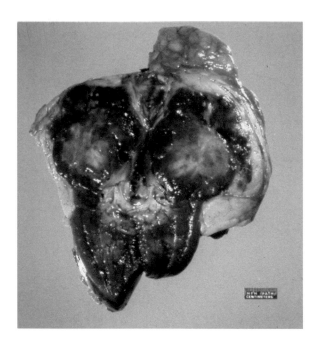

Figure 1-210
RENAL ONCOCYTOMA
This tumor extends outside the kidney into the perirenal fat. (Courtesy of the Henry Ford Hospital, Detroit, MI.)

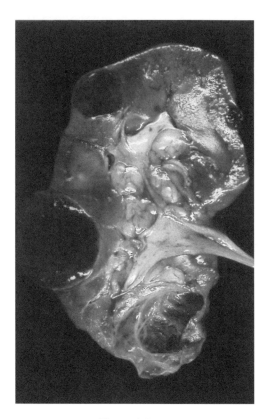

Figure 1-211
RENAL ONCOCYTOMA
This kidney contained nine discrete tumors.

examination. Most oncocytomas are mahogany brown, due to the lipochrome pigment associated with the mitochondria filling the cytoplasm (fig. 1-212). In larger lesions, a stellate scar usually occupies the central portion of the mass, suggesting a slowly progressive central ischemia (see fig. 1-166C) (269,293). There may be more than one scar (fig. 1-213). Cystic degeneration may occur and is usually associated with a scar (fig. 1-214). Central calcification has been identified. Necrosis and hemorrhage are not characteristic features of oncocytomas and these findings should raise the suspicion of RCC.

Histologically, oncocytomas are composed of a uniform population of plump cells arranged in alveolar-type nests (fig. 1-215), trabeculae (fig. 1-216), or even tubules (fig. 1-217). The cytoplasm is granular and acidophilic (see fig. 1-166D). Mixtures of patterns are common but a papillary configuration is not seen (270). Some intermingling of neoplastic and non-neoplastic elements may occur at the tumor interface, but oncocytomas do not manifest an infiltrative growth pattern, or elicit an inflammatory or desmoplastic response. The central scar comprises mature,

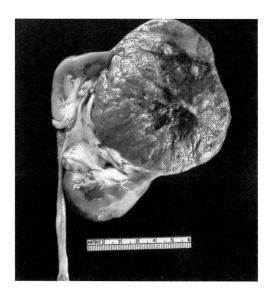

Figure 1-212
RENAL ONCOCYTOMA
The tumors are typically well circumscribed, homogeneous, and mahogany brown. There is a central depressed zone and a scar.

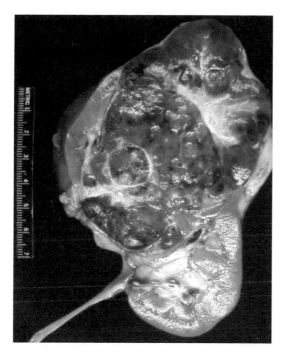

Figure 1-213
RENAL ONCOCYTOMA
This tumor exhibits two stellate scarred zones.

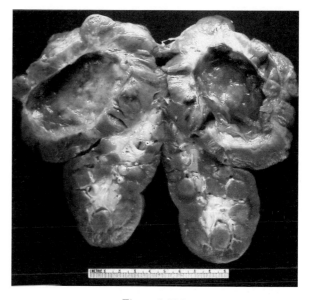

Figure 1-214
RENAL ONCOCYTOMA
There is central cystic change.

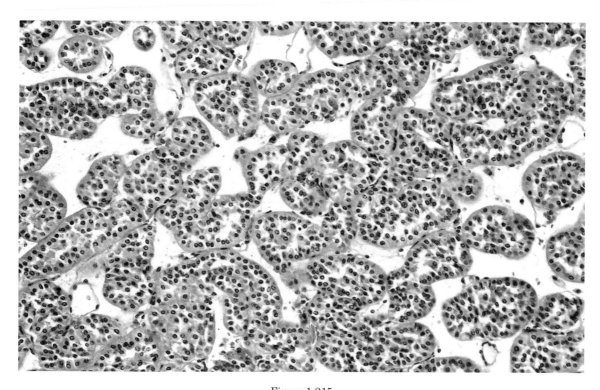

Figure 1-215
RENAL ONCOCYTOMA
The tumor consists of a uniform population of cells arranged in well-formed alveolar nests.

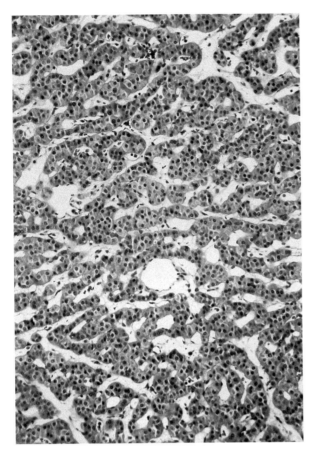

Figure 1-216
RENAL ONCOCYTOMA
This tumor has a trabecular architecture.

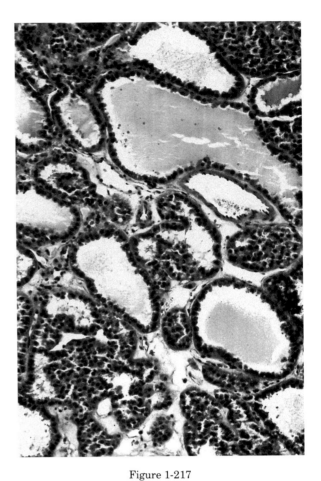

Figure 1-217
RENAL ONCOCYTOMA
In the tubular pattern, a single layer of cells exhibits plump acidophilic cytoplasm.

often hyalinized fibrous tissue entrapping nests of tumor cells (fig. 1-218).

Oncocytoma cells typically have small, round, regular nuclei measuring less than 10 μm in diameter (fig. 1-219). The chromatin is finely granular and evenly dispersed. Nucleoli are inconspicuous and mitoses are rare. The cytoplasm is packed with large mitochondria (fig. 1-220). These structures can be demonstrated by electron microscopy, a phosphotungstic acid stain, or a Sudan B black reaction for lipoproteins.

Although oncocytomas are composed of cytologically uniform cells with nonanaplastic features, there are rare variations. Scattered populations of what appears to be incompletely differentiated oncocytes are seen (fig. 1-221). These cells possess less abundant cytoplasm than ordinary oncocytes and groups may stand

out in tissue sections because of their greater nuclear density. The nuclei of these cells are slightly larger than nuclei of typical oncocytes and occasional mitoses may be found. A gradual morphologic transition into typical oncocytes can be observed. These elements are reminiscent of a blastema and suggest that oncocytes may arise from a precursor "oncoblastic" stem cell. In another variation, there are foci of oncocytes with hyperchromatic, often bizarre nuclei (fig. 1-222). These nuclei may occur singly, but are more often arranged in groups. Wide expanses of the tumor may feature these cells (fig. 1-223). The absence of large nucleoli and mitoses suggests a nonmalignant, symplastic or degenerative change of the type observed in benign endocrine neoplasms. Oncocytomas with atypical features

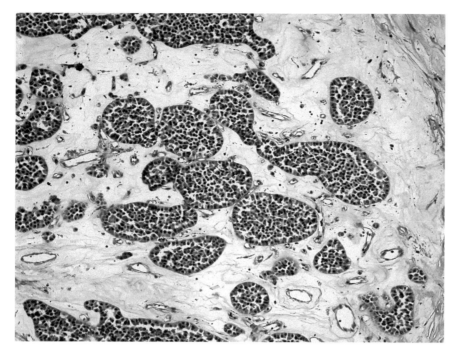

Figure 1-218
RENAL ONCOCYTOMA
In the scarred zone, there is no necrosis, but the tumor cells are separated by mature hyalinized fibrous connective tissue.

must be carefully studied to exclude chromophobe cell carcinoma and granular cell carcinoma (Tables 1-20, 1-21) (274).

Special Techniques. DNA analyses of a large number of renal oncocytomas show conflicting results, reflecting both case selection and sampling (271,276,286). When only cases with a pure population of typical oncocytes were studied by flow cytometry, all were composed of cells with euploid DNA (276). Similar tumors examined by nuclear DNA image cytometry demonstrated aneuploid deviations (271). In a large series of oncocytomas containing some foci of nuclear atypia evaluated by flow cytometry, 39 percent were tetraploid and 11 percent aneuploid (286). Despite foci of aneuploidy, no patient had a recurrence or metastasis after nephrectomy.

Chromosomal abnormalities are common in renal oncocytomas (280,285,291). Deletion of chromosome 1, together with loss of Y, yielding a 44, XY, -1 karyotype is the most frequent. Consistent chromosomal aberrations have not been documented and genotype does not correlate well with biologic behavior.

Differential Diagnosis. Oncocytomas should be differentiated from renal carcinomas with oncocytic and chromophobic features (Tables 1-20, 1-21) (288,289). The distinction rests primarily on

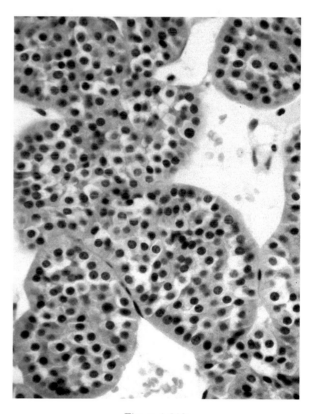

Figure 1-219
RENAL ONCOCYTOMA
The tumor cells have small, round, regular nuclei slightly less than 10 μm in diameter. The cytoplasm is granular and acidophilic.

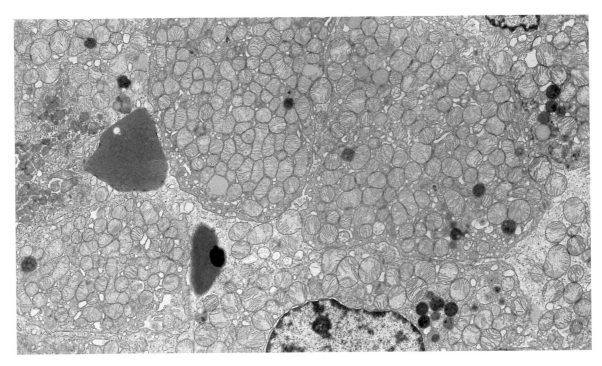

Figure 1-220
RENAL ONCOCYTOMA
The cytoplasm of the oncocyte is packed with large mitochondria (X3000).

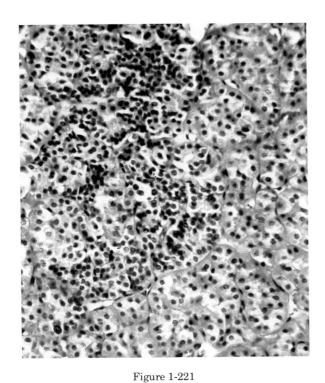

Figure 1-221
RENAL ONCOCYTOMA
Populations of cells with reduced cytoplasm and prominent
nuclear staining represent incompletely differentiated oncocytes.

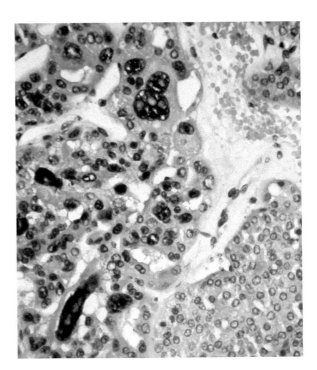

Figure 1-222
RENAL ONCOCYTOMA
Otherwise typical oncocytomas may contain scattered popu-
lations of cells with large, hyperchromatic and bizarre nuclei.

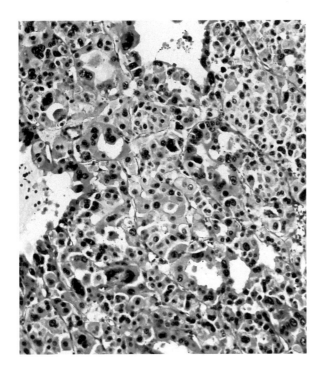

Figure 1-223
RENAL ONCOCYTOMA
Rarely, an oncocytoma may exhibit a large population of bizarre and atypical cells. Nucleoli and mitoses are not found among these cells.

Table 1-28

CLINICAL COURSE OF PATIENTS WITH RENAL ONCOCYTOMA*

Clinical Course	Number of Patients
Patients alive without recurrence	165 (57%)
Patients alive with recurrence**	1 (0%)
Patients dead of unrelated causes	32 (11%)
Patients dead of metastatic renal "oncocytoma"**	2 (1%)
Patients lost to follow-up	3 (1%)
Patients without details of clinical course in reports	89 (30%)
Total	292 (100%)

* From Lieber MM, Hosaka Y, Tsukamato T. Renal oncocytoma. World J Urol 1987; 5:71–9.
**These cases are probably chromophobe cell renal carcinomas.

recognition of anaplastic nuclear changes such as prominent nucleoli and mitoses. A positive reaction using Hale colloidal iron identifies a chromophobe cell carcinoma. Electron microscopy documents the presence of mitochondria and the virtual absence of other organelles. Cells with well-developed rough endoplasmic reticuli, abundant Golgi apparatus, lipid, or glycogen are not oncocytes. Hemorrhage or necrosis in an acidophilic renal tumor should raise doubts about the diagnosis of oncocytoma. The color of the tumor is a less reliable differential feature, although areas that are not homogeneous or appear pale should be examined microscopically.

Prognosis. Renal oncocytomas are benign tumors (Table 1-28). However, adequate survival data are available for only 70 percent of reported cases. Anecdotal reports of aggressive behavior and even death seem to represent chromophobe cell renal carcinomas (281). Patients have survived for many years without progressive disease even though their oncocytomas were not resected (284,287).

RARE TUMORS WITH EPITHELIAL OR RENAL PARENCHYMAL DIFFERENTIATION

Carcinoid Tumor

This was first reported as a primary neoplasm in the kidney in 1966 (304,317,321). By 1993, there were 20 reported cases (309). The histogenesis is unclear, except for carcinoid tumors arising in teratomas; the mechanism is considered analogous to similar tumors arising in the ovary or testis. Neither argyrophilic cells nor other types of neuroendocrine cells have been documented in the normal kidney (307,314). Patients range from 13 to 67 years of age, but most are over 40 years. There is no significant sex predilection. Most patients have symptoms that could be related to a renal mass; only a few are entirely asymptomatic. One patient had carcinoid syndrome, but in several cases symptoms were attributed to other hormonal substances (308,311, 312,317). A patient with Cushing syndrome is the only pediatric case (312).

Carcinoid tumors of the kidney are typically large and solid but occasional cysts have been identified. The histologic features are similar to carcinoid tumors at other sites (figs. 1-224, 1-225). Most are argyrophilic. A few have been so

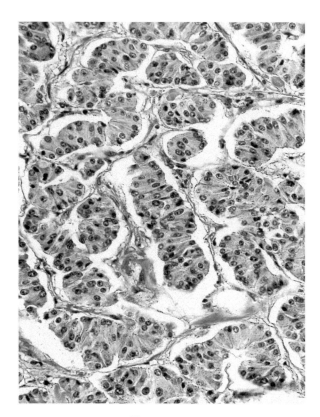

Figure 1-224
RENAL CARCINOID TUMOR
This tumor has an insular pattern.

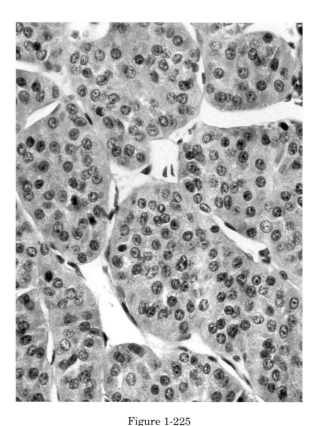

Figure 1-225
RENAL CARCINOID TUMOR
There is an organoid cell arrangement with the typical nuclear features of a carcinoid tumor.

poorly differentiated that the term carcinoid tumor seemed inappropriate and these cases were classified as neuroendocrine carcinomas (fig. 1-226). The immunohistochemical and ultrastructural features are characteristic of neuroendocrine neoplasms. Approximately one third of cases with typical histology metastasize, predominantly to bone (321). Metastases among the more poorly differentiated neuroendocrine tumors are common (304).

Small Cell Carcinoma

This tumor has been observed in the renal parenchyma as well as the renal pelvis (300,304, 305,316,320). Renal pelvic tumors are often associated with more typical transitional cell carcinomas (305). Areas of typical carcinoid tumor rarely occur. Small cell carcinomas are typically large and locally invasive (fig. 1-227). Their histologic features do not differ from those of similar tumors at other sites. Immunohistochemical reactions

have yielded variable results. Intermediate type small cell carcinomas are particularly likely to have antigenic determinants for keratin. Most often, reactions for neurosecretory differentiation are positive and neurosecretory granules can be demonstrated using electron microscopy. Prognosis is poor: nearly all patients develop metastases and die of their tumors.

Juxtaglomerular Cell Tumor

This is a rare neoplasm differentiating toward the specialized paracytic cells adjacent to the afferent arteriole in the hilus of the glomerulus (304,318). Patient age is 8 to 53 years; most are adolescents and young adults. There is no apparent sex predilection. All patients have been hypertensive, often for many years prior to the detection of the tumor. The hypertension is associated with elevated serum levels of renin and, occasionally, with increased aldosterone and

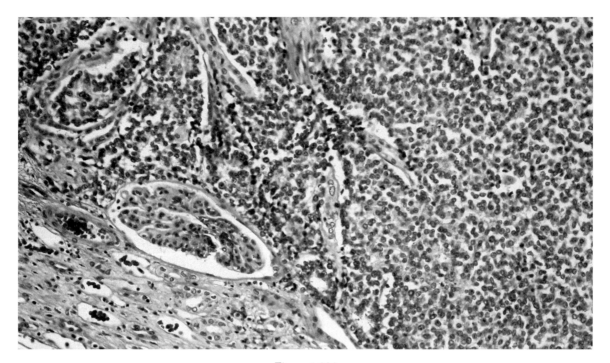

Figure 1-226
NEUROENDOCRINE RENAL CARCINOMA
This tumor is less differentiated than a carcinoid tumor.

hypokalemia. In nearly all cases, surgical removal of the juxtaglomerular tumor has resulted in return to normal blood pressure.

In all reported cases, tumors have been unilateral and solitary. Most have been less than 3 cm in greatest dimension but at least one neoplasm measured 6.5 cm (303). Tumors are usually solid and well circumscribed but scattered small cysts may occur. The cut surface is grey-white to light yellow (304). Tumors are situated in the renal cortex. Microscopically, juxtaglomerular cell tumors are composed of a uniform population of round to polyhedral cells with granular, acidophilic cytoplasm. Cells may be arranged in irregular trabeculae or in organoid patterns (figs. 1-228, 1-229). Tubular structures lined by neoplastic cells have been described as have spindle cell variants. Cytoplasmic granules are characteristic of both normal and neoplastic juxtaglomerular cells (319). These granules react positively with periodic acid-Schiff and Bowie reagents. The nuclei are generally round to oval and there may be a few mitotic figures. Ultrastructurally, cells often contain rhomboid, renin-specific

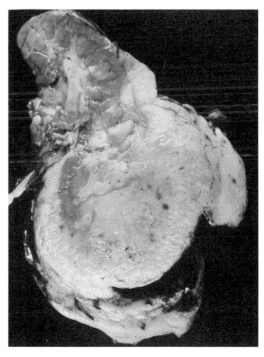

Figure 1-227
SMALL CELL CARCINOMA OF THE KIDNEY
This large invasive tumor is a pale gray. The origin of this tumor could be the renal pelvis or renal parenchyma.

147

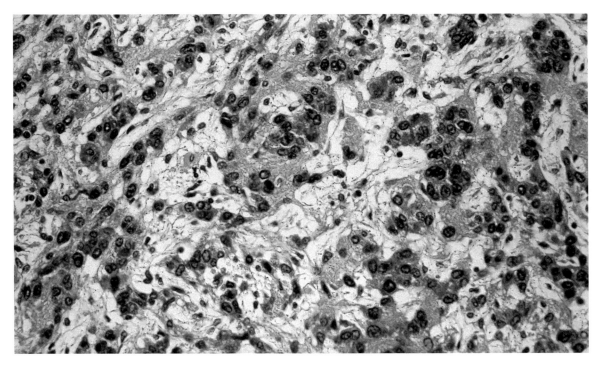

Figure 1-228
JUXTAGLOMERULAR CELL TUMOR
There are collections of epithelial cells with prominently granular cytoplasm.

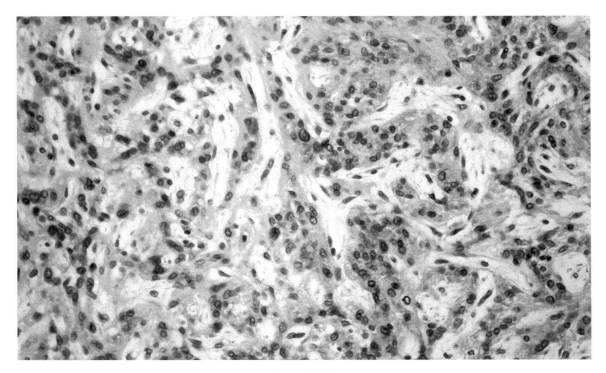

Figure 1-229
JUXTAGLOMERULAR CELL TUMOR
This tumor has an organoid pattern.

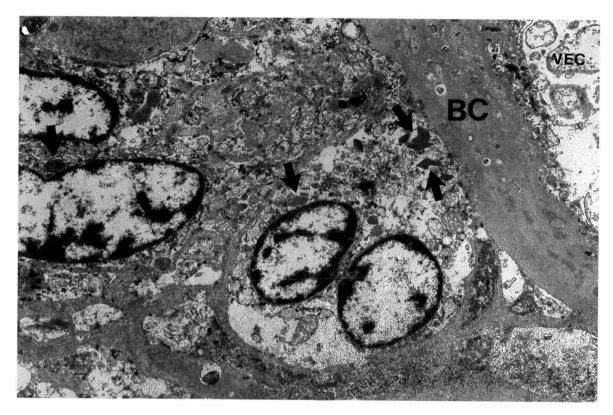

Figure 1-230
JUXTAGLOMERULAR CELL

A juxtaglomerular cell is adjacent to the Bowman capsule (BC). The visceral epithelial cell (VEC) processes are to the right of this. This patient had renal vascular hypertension. The paracrystalline structures of rhomboid shape are renin-specific granules (X9000). (Courtesy of Dr. Praveen Chander, New York, NY.)

crystals (fig. 1-232), which are also found in the normal juxtaglomerular apparatus (figs. 1-230, 1-231) (298). Tumor cells are often associated with nonmyelinated nerve fibers (297). Juxtaglomerular tumors are apparently benign since no local recurrence or metastasis has been reported regardless of the type of surgical resection.

Teratoma

Teratoma rarely occurs as a primary renal tumor (296,307,314). Of the few reported cases, two had areas of carcinoid. One tumor occurred in a dysplastic kidney. With a single exception, renal teratomas have been histologically and clinically benign.

Nephroblastoma

Renal tumors that characteristically arise in children can occur in adults (299,306,310,313). Most are nephroblastomas (see section, Nephroblastoma). Adult nephroblastomas are rare and can

be confused with other mixed malignant tumors. Acceptable cases should contain blastema. Excepting cystic nephroma, nephroblastomas arising in adults have an adverse prognosis. Metastases have occurred in 13 percent of cases at the time of diagnosis and only half of the patients can be expected to be disease free at 5 years despite multimodality therapy.

Cystic Nephroma (Multilocular Cyst)

Although bearing the name "cyst," cystic nephroma (multilocular cyst) is a neoplasm of uncertain histogenesis which exhibits both an epithelial and a stromal component (301,302, 315). In the adult form, cystic nephroma typically is found in middle-aged women. It is characteristically situated in the upper pole of the kidney (figs. 1-233, 1-234). The lesion should always be solitary and unilateral and the cysts multiloculated. The cysts lack any communication

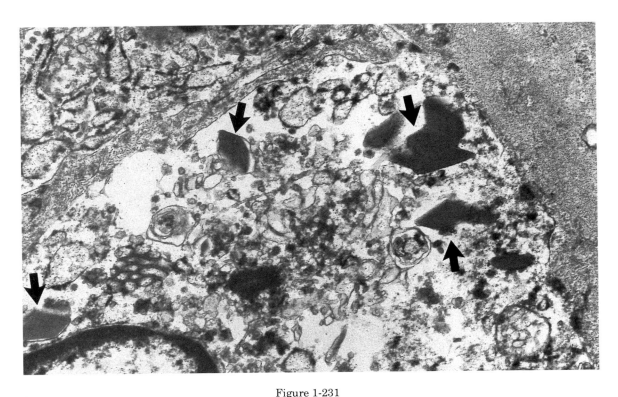

Figure 1-231
JUXTAGLOMERULAR CELL
This is a high-power view of the renin-specific granules (X27,000). (Courtesy of Dr. Praveen Chander, New York, NY.)

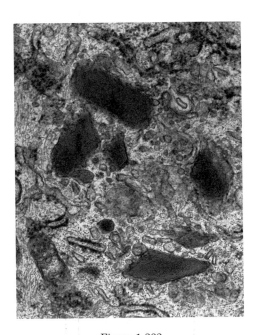

Figure 1-232
JUXTAGLOMERULAR CELL TUMOR
Renin-specific granules are present in the cytoplasm of the tumor cells (X36,000). (Courtesy of Dr. Robert A. Erlandson, New York, NY.)

between locules or between the renal calices or pelvis. The lesions are encapsulated and the adjacent renal parenchyma is normal except for compression-induced changes. All these criteria may not be fulfilled in every case.

The cysts are lined by a single layer of epithelial cells, which vary from flattened to low cuboidal or even columnar (figs. 1-235, 1-236). Stratified zones may be present. Occasional cells exhibit atypical cytologic features including nuclear enlargement and hyperchromasia (fig. 1-237). These cells have mainly eosinophilic cytoplasm. The epithelial cells are strongly positive with antibodies to keratin and exhibit a type of lectin binding suggesting that the epithelium lining the cysts is of distal tubule or collecting duct type. The stromal septa between the cysts consist of dense fibrous connective tissue with scattered loose fascicles of smooth muscle. It is characteristic that no renal nephron elements are found in the stromal septa. Areas of blastema or nephroblastoma almost never occur in adult cystic nephromas. The prognosis after complete excision is excellent.

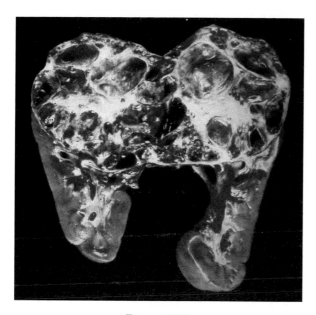

Figure 1-233
RENAL MULTILOCULAR CYST
The lesion is located in the upper pole of the kidney.

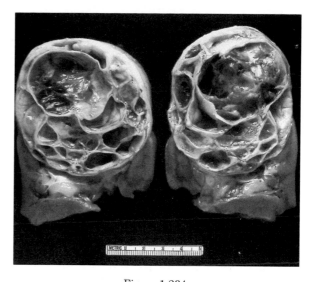

Figure 1-234
RENAL MULTILOCULAR CYST
The lesion contains multiple cystic structures which lack any communication between locules or the renal pelvis.

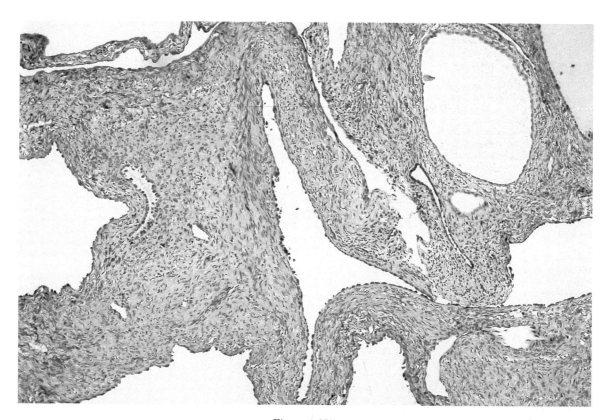

Figure 1-235
RENAL MULTILOCULAR CYST
The epithelial-lined cysts are separated by septa of a distinctive type of fibrous connective tissue. No renal nephron elements are found in the stromal septa.

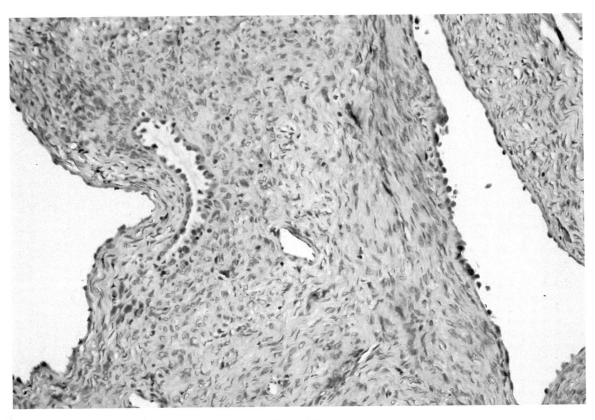

Figure 1-236
RENAL MULTILOCULAR CYST
The epithelial cells lining the cysts vary from flattened to low cuboidal or even columnar.

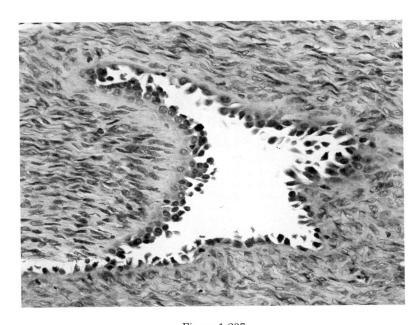

Figure 1-237
RENAL MULTILOCULAR CYST
Occasional lining epithelial cells may exhibit nuclear enlargement and hyperchromasia.

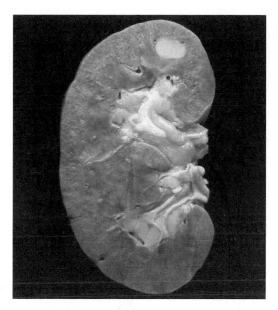

Figure 1-238
MEDULLARY FIBROMA/RENOMEDULLARY
INTERSTITIAL CELL TUMOR
A spade-shaped whitish gray lesion is situated in the medullary pyramid. (Fig. 8-76 from Farrow GM. Diseases of the kidney. In: Murphy WM, ed. Urological pathology. Philadelphia: WB Saunders, 1989:409–82.)

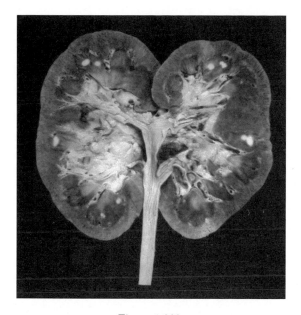

Figure 1-239
MEDULLARY FIBROMA/RENOMEDULLARY
INTERSTITIAL CELL TUMOR
Multiple lesions are all situated in the medullary pyramids.

MESENCHYMAL TUMORS

Medullary Fibroma (Renomedullary Interstitial Cell Tumor)

The interstitium of the renal medulla contains a specialized cell type, the interstitial cell, which produces prostaglandins and is believed to serve in the regulation of intrarenal blood pressure (323–325). Ultrastructurally, these cells contain large numbers of electron-dense granules (lipid droplets); it has been suggested that tumors formerly designated "medullary fibroma" are composed of these renal medullary interstitial cells (323). Interstitial cell tumors are typically small, pale grey, well-circumscribed lesions appearing as incidental findings at autopsy. They have been observed in as many as 50 percent of autopsied kidneys and have been multiple in approximately 50 percent of cases. Lesions usually occur in adults and are rare in individuals less than 18 years of age. Occasionally, an antihypertensive effect has been observed (322). No evidence of systemic function could be found in a study comparing heart weight and blood pressure in autopsied patients with interstitial cell tumors compared to a matched control group without these lesions (325).

Grossly, most interstitial cell tumors are less than 0.3 cm in greatest dimension; lesions measuring more than 0.6 cm are rare (326). The neoplasms tend to be spade shaped and occupy the midportions of medullary pyramids (fig. 1-238). Lesions may be multiple (fig. 1-239). Microscopically, interstitial cell tumors consist of a proliferation of small, stellate or polygonal cells in a loose stromal background with entrapped medullary tubules at the periphery (fig. 1-240). Some lesions are hyalinized and almost acellular; others contain amyloid (326). Histochemical studies demonstrate neutral fat, phospholipid, and acid mucopolysaccharides. Interstitial cell tumors are benign and rarely clinically significant.

Leiomyoma

This is a rare renal neoplasm that occurs in the cortex or capsule (fig. 1-241). Capsular leiomyomas have been identified in approximately 5 percent of autopsies, where they are usually incidental nodules 0.1 to 0.3 cm in greatest dimension. Few patients are symptomatic (329). Some

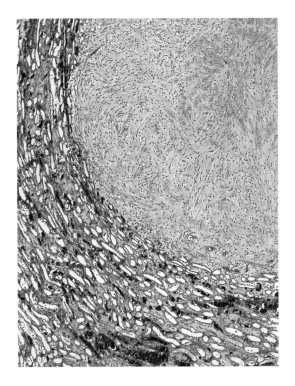

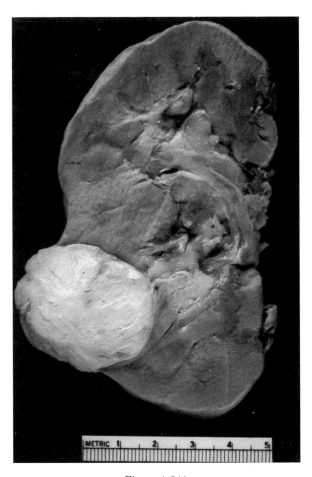

Figure 1-241
RENAL LEIOMYOMA
A firm circumscribed tumor with a whorled appearance to the cut surface.

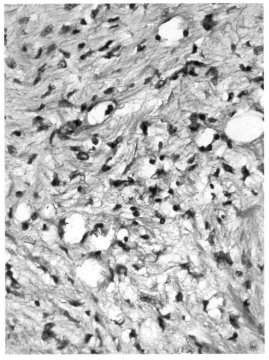

Figure 1-240
MEDULLARY FIBROMA/RENOMEDULLARY
INTERSTITIAL CELL TUMOR

Top: A circumscribed fibrogenic lesion is situated among the collecting tubules.

Bottom: There are small stellate cells, some with vacuolated cytoplasm.

reported cases may actually represent angiomyolipomas. Tumors occur mainly in adults but have been observed in neonates and children (328).

Leiomyomas arising in the kidney do not differ pathologically from similar tumors at other body sites. They may become large (327). Tumors occurring in infants must be differentiated from mesoblastic nephromas.

Lipoma

Renal lipomas are extremely rare tumors which occur in less than 1 percent of autopsied kidneys (330,331). Very few are symptomatic. Most are intrarenal and almost all occur in middle-aged women. Most are found incidentally and appear to

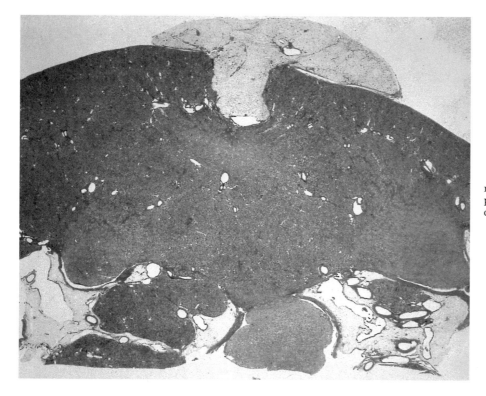

Figure 1-242
RENAL LIPOMA
The tumor is situated peripherally in the cortex and projects beneath the renal capsule.

arise from the renal capsule or the hilar fat (figs. 1-242, 1-243). Intrarenal lipomas must be distinguished from angiomyolipomas. Renal lipomas are true neoplasms and should be differentiated from parapelvic lipomatosis, a condition that occurs following renal cortical atrophy, usually associated with hydronephrosis (fig. 1-244).

Hemangioma

Hemangiomas in the kidney arise in the cortex, medulla, or renal pelvis (332,333). Most occur in young and middle-aged adults. Although lesions are usually single, approximately 12 percent are multifocal and a few are bilateral (fig. 1-245). Among multifocal cases, some patients exhibit features of syndromes associated with vascular lesions, such as Klippel-Trenaunay and Sturge-Weber syndromes (336). Renal hemangiomas are usually small and asymptomatic, and possibly congenital. The most frequent sign is hematuria. Bleeding may be massive, especially in large lesions that involve the renal pelvis (fig. 1-246). Most hemangiomas are cavernous rather than capillary.

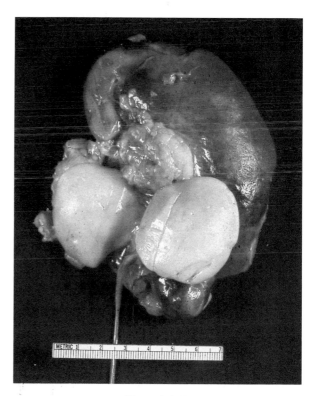

Figure 1-243
RENAL LIPOMA
This tumor appears to arise in the hilar adipose tissue.

155

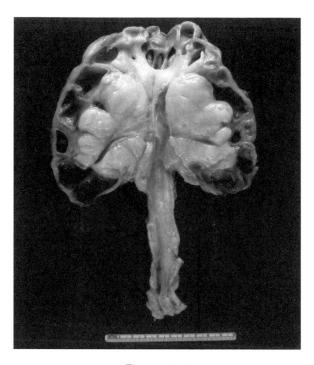

Figure 1-244
PARAPELVIC LIPOMATOSIS
Hydronephrosis and cortical atrophy are associated with an increase in parapelvic adipose tissue.

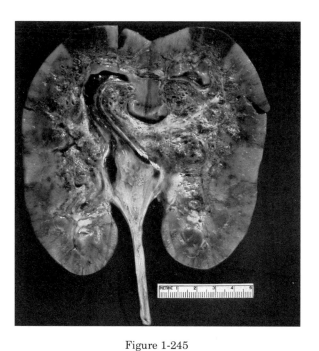

Figure 1-245
RENAL HEMANGIOMA
A sponge-like lesion involves much of the kidney and peripelvic tissues. (Fig. 8-77 from Farrow GM. Diseases of the kidney. In: Murphy WM, ed. Urological pathology. Philadelphia: WB Saunders, 1989:409–82.)

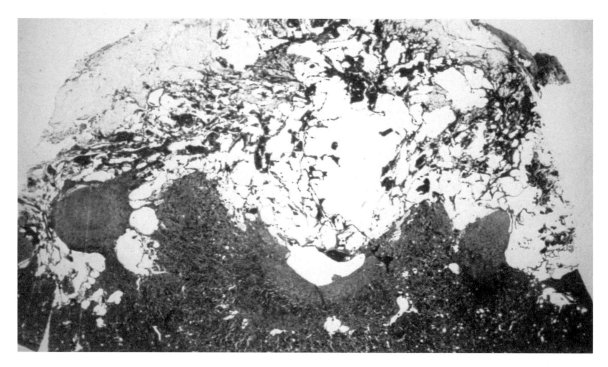

Figure 1-246
RENAL HEMANGIOMA
This massive cavernous hemangioma occupies much of the renal medulla and pelvis.

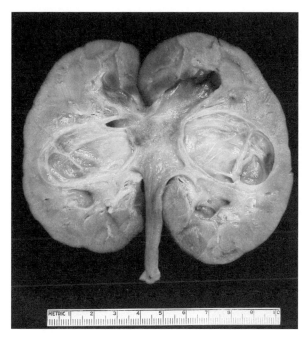

Figure 1-247
PERIPELVIC LYMPHANGIOMA
A large cystic lesion is situated adjacent to the renal pelvis.

Lymphangioma

These tumors are less frequent than hemangiomas and typically occur in young adults complaining of hematuria or a flank mass (334,335,337). Children are affected in approximately one third of cases. Most lymphangiomas are peripelvic and may actually represent lymphangiectasia due to pelvic inflammation with secondary lymphatic obstruction (fig. 1-247). The rare intrarenal lymphangioma has a honeycombed or multicystic gross appearance with cavernous spaces of varying size (fig. 1-248). Histologically, the spaces are lined by flattened endothelial cells on a fibrous septum which may contain elements of smooth muscle. These spaces are filled with lymph. We are aware of no examples of lymphangiosarcoma of the kidney.

Mesoblastic Nephroma

This tumor is primarily a neoplasm of early infancy but has occurred in adults aged 18 to 50 years (338–344). Tumors are solitary and firm, and range in size from 3.8 to 22 cm in greatest dimension. In contrast to the monophasic infan-

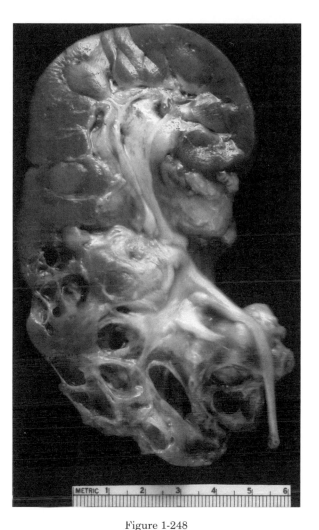

Figure 1-248
RENAL LYMPHANGIOMA
This large intrarenal lesion presents a honeycombed appearance.

tile tumor, two elements have been demonstrated in adult cases: a spindled stromal cell of immature mesenchymal morphology, resembling smooth muscle, and a tubule-forming columnar epithelial cell (fig. 1-249). In some areas, the epithelial tubular structures appear entrapped but in other foci, the tubular elements form confluent zones suggestive of adenomatous transformation. Cystic spaces may occur. In most cases, recurrences and metastases have not developed but at least one exception was recorded in which the tumor recurred 21 years after initial removal (341).

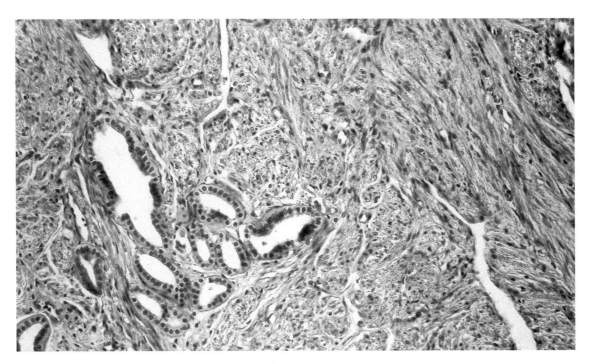

Figure 1-249
ADULT MESOBLASTIC NEPHROMA
There is a spindled myofibroblastic stromal component with tubular elements.

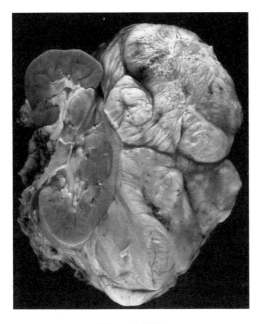

Figure 1-250
RENAL LEIOMYOSARCOMA
This massive tumor is situated peripherally and appears to arise from the renal capsule. (Fig. 1 from Farrow GM, Harrison EG Jr, Utz DC, ReMine WH. Sarcomas and sarcomatoid and mixed malignant tumors of the kidney in adults—Part I. Cancer 1968;22:545–50.)

Leiomyosarcoma

Among primary sarcomas of the kidney, leiomyosarcoma is the most frequent, comprising 40 to 60 percent of reported cases (350,351,356,359). These tumors are usually situated peripherally and appear to arise from the renal capsule (fig. 1-250) or from smooth muscle tissue in the wall of the renal pelvis (fig. 1-251). Leiomyosarcomas may arise in the smooth muscle of large renal blood vessels (fig. 1-252) but as many as one third of tumors are intrarenal (fig. 1-253). These tumors must be distinguished from angiomyolipomas and sarcomatoid renal cell carcinomas. On section, leiomyosarcomas are pale grey, firm, and fleshy, with a nodular or bosselated surface. The histologic features are similar to those of leiomyosarcomas at other sites and various subtypes have been observed (351). Microscopic vascular invasion is common but extension into large renal veins is unusual. Although a few patients have survived for several years, the prognosis is poor: most patients die within the first 2 years following diagnosis. Local recurrence and hematogenous metastases to bone and lung are frequent.

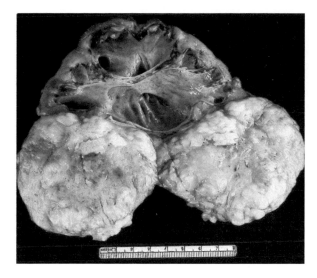

Figure 1-251
RENAL LEIOMYOSARCOMA
This tumor arose in the smooth musculature of the renal pelvis. (Fig. 2 from Farrow GM, Harrison EG Jr, Utz DC, ReMine WH. Sarcomas and sarcomatoid and mixed malignant tumors of the kidney in adults—Part I. Cancer 1968;22:545–50.)

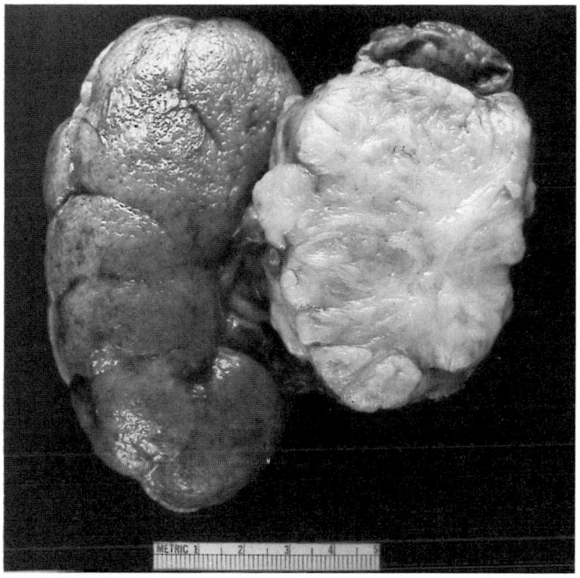

Figure 1-252
LEIOMYOSARCOMA
This tumor arose in the musculature of the renal vein.

Liposarcoma

Liposarcomas typically occur in the retroperitoneum, with secondary involvement of the kidney. Recent reviews have emphasized the difficulty of separating primary renal liposarcoma from secondary involvement by a retroperitoneal tumor (346,351,353). Lesions involving only the renal parenchyma are rare (353). If one accepts the contention that liposarcomas may arise within the inner adipose tissue of the renal capsule and be contained by this structure, then more cases can be included (figs. 1-254, 1-255) (350). Liposarcomas have not always been distinguished from angiomyolipomas in the past.

These cancers do not differ histologically from similar tumors at other body sites. All histologic patterns have been observed, the most common being the myxoid type. Complete surgical excision is extremely difficult to achieve, so that local recurrences and eventual tumor-related deaths are the rule. Intrarenal tumors have a better prognosis than peripheral lesions (353).

Hemangiopericytoma

These tumors have been identified as primary renal neoplasms although about 50 percent of reported cases arose in perirenal tissues or the

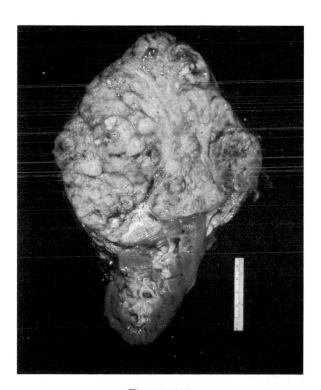

Figure 1-253
RENAL LEIOMYOSARCOMA
This tumor has a large intrarenal component.

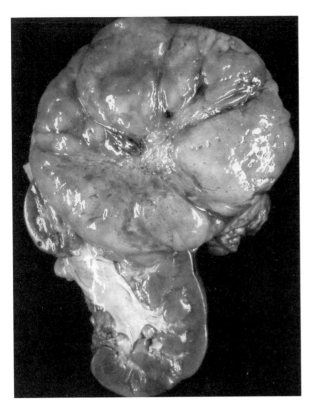

Figure 1-254
RENAL LIPOSARCOMA

This large fatty tumor has an intrarenal component, but projects from the renal surface. (Fig. 8-82 from Farrow GM. Diseases of the kidney. In: Murphy WM, ed. Urological pathology. Philadelphia: WB Saunders, 1989:409–82.)

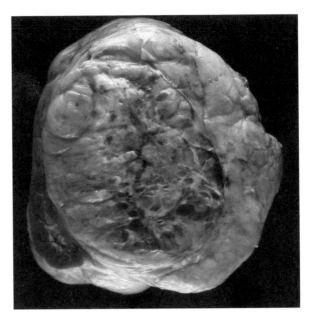

Figure 1-255
RENAL LIPOSARCOMA

The large fatty tumor appears to arise from the inner aspect of the renal capsule and compresses the kidney. (Fig. 7 from Farrow GM, Harrison EG Jr, Utz DC, ReMine WH. Sarcomas and sarcomatoid and mixed malignant tumors of the kidney in adults—Part I. Cancer 1968;22:545–50.)

renal capsule (fig. 1-256) (351,355). Renal lesions are typically large, circumscribed, and fibrous. As with hemangiopericytomas in other sites, criteria for malignancy have not been established. The outlook for long-term survival is better than for most renal sarcomas. Interestingly, three of the reported cases demonstrated a paraneoplastic syndrome of severe hypoglycemia and one patient died in a hypoglycemic coma (345,350).

Fibrosarcoma and Malignant Fibrous Histiocytoma

These tumors may be much less common than the data in Table 1-29 indicate, since many cases of sarcomatoid renal cell carcinoma feature components that closely resemble fibrous histiocytomas and fibrosarcomas (348). The tendency of these lesions to be large and involve perirenal structures further confounds a determination of primary site. Both fibrosarcoma and malignant fibrous histiocytoma are typically solid, fleshy tumors exhibiting hemorrhage and necrosis. Malignant fibrous histiocytomas are characteristically of the storiform-pleomorphic type, but inflammatory types and giant cell variants have been observed (fig. 1-257). Both are aggressive and associated with a poor prognosis (351,352,357).

Rhabdomyosarcoma

These tumors are typically large, solid, fleshy, and pale grey (fig. 1-258) (350). Most are of the pleomorphic variety and do not resemble nephroblastoma, although both nephroblastoma and sarcomatoid carcinoma should be considered before a diagnosis is rendered.

Angiosarcoma

These rare renal tumors are situated in the renal parenchyma where they form multiple, circumscribed, hemorrhagic masses (fig. 1-259) (347, 349,358). Vascular spaces are lined by malignant endothelial cells (fig. 1-260). The outcome has been uniformly fatal.

Table 1-29

SARCOMAS OF THE KIDNEY IN ADULTS

Histologic Type	Number of Cases
Leiomyosarcoma	132
Liposarcoma	46
intrarenal only	(9)
Fibrosarcoma	34
Malignant fibrous histiocytoma	20
Hemangiopericytoma	19
Osteosarcoma	12
Rhabdomyosarcoma	8
Angiosarcoma	6
Mixed sarcoma	6
Spindle cell sarcoma	4
Malignant mesenchymoma	2
Undifferentiated sarcoma	2
Angiomyoliposarcoma	1
Malignant schwannoma	1
Round cell sarcoma	1

Osteosarcoma

This rare tumor consists of osteoid-producing sarcoma cells (fig. 1-261). Varying degrees of chondrosarcomatous differentiation may also be present. Tumors are typically large and invasive. Survival is poor: roughly 80 percent of patients die of their disease (354).

A variety of other malignant mesenchymal tumors have been described in sporadic case reports (Table 1-29). Many are vaguely designated as spindle cell sarcoma or round cell sarcoma.

Angiomyolipoma

Definition. Angiomyolipoma is a tumor composed of varying admixtures of blood vessels, smooth muscle cells, and adipose tissue. The lesion could be considered a choristoma, a disordered arrangement of mature tissue appearing at a site in which that tissue does not normally reside (360). The etiology and pathogenesis are unknown but most previous classifications have included this tumor among mesenchymal neoplasms.

General and Clinical Features. The frequency of angiomyolipomas of the kidney has varied from 0.7 to 2.0 percent of all renal tumors,

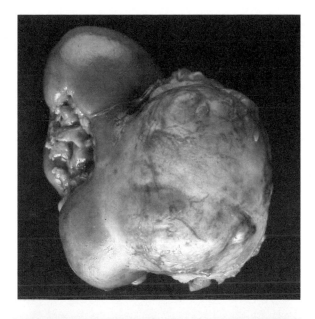

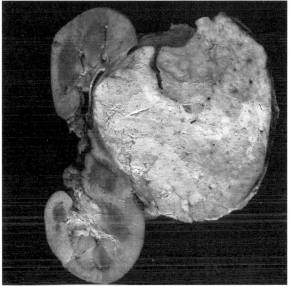

Figure 1-256
HEMANGIOPERICYTOMA

This large circumscribed tumor is situated peripherally, probably arising from the renal capsule. (Fig. 4 from Farrow GM, Harrison EG Jr, Utz DC, ReMine WH. Sarcomas and sarcomatoid and mixed malignant tumors of the kidney in adults—Part I. Cancer 1968;22:545–50.)

depending upon whether cases were observed as incidental findings or as symptomatic tumors with or without associated tuberous sclerosis (361,363,366). Unlike most renal tumors, patients are predominantly women, in a ratio of 2 to 1. The average age at diagnosis is 41 years,

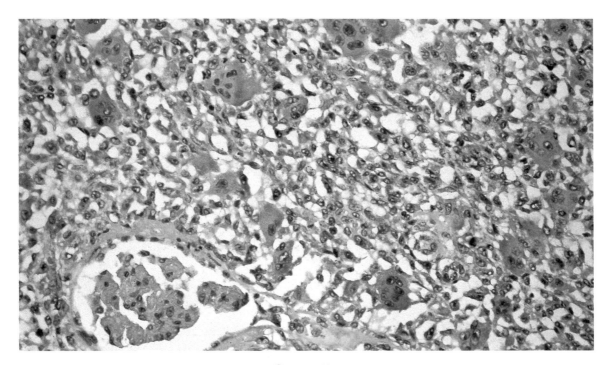

Figure 1-257
MALIGNANT FIBROUS HISTIOCYTOMA
This neoplasm features many multinucleated giant cells.

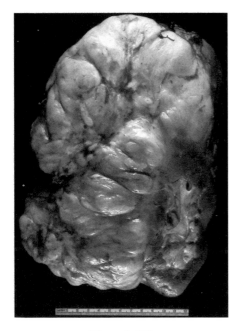

Figure 1-258
RHABDOMYOSARCOMA
This large, fleshy tumor is situated peripherally and appears to arise from the renal capsule. (Fig. 8 from Farrow GM, Harrison EG Jr, Utz DC, ReMine WH. Sarcomas and sarcomatoid and mixed malignant tumors of the kidney in adults—Part I. Cancer 1968;22:545–50.)

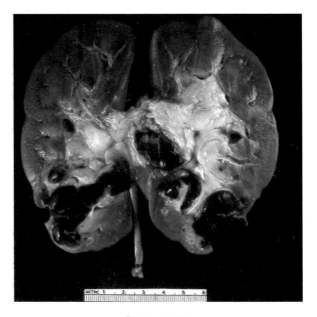

Figure 1-259
ANGIOSARCOMA
There are multiple hemorrhagic masses within the renal parenchyma.

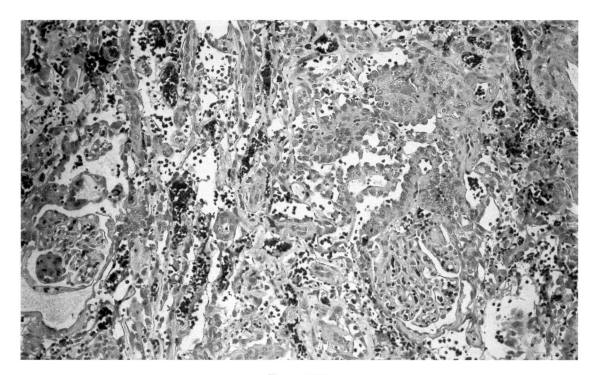

Figure 1-260
ANGIOSARCOMA
Numerous blood-filled vascular spaces are lined by plump endothelial cells.

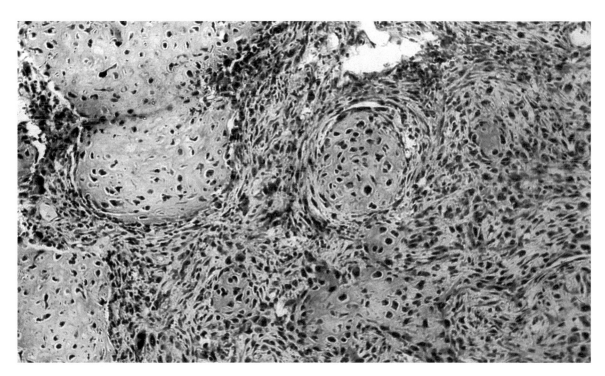

Figure 1-261
RENAL OSTEOSARCOMA
Abundant osteoid is produced by this sarcoma.

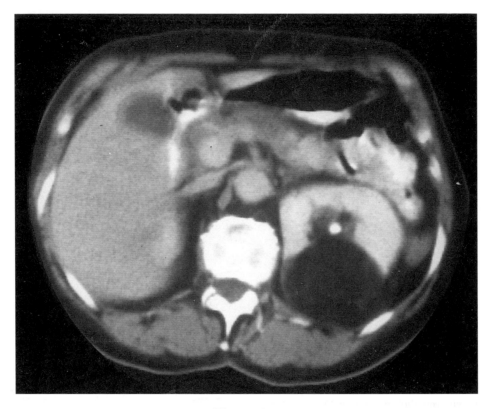

Figure 1-262
RENAL ANGIOMYOLIPOMA
By computerized tomography, an angiomyolipoma is visualized with the same radiodensity as the subcutaneous fat.

although children have been affected (373,375). No racial predilection has been demonstrated. Among symptomatic patients, flank pain related to intratumoral hemorrhage is the most common complaint. Angiomyolipomas are ordinarily detected radiographically, where they can usually be distinguished from other renal tumors (fig. 1-262) (365,370). Fine needle aspiration confirms the diagnosis in many cases.

Angiomyolipomas have been observed in patients with several hereditary disorders including von Recklinghausen disease, von Hippel-Lindau syndrome, and autosomal dominant (adult) polycystic disease. The association is particularly strong with tuberous sclerosis. Whereas angiomyolipomas occur in 80 percent of individuals with tuberous sclerosis, less than half of patients with angiomyolipomas have the tuberous sclerosis syndrome.

Tumors with the histopathologic features of angiomyolipoma have been observed in the renal capsule (capsulomas); attached to the renal capsule but predominantly in the perirenal tissues; localized to the retroperitoneum without renal attachments; and in abdominal organs such as the liver, fallopian tubes, spleen, and regional lymph nodes (362,366–368). Most investigators consider the occurrence of these tumors at extrarenal sites to be evidence of multicentricity rather than metastases.

Pathologic Findings. The typical angiomyolipoma is an intrarenal tumor which replaces a portion of the renal parenchyma (figs. 1-263, 1-264). Lesions may vary considerably in size: capsular lesions rarely measure more than a few millimeters while intrarenal tumors range from 3 to 20 cm (mean, 9.4 cm) in greatest dimension (373). Large masses ordinarily compress the surrounding structures (fig. 1-265). Rarely, they rupture into renal calyces (fig. 1-266) or the renal vein (fig. 1-267) (370) and may extend into the renal collecting system, renal

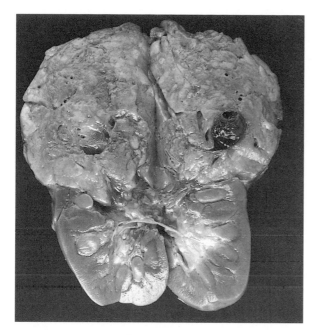

Figure 1-263
RENAL ANGIOMYOLIPOMA
A circumscribed, nonencapsulated fatty tumor is situated in, and replaces, the upper half of the kidney. (Fig. 1A from Farrow GM, Harrison EG Jr, Utz DC, Jones DR. Renal angiomyolipoma: a clinicopathologic study of 32 cases. Cancer 1968;22:564–70.)

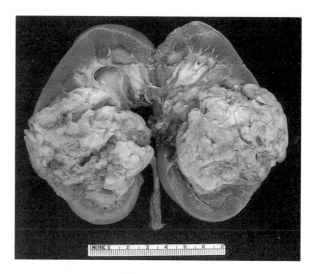

Figure 1-265
RENAL ANGIOMYOLIPOMA
The renal pelvis is compressed and distorted by the tumor.

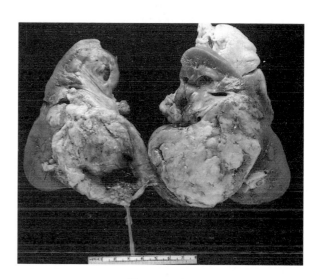

Figure 1-266
RENAL ANGIOMYOLIPOMA
Rarely, angiomyolipomas may extend into the renal pelvis, as in this case. (Fig. 1B from Farrow GM, Harrison EG Jr, Utz DC, Jones DR. Renal angiomyolipoma: a clinicopathologic study of 32 cases. Cancer 1968;22:564–70.)

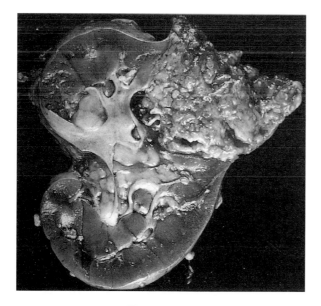

Figure 1-264
RENAL ANGIOMYOLIPOMA
This tumor, composed predominantly of adipose tissue, is situated within the renal parenchyma.

vein, or even the vena cava. Most angiomyolipomas are solitary but multiple tumors have been observed in as many as 20 percent of cases (fig. 1-268). In such situations, a large dominant tumor associated with smaller lesions is typical (fig. 1-269). Massive hemorrhage may occur into an angiomyolipoma (fig. 1-270). Although circumscribed, angiomyolipomas are not encapsulated

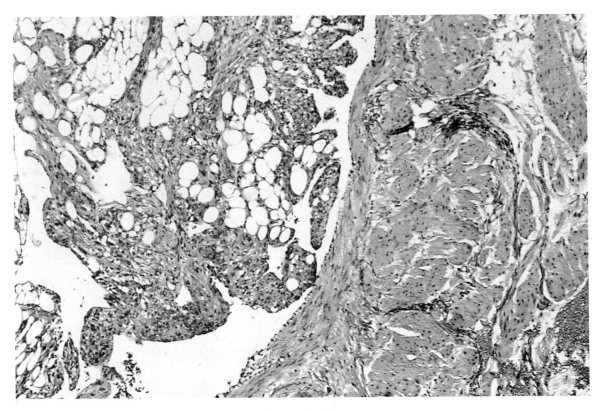

Figure 1-267
ANGIOMYOLIPOMA
This tumor has extended into the main renal vein.

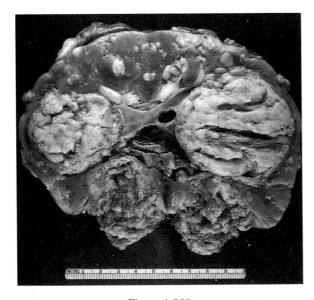

Figure 1-268
ANGIOMYOLIPOMA

This kidney contains innumerable tumors of varying sizes.
(Fig. 2A from Farrow GM, Harrison EG Jr, Utz DC, Jones DR.
Renal angiomyolipoma: a clinicopathologic study of 32 cases.
Cancer 1968;22:564–70.)

and tend to enlarge at the expense of the adjacent renal parenchyma so that elements of normal kidney become surrounded and isolated throughout the tumor (fig. 1-271). Once entrapped, renal tubular elements may dilate and form cysts (fig. 1-272). Rarely, this process is so pronounced that tumors appear polycystic (371,372,374). Most such cases have occurred in patients with tuberous sclerosis.

As previously stated, angiomyolipomas are highly associated with the hereditary disease tuberous sclerosis (mental retardation, epilepsy, cutaneous hamartomas (fig. 1-273), shagreen skin, depigmented spots (fig. 1-274), subungual fibromas of fingers). In most cases, the angiomyolipomas are multiple and bilateral (fig. 1-275). The association is so close that all patients with multiple renal angiomyolipomas should be evaluated for tuberous sclerosis, even though the hereditary syndrome may be only partially expressed (363).

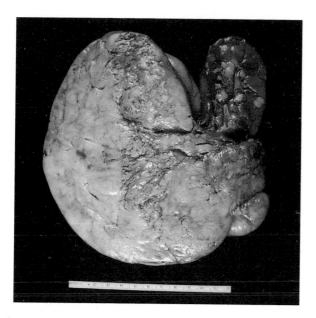

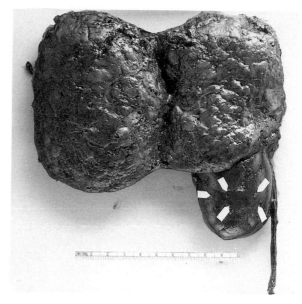

Figure 1-269
ANGIOMYOLIPOMA

In both kidneys, there is a large dominant mass with multiple smaller tumors. (Fig. 8-85 from Farrow GM. Diseases of the kidney. In: Murphy WM, ed. Urological pathology. Philadelphia: WB Saunders, 1989:409–82.)

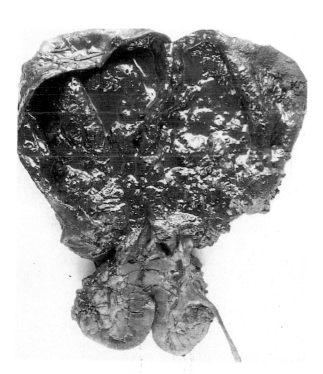

Figure 1-270
ANGIOMYOLIPOMA
Massive intratumoral hemorrhage has occurred in this case.

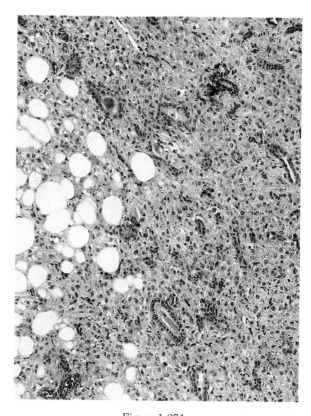

Figure 1-271
ANGIOMYOLIPOMA
Trapped renal tubules are present within the neoplasm.

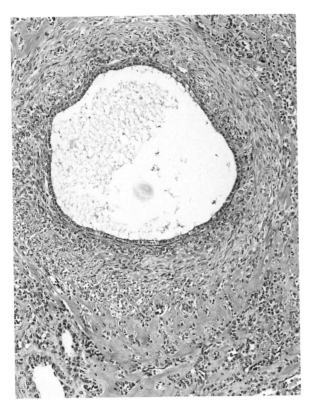

Figure 1-272
ANGIOMYOLIPOMA
This entrapped renal tubule has dilated to form a cyst.

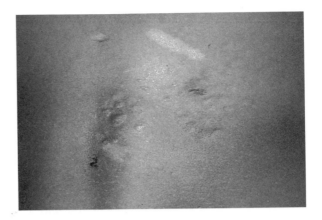

Figure 1-274
TUBEROUS SCLEROSIS
Depigmented spots and shagreen or leathery skin occur typically on the small of the back.

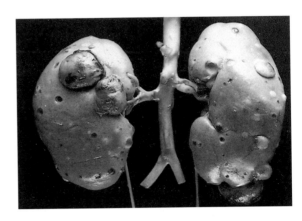

Figure 1-275
RENAL ANGIOMYOLIPOMAS
IN TUBEROUS SCLEROSIS
The tumors are multiple and bilateral. There are also cortical cysts. (Fig. 2C from Farrow GM, Harrison EG Jr, Utz DC, Jones DR. Renal angiomyolipoma: a clinicopathologic study of 32 cases. Cancer 1968;22:564–70.)

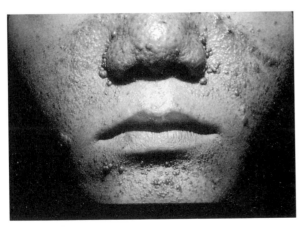

Figure 1-273
TUBEROUS SCLEROSIS
The characteristic cutaneous hamartomas occur about the face and neck. (Fig. 8-93 from Farrow GM. Diseases of the kidney. In: Murphy WM, ed. Urological pathology. Philadelphia: WB Saunders, 1989:409–82.)

Grossly, angiomyolipomas are lobular, yellow, and slightly oily. Tumors consisting primarily of smooth muscle may be pale gray and firm (fig. 1-276). Hemorrhage is a common finding, especially in symptomatic cases, and may be extensive enough to nearly replace the tumor.

Microscopically, angiomyolipomas are composed of mixtures of blood vessels, smooth muscle, and adipose tissue, characteristically admixed in a haphazard fashion (fig. 1-277). Mature adipose tissue, often associated with fat necrosis, lipophages, and giant cells, ordinarily constitutes the bulk of the tumor but any component may predominate (figs. 1-278, 1-279). The smooth muscle cells are often intimately associated with the outer layers of the muscular walls of blood vessels, from which they appear to arise (fig. 1-280). These muscle cells are arranged in a radial configuration with the long axis of their elongated nuclei at perpendicular angles to the vessels, imparting a "hair on end" appearance. The smooth muscle often courses in interlacing fascicles throughout the neoplasm and is punctuated by islands of adipose tissue and vessels. Lesions at extrarenal sites have similar histology (figs. 1-281, 1-282). In some microscopic fields, wide expanses are composed entirely of smooth muscle. There may be nuclear enlargement, hyperchromasia, and scattered mitoses among the smooth muscle cells (fig. 1-283). Some tumors have a sizable population of immature smooth muscle cells or leiomyoblasts with rounded nuclei and cleared cytoplasm, arranged in palisades about a central arteriole (fig. 1-284). The blood vessels are a striking component of the

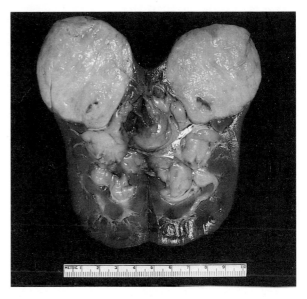

Figure 1-276
ANGIOMYOLIPOMA
The macroscopic appearance suggests that this tumor is predominantly smooth muscle. (Fig. 8-87 from Farrow GM. Diseases of the kidney. In: Murphy WM, ed. Urological pathology. Philadelphia: WB Saunders, 1989:409–82.)

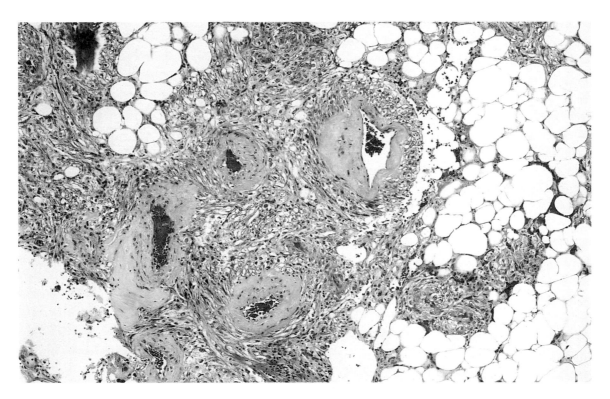

Figure 1-277
ANGIOMYOLIPOMA
There is an intimate mixture of thick-walled blood vessels, smooth muscle, and adipose tissue.

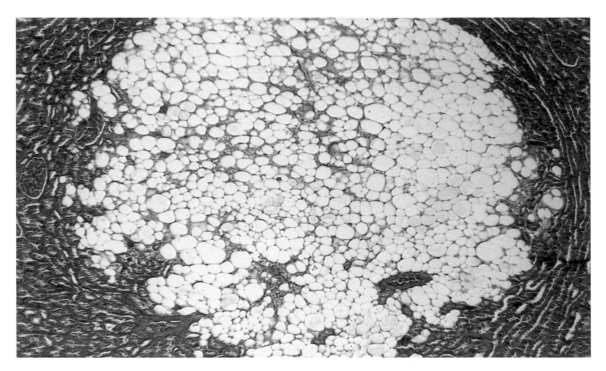

Figure 1-278
ANGIOMYOLIPOMA
This tumor consists principally of adipose tissue.

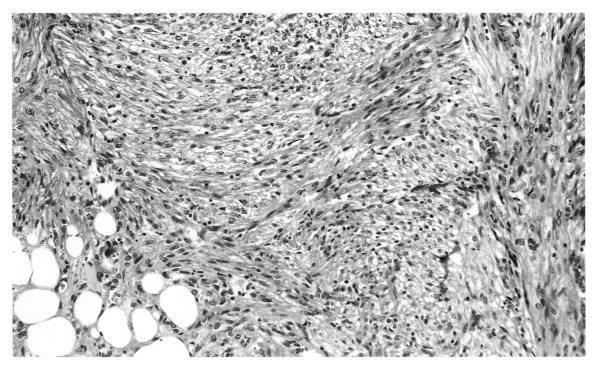

Figure 1-279
ANGIOMYOLIPOMA
This tumor consists principally of smooth muscle.

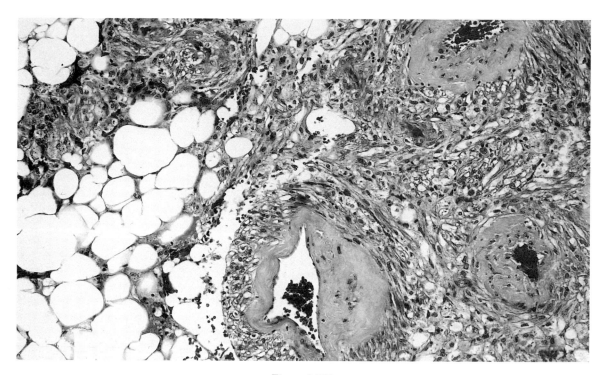

Figure 1-280
ANGIOMYOLIPOMA
The smooth muscle cells appear to arise from the outer walls of blood vessels.

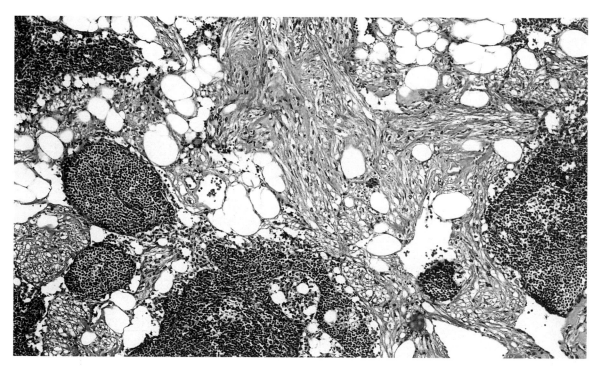

Figure 1-281
ANGIOMYOLIPOMA
This tumor largely replaces a renal hilar lymph node.

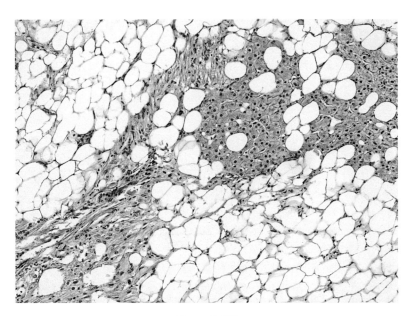

Figure 1-282
ANGIOMYOLIPOMA
This tumor is present within the liver parenchyma.

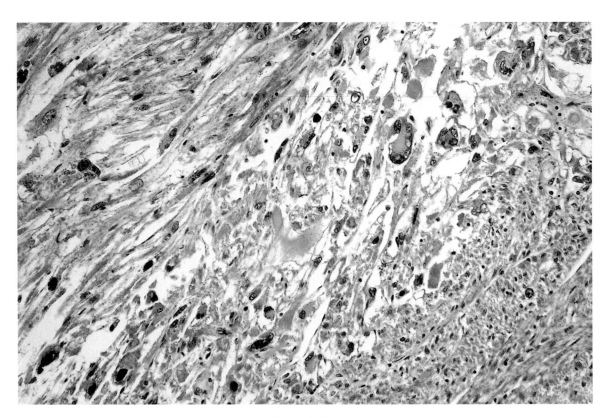

Figure 1-283
ANGIOMYOLIPOMA
Bizarre and atypical changes may be observed in the smooth muscle component.

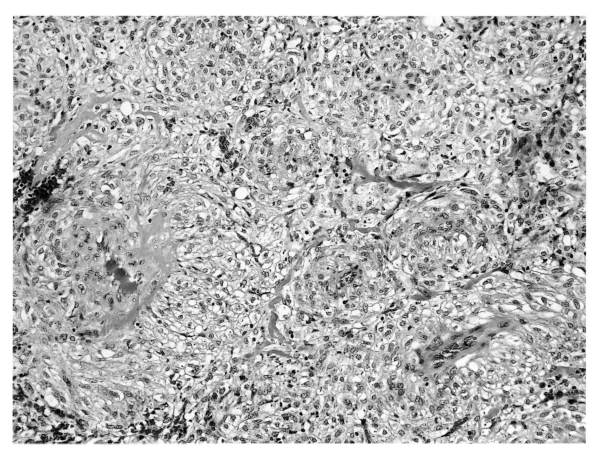

Figure 1-284
ANGIOMYOLIPOMA
Immature smooth muscle cells (leiomyoblasts) may be abundant.

tumor and typically have very thick, abnormally formed walls. In many areas, the muscular tissue of blood vessels is replaced by dense fibrous connective tissue of irregular thickness. These vessels resemble arterialized veins like those found in arteriovenous malformations (fig. 1-285). The internal elastic laminae are generally absent from vascular walls or, when present, are fragmented, reduplicated, and frayed. The blood vessels of angiomyolipomas may be extremely tortuous and their walls may be focally thinned and dilated, creating small cirsoid aneurysms (fig. 1-286). Specimens obtained by aspiration cytology typically have a mixture of adipose tissue and smooth muscle (fig. 1-287).

Prognosis. Despite a heterologous composition and lack of cellular anaplasia, angiomyoli-

poma represents a significant aberration in normal development which can predispose to life-threatening complications. The first satisfactorily documented case of malignancy developing in an angiomyolipoma appeared in 1991 (364). In this case, a renal tumor that had extended into the liver and metastasized to the lung exhibited areas of typical angiomyolipoma, along with other foci of transformation, into a high-grade spindle cell sarcoma. Patients with tuberous sclerosis have a number of abnormalities that may be life-threatening. Even individuals lacking associated syndromes or malignant transformation may develop progressive renal failure and massive hemorrhage (363,369). New angiomyolipomas have appeared in the remaining kidney after nephrectomy for a contralateral lesion.

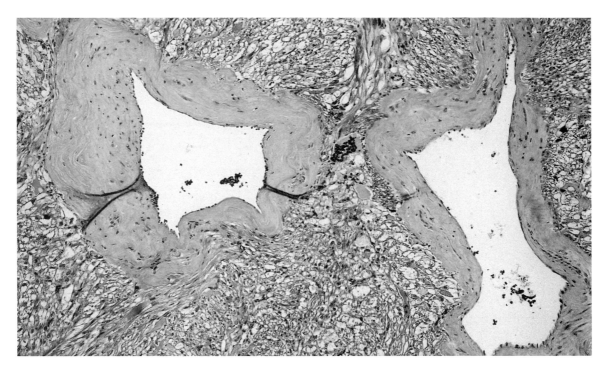

Figure 1-285
ANGIOMYOLIPOMA
Thick-walled blood vessels resembling arterialized veins are characteristic.

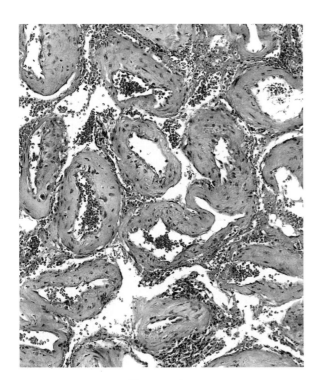

Figure 1-286
ANGIOMYOLIPOMA
Abnormal tumor vessels may form aneurysms.

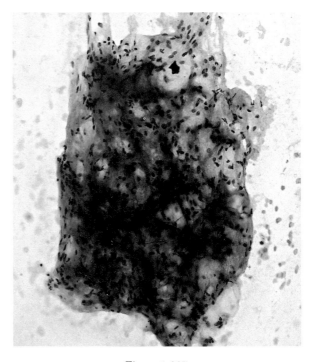

Figure 1-287
ANGIOMYOLIPOMA
In this aspiration cytology preparation, a mixture of smooth muscle and adipose tissue is present.

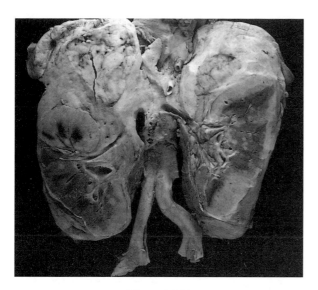

Figure 1-288
MALIGNANT LYMPHOMA
Massive retroperitoneal lymphoma engulfs both kidneys and adrenal glands.

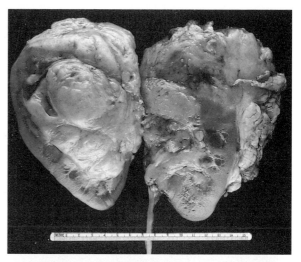

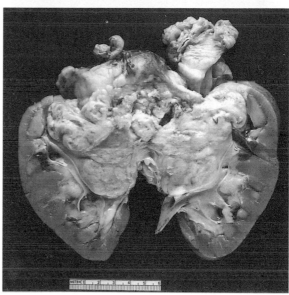

Figure 1-289
MALIGNANT LYMPHOMA
The main mass of tumor is situated principally in the hilar region in both cases.

LYMPHOID TUMORS

Lymphoma

Involvement of the kidneys by malignant lymphoma is common in patients with late-stage lesions, particularly among those with non-Hodgkin lymphomas having extensive retroperitoneal involvement (fig. 1-288). Clinical evidence of genitourinary involvement is found in about 7.5 percent of cases but this figure increases to nearly 70 percent among autopsy series (380,383). Radiographic studies have also demonstrated a high frequency of renal involvement in late-stage lymphoma. Conversely, primary renal lymphoma without evidence of systemic disease is rare (376,382). In such cases, the lymphoma is usually localized to the hilus (fig. 1-289) but may appear as discreet, solitary or multiple nodular renal parenchymal masses (figs. 1-290, 1-291). Diffuse infiltration of the kidneys usually occurs bilaterally and is more characteristic of leukemia than lymphoma. Hilar lymphomas tend to be 6 to 11 cm in greatest dimension and encompass the hilar lymph nodes so that a possible nodal origin cannot be completely excluded. Parenchymal nodules measure up to 15 cm in greatest dimension and are distributed throughout both the cortex and medulla.

Histologically, primary renal lymphomas are usually of the large cell, diffuse type (fig. 1-292).

Renal involvement occurs in an unusual form of malignant lymphoma originally described as "lymphomatoid granulomatosis" (378). This lesion is an angiocentric form of peripheral T-cell lymphoma in which lesions typically are present in the lungs and skin, as well as the kidneys (fig. 1-293) (377,379, 381). The microscopic features of T-cell lymphoma of the kidney are similar to those in other involved organs (figs. 1-294, 1-295).

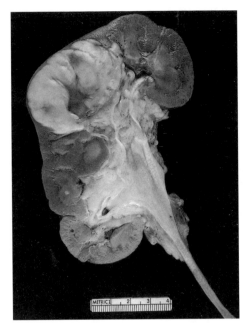

Figure 1-290
MALIGNANT LYMPHOMA

This tumor presents as a solitary mass in the kidney. (Fig. 8-84 from Farrow GM. Diseases of the kidney. In: Murphy WM, ed. Urological pathology. Philadelphia: WB Saunders, 1989:409–82.)

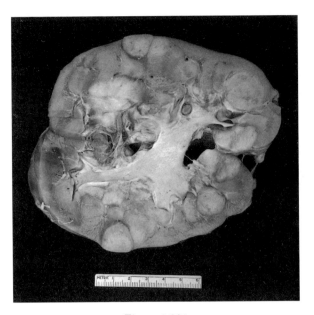

Figure 1-291
MALIGNANT LYMPHOMA

There are multiple tumor nodules in the kidney. (Fig. 2B from Farrow GM, Harrison EG Jr, Utz DC. Sarcomas and sarcomatoid and mixed malignant tumors of the kidney in adults—Part II. Cancer 1968;22:551–55.)

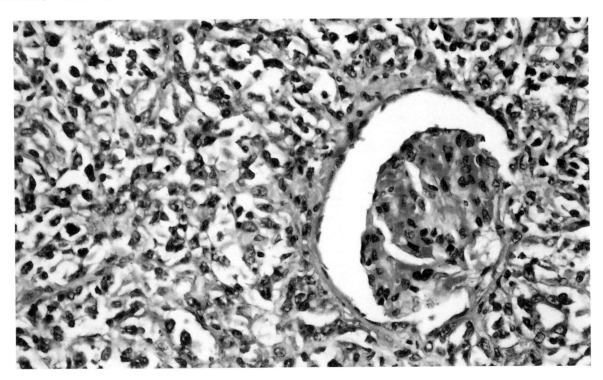

Figure 1-292
MALIGNANT LYMPHOMA
This is a large cell type diffuse lymphoma.

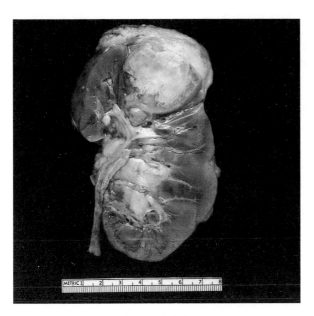

Figure 1-293
ANGIOCENTRIC T-CELL LYMPHOMA
(LYMPHOMATOID GRANULOMATOSIS)

A largely necrotic solitary mass is present in the upper pole of the kidney. (Fig. 2A from Farrow GM, Harrison EG Jr, Utz DC. Sarcomas and sarcomatoid and mixed malignant tumors of the kidney in adults—Part II. Cancer 1968;22:551–55.)

Plasmacytoma

This lesion is rarely found in the kidney (376). Most recorded cases have been associated with disease in the bones. Amyloidosis has been observed in at least one case. Renal plasmacytomas tend to be solitary mass lesions (fig. 1-296). A few long-term survivals have followed resection of the tumor.

METASTATIC TUMORS TO THE KIDNEY

In the later stages of evolution of malignant tumors at other locations, metastatic deposits may occur in the kidneys. Differential diagnosis is ordinarily not a problem since metastatic tumors masquerading as primary renal neoplasms are unusual in well-evaluated patients. The most common primary sites are lung, skin (malignant melanoma), the contralateral kidney, the gastrointestinal tract, ovary, and testis (figs. 1-297, 1-298) (384).

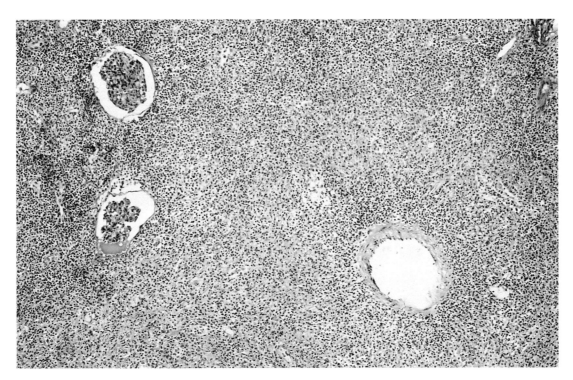

Figure 1-294
ANGIOCENTRIC T-CELL LYMPHOMA (LYMPHOMATOID GRANULOMATOSIS)
There is a massive lymphoid infiltrate with an angiocentric distribution.

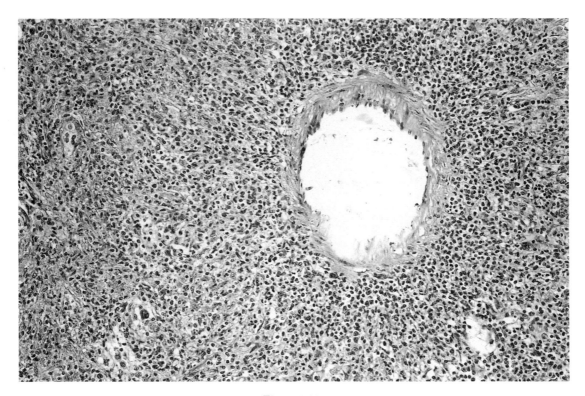

Figure 1-295
ANGIOCENTRIC T-CELL LYMPHOMA (LYMPHOMATOID GRANULOMATOSIS)
This type of T-cell lymphoma features a mixed inflammatory cell population with scattered, large, atypical lymphoid cells. There is angiocentricity of the infiltrate with destruction of the vessel wall.

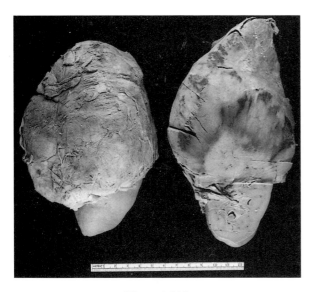

Figure 1-296
PLASMACYTOMA
This large renal mass replaces a large portion of the kidney. The patient died 16 years following nephrectomy from unrelated causes. (Fig. 5A from Farrow GM, Harrison EG Jr, Utz DC. Sarcomas and sarcomatoid and mixed malignant tumors of the kidney in adults—Part II. Cancer 1968;22:551–55.)

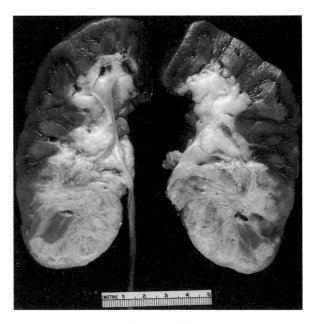

Figure 1-297
METASTATIC SQUAMOUS CELL CARCINOMA
The primary tumor was in the lung.

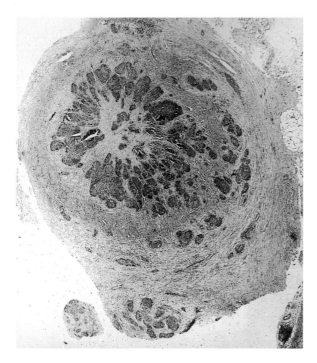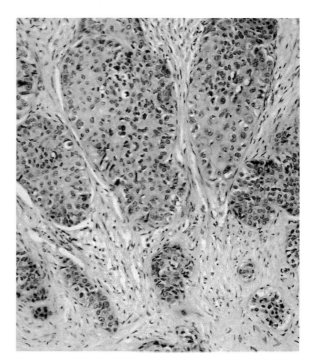

Figure 1-298
METASTATIC SQUAMOUS CELL CARCINOMA
Left: Metastatic tumor occludes the lumen of the renal artery.
Right: The squamous cell nature of the tumor is evident.

NON-NEOPLASTIC TUMOROUS CONDITIONS

In its broadest sense, the word "tumor" includes any localized enlargement of an anatomic structure. Thus, there are tumors that are not neoplastic but simulate neoplasms clinically and radiologically.

Xanthogranulomatous Pyelonephritis

This is a distinctive form of subacute and chronic renal inflammation prone to form a mass lesion that may mimic a renal neoplasm. Several collected series have appeared in the literature since the first description in 1916 (387,393,394, 397). Most patients are women in the fourth to sixth decades of life. The most common presenting complaints are fever, flank pain, and a tender flank mass (388,391,393,398). Nephrolithiasis is a characteristic associated feature, present in up to 70 percent of cases. As determined by excretory urography, the affected kidney is nonfunctioning in 50 to 70 percent of cases. Common urinary tract bacteria such as *Proteus* and *Escherichia* species can be isolated from the urine but the

urine culture is negative in as much as 30 percent of cases, even though organisms can be isolated from the lesion itself in 95 percent of cases (390). Because of the mass effect, radiologic findings mimic those of a renal neoplasm (386, 389,399). The disease is almost always unilateral but may involve any part or all of the kidney.

In its early stages, xanthogranulomatous pyelonephritis is usually confined to the kidney and appears grossly as golden yellow nodules ranging from a few millimeters to several centimeters in greatest dimension. By the time of clinical detection, however, the inflammatory mass is usually very large and may penetrate the Gerota fascia (fig. 1-299).

Microscopically, the histologic features of xanthogranulomatous pyelonephritis are variable. Frankly purulent foci with micro-abscesses and numerous neutrophils may coexist with the more classic histopathology of abundant, lipid-laden macrophages intermixed with lymphocytes and plasma cells (fig. 1-300). The lipid-laden macrophages (xanthoma cells) may mimic the cells of well-differentiated clear cell renal

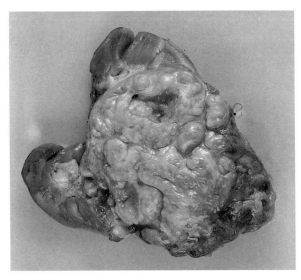

Figure 1-299
XANTHOGRANULOMATOUS PYELONEPHRITIS
A large golden yellow mass replaces a large portion of the kidney and extends into the perirenal tissues. (Fig. 8-23 from Farrow GM. Diseases of the kidney. In: Murphy WM, ed. Urological pathology. Philadelphia: WB Saunders, 1989:409–82.)

carcinoma. Multinucleated giant cells and spindled fibroblasts may be abundant and such areas can resemble the spindle cell component of a sarcomatoid renal cell carcinoma (fig. 1-301). In a small proportion of cases, Michaelis-Gutmann bodies are found, and when this occurs the designation *malakoplakia* is appropriate.

Ask-Upmark Kidney

This is a rare form of unilateral congenital renal hypoplasia that may mimic the radiographic appearance of a renal neoplasm. The abnormality was first reported by Ask-Upmark in 1929 and was observed mainly among adolescents presenting with hypertension (385). In one autopsy study, the abnormality was found in 2 of 1000 subjects (392), but in another series of 2153 pediatric autopsies, no cases were observed (396).

On radiologic or ultrasonic examination, the capsular surface of the Ask-Upmark kidney is distorted by one or several grooves. The segments

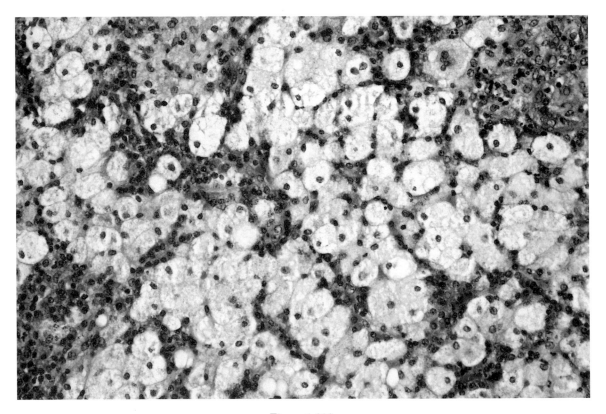

Figure 1-300
XANTHOGRANULOMATOUS PYELONEPHRITIS
There is a mixture of lipid-laden macrophages (xanthoma cells) with lymphocytes and plasma cells.

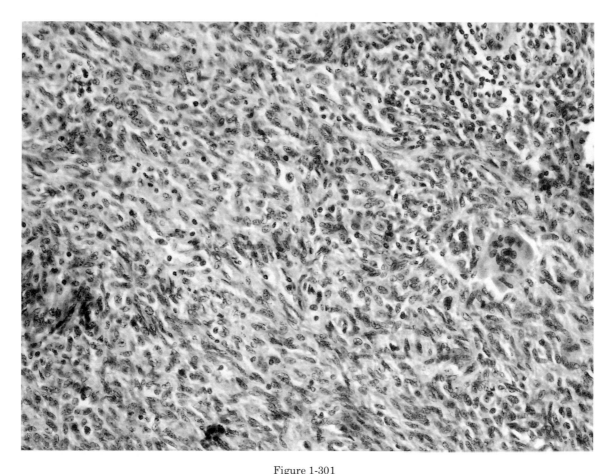

Figure 1-301
XANTHOGRANULOMATOUS PYELONEPHRITIS
Spindled fibroblasts with only scattered multinucleated giant cells may mimic a sarcoma or sarcomatoid carcinoma.

of renal parenchyma demarcated by the grooves may become distorted, mimicking a renal neoplasm (figs. 1-302, 1-303).

Pathologically, there is a reduced number of medullary pyramids. Hypoplastic and normal areas are juxtaposed, and there may be a pseudo-diverticular dilatation of the renal pelvis (395). The arcuate and interlobular arteries in Ask-Upmark lesions are stenotic and renal ischemia is a likely cause for the characteristic hypertension.

A wide variety of cystic and dysplastic renal lesions could be included in this section. Fortunately, most lack the clinical and pathologic features that might be confused with those of neoplasia. Those that must be considered in the differential diagnosis of renal neoplasms have already been discussed. The subject is extremely complex and beyond the scope of this atlas.

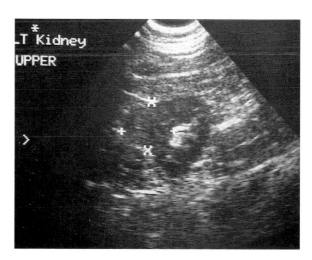

Figure 1-302
ASK-UPMARK KIDNEY
In this ultrasound image, a mass (outlined by cursors) projects from the kidney surface.

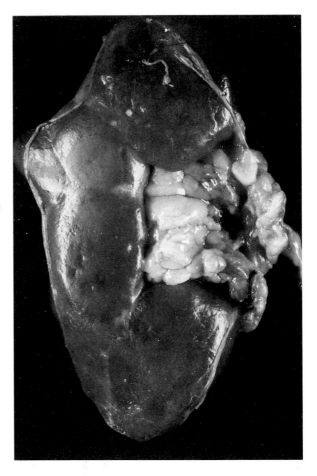

Figure 1-303
ASK-UPMARK KIDNEY
Segments of kidney from the case illustrated in figure 1-302 are demarcated by grooves, creating a mass-like effect.

REFERENCES

Normal Anatomy

1. Bander NH, Cordon-Cardo C, Finstad CL, et al. Immunohistologic dissection of the human kidney using monoclonal antibodies. J Urol 1985;133:502–5.
2. Clapp WL. Adult kidney. In: Sternberg SS, ed. Histology for pathologists. New York: Raven Press, 1992:677–707.
3. Cohen C, McCue PA, Derose PB. Histogenesis of renal cell carcinoma and oncocytoma. An immunohistochemical study. Cancer 1988;62:1946–51.
4. Hennigar RA, Spicer SA, Sens DA, Othersen HB Jr, Garvin AJ. Histochemical evidence for tubule segmentation in a case of Wilms' tumor. Am J Clin Pathol 1986;85:724–31.
5. Inke G. The protolobar structure of the kidney. Its biologic and clinical significance. New York: Alan R. Liss, 1988.
6. Kissane JM. Development and structure of the urogenital system. In: Murphy WM, ed. Urological pathology. Philadelphia: WB Saunders, 1989:1–12.
7. Kriz W, Dieterich HJ. Das Lymphgefäßystem der Niere bei einigen Säugetieren: Licht- und Elektronenmikro-skopsche Untersuchungen. Z Anat Entwicklungsgesch 1970;131:111–47.
8. Medeiros LJ, Michie SA, Johnson DE, Warnke RA, Weiss LM. An immunoperoxidase study of renal cell carcinomas: correlation with nuclear grade, cell type, and histologic pattern. Hum Pathol 1988;19:980–7.
9. Mitchell GA. The nerve supply of the kidneys. Acta Anat 1950;10:1–37.
10. Pierce EC. Renal lymphatics. Anat Rec 1944;90:315–35.
11. Pirani CL. Evaluation of kidney biopsy specimens. In: Tisher CC, Brenner BM, eds. Renal pathology. Philadelphia: JB Lippincott, 1989:11–42.
12. Potter EL. Normal and abnormal development of the kidney. Chicago: Year Book Medical Publishers, 1972.
13. Schenk EA, Schwartz RH, Lewis RA. Tamm-Horsfall mucoprotein. I. Localization in the kidney. Lab Invest 1971;25:92–5.
14. Tisher CC, Madsen KM. Anatomy of the kidney. In: Brenner BM, Rector FC Jr, eds. The kidney. 3rd ed. Philadelphia: WB Saunders, 1986:3–60.

Nephroblastoma and Nephroblastomatosis

15. Allsbrook WC, Boswell WC, Takahashi H, et al. Recurrent renal cell carcinoma arising in Wilms' tumor. Cancer 1991;67:690–5.

16. Arrigo S, Beckwith JB, Sharples K, D'Angio G, Haase G. Better survival after combined modality care for adults with Wilms' tumor. Cancer 1990;66:827–30.

17. Aterman K. Extrarenal nephroblastomas. J Cancer Res Clin Oncol 1989;115:409–17.

18. Babaian RJ, Skinner DG, Waisman J. Wilms' tumor in the adult patient: diagnosis, management, and review of the world medical literature. Cancer 1980;45:1713–9.

19. Beckwith JB. Precursor lesions of Wilms' tumor: clinical and biological implications. Med Pediatr Oncol 1993;21:158–68.

20. _____. Staging designation for bilateral Wilms' tumours [Letter]. Med Pediatr Oncol 1991;19:334.

21. _____. Wilms' tumor and other renal tumors of childhood. In: Finegold M, ed. Pathology of neoplasia in children and adolescents. Philadelphia: WB Saunders, 1986:313–32.

22. _____, Kiviat NB, Bonadio FJ. Nephrogenic rests, nephroblastomatosis, and the pathogenesis of Wilms' tumor. Pediatr Pathol 1990;10:1–30.

23. _____, Palmer NF. Histopathology and prognosis of Wilms' tumors: results from the National Wilms' Tumor Study. Cancer 1978;41:1937–48.

24. Bennington JL, Beckwith JB. Tumors of the kidney, renal pelvis, and ureter. Atlas of Tumor Pathology, 2nd Series, Fascicle 12. Washington, D.C.: Armed Forces Institute of Pathology, 1975, 31–78.

25. Bever CT, Koenigsberger R, Antunes JL, Wolff J. Epidural metastasis by Wilms' tumor. Am J Dis Child 1981;135:644–6.

26. Blute ML, Kelalis PP, Offord KP, Breslow N, Beckwith JB, D'Angio GJ. Bilateral Wilms' tumor. J Urol 1987;138(4 Pt 2):968–73.

27. Bove KE, McAdams AJ. The nephroblastomatosis complex and its relationship to Wilms' tumor. A clinicopathologic treatise. Perspect Pediatr Pathol 1976;3:185–223.

28. Breslow NE, Beckwith JB. Epidemiological features of Wilms' tumor: results of the National Wilms' Tumor Study. JNCI 1982;68:429–36.

29. _____, Churchill G, Nesmith B, et al. Clinicopathologic features and prognosis for Wilms' tumor patients with metastases at diagnosis. Cancer 1986;58:2501–11.

30. Breslow N, Beckwith JB, Ciol M, Sharples K. Age distribution of Wilms' tumor: report from the National Wilms' Tumor Study. Cancer Res 1988;48:1653–7.

31. Call KM, Glaser T, Ito CY, et al. Isolation and characterization of a zinc finger polypeptide gene at the human chromosome 11 Wilms' tumor locus. Cell 1990;60:509–20.

32. Chatten J. Epithelial differentiation in Wilms' tumor: a clinico-pathologic appraisal. Perspect Pediatr Pathol 1976;3:225–54.

33. Coppes MJ. Serum biological markers and paraneoplastic syndromes in Wilms tumor. Med Pediatr Oncol 1993;21:213–21.

34. _____, Beckwith B. Eponyms in medicine: possessive or nonpossesive? J Pediatr 1993;122:165.

35. _____, Zandvoort SW, Sparling CR, Poon AO, Weitzman S, Blanchette VS. Acquired von Willebrand disease in Wilms' tumor patients. J Clin Oncol 1992;10:422–7.

36. D'Angio GJ, Evans AE, Breslow N, et al. Treatment of Wilms' tumor: results of the National Wilms' Tumor Study. Cancer 1986;38:633–46.

37. Delemarre JF, Sandstedt B, Gerard-Marchant G, Tournade MF. SIOP nephroblastoma trials and studies, morphological aspects. In: Raybaud C, Clement C, Lebreuil G, Bernard JL, eds. Pediatric oncology. Amsterdam, Oxford, Princeton: Excerpta Medica, 1982:261–72.

38. Douglass EC, Look AT, Webber B, et al. Hyperdiploidy and chromosomal rearrangements define the anaplastic variant of Wilms' tumor. J Clin Oncol 1986;4:975–81.

39. Droz D, Rousseau-Merck MF, Jaubert F, et al. Cell differentiation in Wilms' tumor (nephroblastoma): an immunohistochemical study. Hum Pathol 1990;21:536–44.

40. Faria P, Beckwith JB. A new definition of focal anaplasia identifies cases with good outcome. A report from the National Wilms' Tumor Study [Abstract]. Mod Pathol 1993;6:3P.

41. Fernandes ET, Parham DM, Ribeiro RC, Douglass EC, Kumar AP, Wilimas J. Teratoid Wilms' tumor: the St. Jude experience. J Pediatr Surg 1988;23:1131–4.

42. Gearhart JP, Partin AW, Leventhal B, Beckwith JB, Epstein JI. The use of nuclear morphometry to predict response to therapy in Wilms' tumor. Cancer 1992;69:804–8.

43. Gerald WL, Miller HK, Battifora H, Miettinen M, Silva EG, Rosai J. Intraabdominal desmoplastic small round-cell tumor. Report of 19 cases of a distinctive type of high-grade polyphenotypic malignancy affecting young individuals. Am J Surg Pathol 1991;15:499–513.

44. Gessler M, Poustka A, Cavenee W, Neve RL, Orkin SH, Bruns GA. Homozygous deletion in Wilms tumours of a zinc-finger gene identified by chromosome jumping. Nature 1990;343:774–8.

45. Gonzalez-Crussi F. Wilms' tumor (nephroblastoma) and related renal neoplasms of childhood. Boca Raton, Fla.: CRC Press, 1984.

46. Green DM, Breslow NE, Beckwith JB, Norkool P. Screening of children with hemihypertrophy, aniridia, and Beckwith-Wiedemann syndrome in patients with Wilms' tumor: a report from the National Wilms' Tumor Study. Med Pediatr Oncol 1993;21:188–92.

47. Haber DA, Buckler AJ, Glaser T, et al. An internal deletion within an 11p13 zinc finger gene contributes to the development of Wilms' tumor. Cell 1990;61:1257–69.

48. Heppe RK, Koyle MA, Beckwith JB. Nephrogenic rests in Wilms tumor patients with the Drash syndrome. J Urol 1991;145:1225–8.

49. Hou LT, Holman RL. Bilateral nephroblastomatosis in a premature infant. J Pathol 1961;82:249–55.

50. Huser J, Grignon DJ, Ro JY, Ayala AG, Shannon RL, Papadopoulos NJ. Adult Wilms tumor: a clinicopathologic study of 11 cases. Mod Pathol 1990;3:321–6.

51. Johnston MA, Carachi R, Lindop GB, Leckie B. Inactive renin levels in recurrent nephroblastoma. J Pediatr Surg 1991;26:613–4.

52. Koufos A, Grundy P, Morgan K, et al. Familial Wiedemann-Beckwith syndrome and a second Wilms tumor locus both map to 11p15.5. Am J Hum Genet 1989;44:711–9.

53. Lawler W, Marsden HB, Palmer MK. Wilms' tumor: histologic variation and prognosis. Cancer 1975;36:1122–6.

54. Layfield LJ, Ritchie AW, Ehrlich R. The relationship of deoxyribonucleic acid content to conventional prognostic factors in Wilms tumor. J Urol 1989;142:1040–3.

55. Li FP, Gimbrere K, Gelber RD, et al. Outcome of pregnancy in survivors of Wilms' tumor. JAMA 1987; 257:216–9.

56. Llombart-Bosch A, Pedro-Olaya A, Cerda-Nicolas M. Presence of ganglion cells in Wilms' tumors: a review of the possible neuroepithelial origin of nephroblastoma. Histopathology 1980;4:321–30.

57. Longaker MT, Adzick NS, Sadigh D, et al. Hyaluronic acid-stimulating activity in the pathophysiology of Wilms' tumors. JNCI 1990;82:135–9.

58. Machin GA. Persistent renal blastema (nephroblastomatosis) as a frequent precursor of Wilms' tumor: a pathological and clinical review. Part 1. Nephroblastomatosis in context of embryology and genetics. Am J Pediatr Hematol Oncol 1980;2:165–72.

59. Magee F, Mah RG, Taylor GP, Dimmick JE. Neural differentiation in Wilms' tumor. Hum Pathol 1987; 18:33–7.

60. Mahoney JP, Saffos RO. Fetal rhabdomyomatous nephroblastoma with a renal pelvic mass simulating sarcoma botryoides. Am J Surg Pathol 1981;5:297–306.

61. Masson P. Le constituent nerveux des tumeurs de Wilms. Ann Pathol 1957;2:133–49.

62. Matsunaga E. Genetics of Wilms' tumor. Hum Genet 1981;57:231–46.

63. Maw MA, Grundy PE, Millow LJ, et al. A third Wilms' tumor locus on chromosome 16q. Cancer Res 1992; 52:3094–8.

64. Mierau GW, Beckwith JB, Weeks DA. Ultrastructure and histogenesis of the renal tumors of childhood: an overview. Ultrastruct Pathol 1987;11:313–33.

65. Murphy GP, Mirand EA, Johnston GS, Gibbons RP, Jones RL, Scott WW. Erythropoietin release associated with Wilms' tumor. Johns Hopkins Med J 1967;120:26–32.

66. Oppedal BR, Glomstein A, Zetterberg A. Feulgen DNA values in Wilms' tumour in relation to prognosis. Pathol Res Pract 1988;183:756–60.

67. Orlowski JP, Levin HS, Dyment PG. Intrascrotal Wilms' tumor developing in a heterotopic anlage of probable mesonephric origin. J Pediatr Surg 1980;15:679–82.

68. Pal N, Wadey RB, Buckle B, Yeomans E, Pritchard J, Cowell JK. Preferential loss of maternal alleles in sporadic Wilms' tumour. Oncogene 1990;5:1665–8.

69. Pochedly C, Baum ES, eds. Wilms' tumor. Clinical and biological manifestations. New York: Elsevier, 1984.

70. Posalaky Z, Drake RM, Mawk JR, et al. Ectopic immature renal tissue over the dorsum of lumbar and sacral area in two infants. Pediatrics 1982;69:336–9.

71. Riccardi VM, Sujansky E, Smith AC, Francke U. Chromosomal imbalance in the aniridia-Wilms' tumor association: 11p interstitial deletion. Pediatrics 1978;61:604–10.

72. Sawyer JR, Tryka AF, Lewis JM. A novel reciprocal chromosome translocation t(11:22)(p13;q12) in an intraabdominal desmoplastic small round-cell tumor. Am J Surg Pathol 1992;16:411–6.

73. Schmidt D. Nephroblastome (Wilms-tumoren) und Nephroblastom-Sondervarianten. Pathologie, Klassifikation, differential Diagnose. Stuttgart: Gustav Fischer Verlag, 1989.

74. Sheng WW, Soukup S, Bove K, Gotwals G, Lampkin B. Chromosome analysis of 31 Wilms' tumors. Cancer Res 1990;50:2786–93.

75. Sotelo-Avila C. Nephroblastoma and other pediatric renal cancers. In: Eble JN, ed. Tumors and tumor-like conditions of the kidneys and ureters. New York: Churchill Livingstone, 1990:71–121.

76. Stern M, Longaker MT, Adzick NS, Harrison MR, Stern R. Hyaluronidase levels in urine from Wilms' tumor patients. JNCI 1991;83:1569–74.

77. Tsuchida Y, Mochida Y, Kamii Y, et al. Determination of plasma total renin level by RIA with a monoclonal antibody: value as a marker for nephroblastoma. J Pediatr Surg 1990;25:1092–4.

78. Variend S, Spincer RD, Mackinnon AE. Teratoid Wilms' tumor. Cancer 1984;53:1936–42.

79. Wakely PE Jr, Sprague RI, Kornstein MJ. Extrarenal Wilms' tumor: an analysis of four cases. Hum Pathol 1989;20:691–5.

80. Webber B, Parham DM, Drake LG, Wilimas JA. Renal tumors in childhood. Pathol Annu 1992;27:191–232.

81. Weeks DA, Beckwith JB, Luckey DW. Relapse-associated variables in stage I favorable histology Wilms' tumor. A report of the National Wilms' Tumor Study. Cancer 1987;60:1204–12.

82. Wick MR, Cherwitz DL, Manivel JC, Sibley R. Immunohistochemical findings in tumors of the kidney. In: Eble JN, ed. Tumors and tumor-like conditions of the kidneys and ureters. New York: Churchill Livingstone, 1990:207–47.

83. Wigger HJ. Fetal rhabdomyomatous nephroblastoma — a variant of Wilms' tumor. Hum Pathol 1976;7:613–23.

84. Wilms M. Die Mischgeschwülste der Niere. In: Die Mischgeschwülste. Leipzig: A. Georgi, 1899:5–90.

85. Zuppan CW, Beckwith JB, Luckey DW. Anaplasia in unilateral Wilms' tumor. a report from the National Wilms' Tumor Study pathology center. Hum Pathol 1988;19:1199–209.

86. _____, Beckwith JB, Weeks DA, Luckey DW, Pringle KC. The effect of preoperative therapy on the histologic features of Wilms' tumor: an analysis of cases from the Third National Wilms' Tumor Study. Cancer 1991;68:385–94.

Cystic Nephroma and Cystic, Partially Differentiated Nephroblastoma

87. Beckwith JB, Kiviat NB. Multilocular renal cysts and cystic renal tumors. AJR Am J Roentgenol 1981; 136:435–6.

88. Joshi VV. Cystic partially differentiated nephroblastoma: an entity in the spectrum of pediatric renal neoplasia. Perspect Pediatr Pathol 1979;5:217–35.

89. _____, Beckwith JB. Multilocular cyst of the kidney (cystic nephroma) and cystic, partially differentiated nephroblastoma: terminology and criteria for diagnosis. Cancer 1989;64:466–79.

90. Shimokama T, Watanabe T. Multilocular renal cyst. Scanning and transmission electron microscopic observations. Pathol Res Pract 1989;184:255–62.

Mesoblastic Nephroma

91. Angulo JC, Lopez JI, Ereno C, Unda M, Flores N. Hydrops fetalis and congenital mesoblastic nephroma. Child Nephrol Urol 1991;11:115–6.

92. Argyle JC, Tomlinson GE, Steward D, Schneider NR. Ultrastructural, immunocytochemical, and cytogenetic characterization of a large congenital fibrosarcoma. Arch Pathol Lab Med 1992;116:972–5.

93. Barrantes JC, Toyn C, Muir KR, et al. Congenital mesoblastic nephroma: possible prognostic and management value of assessing DNA content. J Clin Pathol 1991;44:317–20.

94. Beckwith JB, Weeks DA. Congenital mesoblastic nephroma. When should we worry? [Editorial] Arch Pathol Lab Med 1986;110:98–9.

95. Bolande RP. Congenital mesoblastic nephroma of infancy. Perspect Pediatr Pathol 1973;1:227–50.

96. _____, Brough AJ, Izant RJ Jr. Congenital mesoblastic nephroma of infancy. A report of eight cases and the relationship to Wilms' tumor. Pediatrics 1967; 40:272–8.

97. Chan HS, Cheng MY, Mancer K, et al. Congenital mesoblastic nephroma: a clinicoradiologic study of 17 cases representing the pathologic spectrum of the disease. J Pediatr 1987;111:64–70.

98. Cook HT, Taylor GM, Malone P, Risdon RA. Renin in mesoblastic nephroma: an immunohistochemical study. Hum Pathol 1988;19:1347–51.

99. Favara BE, Johnson W, Ito J. Renal tumors in the neonatal period. Cancer 1968;22:845–55.

100. Ganick DJ, Gilbert EF, Beckwith JB, Kiviat N. Congenital cystic mesoblastic nephroma. Hum Pathol 1981; 12:1039–43.

101. Gonzalez-Crussi F, Sotelo-Avila C, Kidd JM. Malignant mesenchymal nephroma of infancy. Report of a case with pulmonary metastases. Am J Surg Pathol 1980;4:185–90.

102. Gormley TS, Skoog SJ, Jones RV, Maybee D. Cellular congenital mesoblastic nephroma: what are the options? J Urol 1989;142(2 Pt 2):479–83.

103. Gray ES. Mesoblastic nephroma and non-immunological hydrops fetalis. Pediatr Pathol 1989;9:607–9.

104. Howell CG, Othersen HB, Kiviat NE, Norkool P, Beckwith JB, DAngio GJ. Therapy and outcome in 51 children with mesoblastic nephroma: a report of the National Wilms' Tumor Study. J Pediatr Surg 1982; 17:826–31.

105. Joshi VV, Kaznicka J, Walters TR. Atypical mesoblastic nephroma: pathologic characterization of a potentially aggressive variant of conventional mesoblastic nephroma. Arch Pathol Lab Med 1986;110:100–6.

106. Kumar S, Marsden HB, Carr T, Kodet R. Mesoblastic nephroma contains fibronectin but lacks laminin. J Clin Pathol 1985;38:507–11.

107. Malone PS, Duffy PG, Ransley PG, Risdon RA, Cook T, Taylor M. Congenital mesoblastic nephroma, renin production, and hypertension. J Pediatr Surg 1989;24:599–600.

108. Marsden HB, Newton WA. New look at mesoblastic nephroma. J Clin Pathol 1986;39:508–13.

109. Mierau GW, Beckwith JB, Weeks DA. Ultrastructure and histogenesis of the renal tumors of childhood: an overview. Ultrastruct Pathol 1987;11:313–33.

110. Pettinato G, Manivel JC, Wick MR, Dehner LP. Classical and cellular (atypical) congenital mesoblastic nephroma. A clinicopathologic, ultrastructural, immunohistochemical, and flow cytometric study. Hum Pathol 1989;20:682–90.

111. Potter EL. Normal and abnormal development of the kidney. Chicago: Year Book Medical Publishers, 1972.

112. Schmidt D. Nephroblastome (Wilms-tumoren) und nephroblastom-sondervarianten. Pathologie, klassifikation, differential diagnose. Stuttgart: Gustav Fischer Verlag, 1989:62.

113. Shanbhogue LK, Gray E, Miller SS. Congenital mesoblastic nephroma of infancy associated with hypercalcemia. J Urol 1986;135:771–2.

114. Teyssier JR, Ferre D. Frequent clonal chromosomal changes in human non-malignant tumors. Int J Cancer 1989;44:828–32.

115. Varsa EW, McConnell TS, Dressler LG, Duncan M. Atypical congenital mesoblastic nephroma. Report of a case with karyotypic and flow cytometric analysis. Arch Pathol Lab Med 1989;113:1078–80.

116. Vido L, Carli M, Rizzoni G, et al. Congenital mesoblastic nephroma with hypercalcemia. Pathogenetic role of prostaglandins. Am J Pediatr Hematol Oncol 1986;8:149–52.

117. Wick MR, Cherwitz DL, Manivel JC, Sibley R. Immunohistochemical findings in tumors of the kidney. In: Eble JN, ed. Tumors and tumor-like conditions of the kidneys and ureters. New York: Churchill Livingstone, 1990:207–47.

118. Wigger HJ. Fetal mesenchymal hamartoma of infancy. A tumor of secondary mesenchyme. Cancer 1975;36:1002–8.

119. Wöckel W, Scheibner K, Lageman A. A variant of Wiedemann-Beckwith syndrome. Eur J Pediatr 1981;135:319–24.

120. Yokomori K, Hori T, Takemura T, Tsuchida Y. Demonstration of both primary and secondary reninism in renal tumors in children. J Pediatr Surg 1988;23:403–9.

Clear Cell Sarcoma

121. Altmannsberger M, Osborn M, Schäfer H, Shauer A, Weber K. Distinction of nephroblastomas from other childhood tumors using antibodies to intermediate filaments. Virchows Arch [Cell Pathol] 1984;45:113–24.

122. Beckwith JB, Palmer NF. Histopathology and prognosis of Wilms' tumor: results from the first National Wilms' Tumor Study. Cancer 1978;41:1937–48.

123. Drut R, Pomar M. Cytologic characteristics of clear-cell sarcoma of the kidney (CCSK) in fine-needle aspiration biopsy (FNAB): a report of four cases. Diagn Cytopathol 1991;7:611–4.

124. Haas JE, Bonadio JF, Beckwith JB. Clear cell sarcoma of the kidney with emphasis on ultrastructural studies. Cancer 1984;54:2978–87.

125. Hennigar RA, Sens DA, Spicer SS, et al. Lectin histochemistry of nephroblastoma (Wilms' tumor). Histochem J 1985;17:1091–100.

126. Kumar S, Carr T, Marsden HB, Calabuig-Crespo MC. Study of childhood renal tumours using antisera to fibronectin, laminin, and epithelial membrane antigen. J Clin Pathol 1986;39:51–7.

127. Marsden HB, Lawler W. Bone metastasizing renal tumour of childhood. Histopathological and clinical review of 38 cases. Virchows Arch [A] 1980;387:341–51.

128. _____, Lawler W, Kumar PM. Bone metastasizing renal tumor of childhood. Morphological and clinical features, and differences from Wilms' tumor. Cancer 1978;42:1922–8.

129. Mierau GW, Weeks DA, Beckwith JB. Anaplastic Wilms' tumor and other clinically aggressive childhood renal neoplasms: ultrastructural and immunocytochemical features. Ultrastruct Pathol 1989;13:225–48.

130. Morgan E, Kidd JM. Undifferentiated sarcoma of the kidney. A tumor of childhood with histopathologic and clinical characteristics distinct from Wilms' tumor. Cancer 1978;42:1916–21.

131. Novak RW, Caces JN, Johnson WW. Sarcomatous renal tumor of childhood. An electron microscopic study. Am J Clin Pathol 1980;73:622–5.

132. Punnett HH, Halligan GE, Zaeri N, Karmazin N. Translocation 10;17 in clear cell sarcoma of the kidney. A first report. Cancer Genet Cytogenet 1989;41:123–8.
133. Sandstedt BE, Delemarre JF, Harms D, Tournade MF. Sarcomatous Wilms tumour with clear cells and hyalinization. A study of 38 tumours in children from the SIOP nephroblastoma file. Histopathology 1987; 11:273–85.
134. Schmidt D. Nephroblastome (Wilms-tumoren) und nephroblastom-sondervarianten. Stuttgart: Gustav Fischer Verlag, 1989:133–8.

135. _____, Harms D, Evers KG, Bliesener JA, Beckwith JB. Bone-metastasizing renal tumor (clear cell sarcoma) of childhood with epithelioid elements. Cancer 1985;56:609–13.
136. Sotelo-Avila C, Gonzalez-Crussi F, Sadowinski S, Gooch WM III, Pena R. Clear cell sarcoma of the kidney: a clinicopathologic study of 21 patients with long-term follow-up evaluation. Hum Pathol 1985;16:1219–30.
137. Wick MR, Cherwitz DL, Manivel JC, Sibley R. Immunohistochemical findings in tumors of the kidney. In: Eble JN, ed. Tumors and tumor-like conditions of the kidneys and ureters. New York: Churchill Livingstone, 1990:207–47.

Rhabdoid Tumor

138. Akhtar M, Ali MA, Sackey K, Bakry M, Burgess A. Fine-needle aspiration biopsy diagnosis of malignant rhabdoid tumor of the kidney. Diagn Cytopathol 1991;7:36–40.
139. Beckwith JB, Palmer NF. Histopathology and prognosis of Wilms' tumor: results from the First National Wilms' Tumor Study. Cancer 1978;41:1937–48.
140. Bonnin JM, Rubinstein LJ, Palmer NF, Beckwith JB. The association of embryonal tumors originating in the kidney and in the brain. A report of seven cases. Cancer 1984;54:2137–46.
141. Biegel JA, Rorke LB, Packer RJ, Emanuel BS. Monosomy 22 in rhabdoid or atypical tumors of the brain. J Neurosurg 1990;73:710–4.
142. Chang CH, Ramirez N. Primitive neuroectodermal tumor of the brain associated with malignant rhabdoid tumor of the liver: a histologic, immunohistochemical, and electron microscopic study. Pediatr Pathol 1989;9:307–19.
143. Douglass EC, Valentine M, Rowe ST, et al. Malignant rhabdoid tumor: a highly malignant childhood tumor with minimal karyotypic changes. Genes Chromosom Cancer 1990;2:210–6.
144. Drut R. Malignant rhabdoid tumor of the kidney diagnosed by fine-needle aspiration cytology. Diagn Cytopathol 1990;6:124–6.
145. Gaffney EF, Breatnach F. Diverse immunoreactivity and metachronous ultrastructural variability in fatal primitive childhood tumor with rhabdoid features [Letter]. Arch Pathol Lab Med 1989;113:1322.
146. Gerald WL, Miller HK, Battifora H, Miettinen M, Silva EG, Rosai J. Intra-abdominal desmoplastic small round-cell tumor. Report of 19 cases of a distinctive type of high-grade polyphenotypic malignancy affecting young individuals. Am J Surg Pathol 1991;15:499–513.
147. Gonzalez-Crussi F, Goldschmidt RA, Hsueh W, Trujillo YP. Infantile sarcoma with intracytoplasmic filamentous inclusions: distinctive tumor of possible histiocytic origin. Cancer 1982;49:2365–75.
148. Haas JE, Palmer NF, Weinberg AG, Beckwith JB. Ultrastructure of malignant rhabdoid tumor of the kidney. A distinctive renal tumor of children. Hum Pathol 1981;12:646–57.
149. Lynch HT, Shurin SB, Dahms BB, Izant RJ, Lynch J, Danes BS. Paravertebral malignant rhabdoid tumor in infancy: in vitro studies of a familial tumor. Cancer 1983;52:290–6.
150. Mayes LC, Kasselberg AG, Roloff JG, Lukens JN. Hypercalcemia associated with immunoreactive parathy-

roid hormone in a malignant rhabdoid tumor of the kidney (rhabdoid Wilms' tumor). Cancer 1984;54:882–4.
151. Mierau GW, Weeks DA, Beckwith JB. Anaplastic Wilms' tumor and other clinically aggressive childhood renal neoplasms: ultrastructural and immunocytochemical features. Ultrastruct Pathol 1989;13:225–48.
152. Sawyer JR, Tryka AF, Lewis JM. A novel reciprocal chromosome translocation t(11;22)(p13;q12) in an intraabdominal desmoplastic small round-cell tumor. Am J Surg Pathol 1992;16:411–6.
153. Schmidt D, Leuschner I, Harms D, Sprenger E, Schafer HJ. Malignant rhabdoid tumor. A morphological and flow cytometric study. Pathol Res Pract 1989;184:202–10.
154. Seo IS, Min KW, Brodhecker C, Mirkin LD. Malignant renal rhabdoid tumor: immunohistochemical and ultrastructural studies. Histopathology 1988;13;657–66.
155. Sotelo-Avila C, Gonzalez-Crussi F, deMello D, et al. Renal and extrarenal rhabdoid tumors in children: a clinicopathological study of 14 patients. Semin Diagn Pathol 1986;3:151–63.
156. Takagi M, Takakuwa T, Ushigome S, Nakata K, Fujioka T, Watanabe A. Sarcomatous variants of Wilms' tumor. Immunohistochemical and ultrastructural comparison with classical Wilms' tumor. Cancer 1987;59:963–71.
157. Tsokos M, Kouraklis G, Chandra RS, Bhagavan BS, Triche TJ. Malignant rhabdoid tumor of the kidney and soft tissues: evidence for a diverse morphological and immunocytochemical phenotype. Arch Pathol Lab Med 1989;113:115–20.
158. Vogel AM, Gown AM, Caughlin J, Haas JE, Beckwith JB. Rhabdoid tumors of the kidney contain mesenchymal specific and epithelial specific intermediate filament proteins. Lab Invest 1984;50:232–8.
159. Weeks DA, Beckwith JB, Mierau GW. Rhabdoid tumor. An entity or a phenotype? Arch Pathol Lab Med 1989;113:113–4.
160. _____, Beckwith JB, Mierau GW, Luckey DW. Rhabdoid tumor of kidney: a report of 111 cases from the National Wilms' Tumor Study pathology center. Am J Surg Pathol 1989;13:439–58.
161. _____, Beckwith JB, Mierau GW, Zuppan CW. Renal neoplasms mimicking rhabdoid tumor of kidney. A report from the National Wilms' Tumor Study pathology center. Am J Surg Pathol 1991;15:1042–54.
162. Wick MR, Cherwitz DL, Manivel JC, Sibley R. Immunohistochemical findings in tumors of the kidney. In: Eble JN, ed. Tumors and tumor-like conditions of the kidneys and ureters. New York: Churchill Livingstone, 1990:207–47.

Other Renal Tumors

163. Chatten J, Cromie WJ, Duckett JW. Ossifying tumor of infantile kidney. Report of two cases. Cancer 1980; 45:609–12.

164. Dehner LP. Intrarenal teratoma occurring in infancy: report of a case with discussion of extragonadal germ cell tumors in infancy. J Pediatr Surg 1973;8:369–78.

165. Edwards O, Chatten J. Hydropic cell variant (clear cell variant) of Wilms' tumor. Arch Pathol Lab Med 1985; 109:956–8.

166. Glick AD, Leung NK, Tham KT, Wong SW. Unusual clear cell tumor of the kidney in infancy. Am J Surg Pathol 1981;5:581–5.

167. Hennigar RA, Beckwith JB. Nephrogenic adenofibroma. A novel kidney tumor of young people. Am J Surg Pathol 1992;16:325–34.

168. Jerkins GR, Callihan TR. Ossifying renal tumor of infancy. J Urol 1986;135:120–1.

169. Leuschner I, Harms D, Schmidt D. Renal cell carcinoma in children: histology, immunohistochemistry, and follow-up of 10 cases. Med Pediatr Oncol 1991; 19:33–41.

170. Pickering SP, Fletcher BD, Bryan PJ, Abramowsky CR. Renal lymphangioma: a cause of neonatal nephromegaly. Pediatr Radiol 1984;14:445–8.

Renal Cell Carcinoma and Adenoma

171. Arner O, Blanck C, Schreeb TV. Renal adenocarcinoma — grading of malignancy — prognosis. A study of 197 cases. Acta Chir Scan 1965;346(Suppl):1–51.

172. Bannasch P, Krech R, Zerban H. Morphogenese und mikromorphologie epitheliar nierentumoren bei nitrosomorpholin-vergifteten rattan. IV. Tubulära läsionen und basophile tumoren. J Cancer Res Clin Oncol 1980;98:243–65.

173. _____, Zerban H. Animal models and renal carcinogenesis. In: Eble JN, ed. Tumors and tumor like conditions of the kidneys and ureters. New York: Churchill Livingstone, 1990.

174. Bard RH, Lord B, Fromowitz F. Papillary adenocarcinoma of kidney. II. Radiographic and biologic characteristics. Urology 1982;19:16–20.

175. Bell ET. A classification of renal tumors with observations on the frequencies of various types. J Urol 1938; 39:238–43.

176. Bennington JL. Specimen of renal adenoma and carcinoma [Abstract]. Am J Surg Pathol 1981;5:194.

177. _____. Tumors of the kidney. In: Javadpour N, Barsky SH, eds. Baltimore: Williams & Wilkins, 1987: 106–37.

178. _____, Beckwith JB. Tumors of the kidney, renal pelvis and ureter. Atlas of Tumor Pathology, 2nd Series, Fascicle 12. Washington, D.C.: Armed Forces Institute of Pathology, 1975.

179. Blei CL, Hartman, DS, Friedman AC, Davis CJ Jr. Papillary renal cell carcinoma: ultrasonic/pathologic correlation. JCU J Clin Ultrasound 1982;10:429–34.

180. Boczko S, Fromowitz FB, Bard RH. Papillary adenocarcinoma of the kidney: a new perspective. Urology 1979;14:491–5.

181. Bonsib SM, Lager DJ. Chromophobe cell carcinoma: analysis of 5 cases. Am J Surg Pathol 1990;14:260–7.

182. Boring CC, Squires TS, Tong T. Cancer statistics, 1993. CA Cancer J Clin 1993;43:7–26.

183. Borowitz MJ, Weiss MA, Bossen EH, Metzgar RS. Characterization of renal neoplasms with monoclonal antibodies to leukocyte differentiation antigens. Cancer 1986;57:251–6.

184. Boxer RJ, Waisman J, Lieber MM, Mampaso FM, Skinner DG. Non-metastatic hepatic dysfunction associated with renal cell carcinoma. J Urol 1978;119:468–71.

185. Bretan PN Jr, Busch MP, Hricak H, Williams RD. Chronic renal failure: a significant risk factor in the development of acquired renal cysts and renal cell carcinoma. Case reports and review of the literature. Cancer 1986;57:1871–9.

186. Browne MK, Glashan RW. Multiple pathology in unilateral supernumerary kidney. Br J Surg 1971;58:73–6.

187. Carney JA. Wilms' tumor and renal cell carcinoma in a retroperitoneal teratoma. Cancer 1975;35:1179–83.

188. Chatelain C, Jardin A, Bitker O, Hammoudi Y. Treatment of renal cell carcinoma involving the vena cava and the right atrium. In: de Kernion JB, Pavone-Macaluso M, eds. Tumors of the kidney. Baltimore: Williams & Wilkins, 1986:98–110.

189. Christenson PJ, Craig JP, Bibro MC, O'Connell KJ. Cysts containing renal cell carcinoma in von Hippel-Lindau disease. J Urol 1982;128:798–800.

190. Chung-Park M, Ricanati E, Lankerani M, Kedia K. Acquired renal cysts and multiple renal cell and urothelial tumors. Am J Clin Pathol 1983;79:238–42.

191. Cohen AJ, Li FP, Berg S, et al. Hereditary renal-cell carcinoma associated with a chromosomal translocation. N Engl J Med 1979;301:592–5.

192. Cohen C, McCue PA, Derose PB. Histogenesis of renal cell carcinoma and renal oncocytoma. An immunohistochemical study. Cancer 1988;62:1946–51.

193. Cohnheim J. Lectures on general pathology. Handbook for practitioners and students. Translated from 2nd German ed. by McKee AB. London: New Sydenham Society, 1989.

194. Cromie WJ, Davis CJ, DeTure FA. Atypical carcinoma of kidney, possibly originating from collecting duct epithelium. Urology 1979;13:315–7.

195. Datta BN. Hyaline intracytoplasmic globules in renal carcinoma [Letter]. Arch Pathol Lab Med 1977;101:301.

196. Deitchman B, Sidhu GS. Ultrastructural study of a sarcomatoid variant of renal cell carcinoma. Cancer 1980;46:1152–7.

197. de Kernion JB. Renal tumors. In: Walsh PC, Gittes RF, Perlmutter AD, Stamey TA, eds. Campbell's urology. 5th ed. Philadelphia: WB Saunders, 1986:1053–93.

198. Dunnill MS, Millard PR, Oliver D. Acquired cystic disease of the kidneys: a hazard of long-term intermittent maintenance haemodialysis. J Clin Pathol 1977;30:868–77.

199. Ekblom P, Miettinen A, Saxén L. Induction of brush border antigens of the proximal tubule in the developing kidney. Dev Biol 1980;74:263–74.

200. Farrow GM, Harrison EG Jr, Utz DC. Sarcomas and the sarcomatoid and mixed malignant tumors of the kidney in adults — Part III. Cancer 1968;22:556–63.

201. Fisher ER, Horvat B. Comparative ultrastructural study of so-called renal adenoma and carcinoma. J Urol 1972;108:382–6.

202. Fleming S, Lewi HJ. Collecting duct carcinoma of the kidney. Histopathology 1986;10:1131–41.

203. _____, Symes CE. The distribution of cytokeratin antigens in the kidney and in renal tumors. Histopathology 1987;11:157–70.

204. Flint A, Cookingham C. Cytologic diagnosis of the papillary variant of renal-cell carcinoma. Acta Cytol 1987;31:325–9.

205. Frohmuller HG, Grups JW, Heller V. Comparative value of ultrasonography, computerized tomography, angiography and excretory urography in the staging of renal cell carcinoma. J Urol 1987;138:482–4.

206. Fuhrman SA, Lasky LC, Limas C. Prognostic significance of morphologic parameters in renal cell carcinoma. Am J Surg Pathol 1982;6:655–63.

207. Gardner KD. Acquired renal cystic disease and renal adenocarcinoma in patients on long term hemodialysis. N Engl J Med 1984;310–90.

208. Golimbu M, Joshi P, Sperber A, Tessler A, Al-Askari S, Morales P. Renal cell carcinoma: survival and prognostic factors. Urology 1986;27:291–301.

209. Gondos B. Diagnosis of tumors of the kidney: ultrastructural classification. Ann Clin Lab Sci 1981;11:308–15.

210. Gorey T, Spees EK, Sapier D. Renal malignancies are increased in transplantation candidates [Abstract]. J Urol 1984;131:230A.

211. Grawitz PA. Die sogennanten lipoma der niere. Virchows Arch Pathol Anat 1883;93:39–63.

212. Gregoire JR, Torres VE, Holley KE, Farrow GM. Renal epithelial hyperplastic and neoplastic proliferation in autosomal dominant polycystic kidney disease. Am J Kidney Dis 1987;9:27–38.

213. Hai MA, Diaz-Perez R. Atypical carcinoma of kidney originating from collecting duct epithelium. Urology 1982;19:89–92.

214. Hoehn W, Hermanek P. Invasion of veins in renal cell carcinoma — frequency, correlation and prognosis. Eur Urol 1983;9:276–80.

215. Hofstädter F, Jaksc G, Rauschmeier II, Delgado R. The value of DNA cytophotometry for the prognostic evaluation of renal adenocarcinoma. In: deKernion JB, Pavone-Macaluso M, eds. Tumors of the kidney. Baltimore: Williams & Wilkins, 1984:34–50.

216. Hosoe S, Brauch H, Latif F, et al. Localization of the von Hippel-Lindau disease gene to a small region of chromosome 3. Genomics 1990;8:634–40.

217. Jacobs SC, Berg SI, Lawson RK. Synchronous bilateral renal cell carcinoma: total surgical excision. Cancer 1980;46:2341–5.

218. Jagirdar J, Irie T, French SW, Patil J, Schwarz R, Paronetto F. Globular Mallory-like bodies in renal cell carcinoma: report of a case and review of cytoplasmic eosinophilic globules. Hum Pathol 1985;16:949–52.

219. Johnson WF. Carcinoma in a polycystic kidney. J Urol 1953;69:10–2.

220. Juul N, Torp-Pedersen S, Grnvall S, Holm HH, Koch F, Larsen S. Ultrasonically guided fine needle aspiration biopsy of renal masses. J Urol 1985;133:579–81.

221. Karstaedt N, McCullough DL, Wolfman NT, Dyer RB. Magnetic resonance imaging of the renal mass. J Urol 1986;136:566–70.

222. Kennedy S, Merino M, Linehan WM, Roberts JR, Robertson CN, Neumann RD. Collecting duct carcinoma of the kidney. Hum Pathol 1990;21:449–56.

223. Khorsand J, Ro JY, Mackay B, Ayala HG, Ordonez NG. Sarcomatoid renal cell carcinoma. An immunocytochemical and ultrastructural study of 26 cases [Abstract]. Lab Invest 1986;54:31A.

224. Kim JK, Frohnert PP, Hui YS, Barnes LD, Farrow GM, Dousa TP. Enzymes of the 3', 5'-nucleotide metabolism in human renal cortex and renal adenocarcinoma. Possible role in growth and metabolic behavior of tumor cells. Kidney Int 1977;12:172–83.

225. Kolonel LN. Association of cadmium with renal cancer. Cancer 1976;37:1782–7.

226. Kovacs G. Papillary renal cell carcinoma. A morphologic and cytogenetic study of 11 cases. Am J Pathol 1989;134:27–34.

227. _____, Szucs S, De Reise W, Baumgärtel H. Specific chromosome aberration in human renal cell carcinoma. Int J Cancer 1987;40:171–8.

228. Kumar S, Cederbaum AI, Pletka PG. Renal cell carcinoma in polycystic kidneys: case report and review of the literature. J Urol 1980;24:708–9.

229. Lack EE, Cassady JR, Sallan SE. Renal cell carcinoma in childhood and adolescence: a clinical and pathological study of 17 cases. J Urol 1985;133:822–8.

230. Landier E, Desligneres S, Debre B, Boccon-Gibod L, Steg A. Papillary renal cell carcinoma. Ann Urol (Paris) 1980;14:205–8.

231. Lang EK. Angio-computed tomography and dynamic computed tomography in staging of renal cell carcinoma. Radiology 1984;151:149–55.

232. Leary T. Crystalline ester cholesterol and adult renal tumors. Arch Pathol 1950;50:151–78.

233. Mack RA, Hussain MB, Imray TJ, Wilson RB, Cohen SM. Osteogenic and sarcomatoid differentiation of a renal cell carcinoma. Cancer 1985;56:2452–7.

234. Mancilla-Jimenez R, Stanley RJ, Blath RA. Papillary renal cell carcinoma: a clinical, radiologic, and pathologic study of 34 cases. Cancer 1976;38:2469–80.

235. Marcus PB, Kemp CB. Ectopic renal cell carcinoma: pathologist's problem. Urology 1978;12:453–7.

236. Mauro MA, Wadsworth DE, Stanley RJ, McClennan BL. Renal cell carcinoma: angiography in the CT era. AJR Am J Roentgenol 1982;139:1135–8.

237. McDonald JR, Priestly JT. Malignant tumors of the kidney — surgical and prognostic significance of tumor thrombosis of the renal vein. Surg Gynecol Obstet 1943;77:295–306.

238. McNichols DW, Segura JW, DeWeerd JH. Renal cell carcinoma: long-term survival and late recurrence. J Urol 1981;126:17–23.

239. Medeiros LJ, Gelb AB, Weiss LM. Renal cell carcinoma: prognostic significance of morphologic parameters in 121 cases. Cancer 1988;61:1639–51.

240. Moon TD, Dexter DF, Morales A. Synchronous independent primary osteosarcoma and adenocarcinoma of kidney. Urology 1983;21:608–10.

241. Murad T, Komaiko W, Oyasu R, Bauer K. Multilocular cystic renal cell carcinoma. Am J Clin Pathol 1991;95:633–7.

242. Murphy WM, Zambroni BR, Emerson LD, Moinuddin S, Lee LH. Aspiration biopsy of the kidney: simultaneous collection of cytologic and histologic specimens. Cancer 1985;56:200–5.

243. Myers GH, Fehrenbaker LG, Kelalis P. Prognostic significance of renal vein invasion by hypernephroma. J Urol 1968;100:420–3.

244. Pathak S, Strong LC, Ferrell RE, Trindade A. Familial renal cell carcinoma with a 3:11 chromosome translocation limited to tumor cells. Science 1982;217:939–41.

245. Pilotti S, Rilke F, Alasio L, Garbagnati F. The role of fine needle aspiration in the assessment of renal masses. Acta Cytol 1988;32:1–10.

246. Press GA, McClennan BL, Melson GL, Weyman PJ, Mauro MA, Lee JK. Papillary renal cell carcinoma: CT and sonographic evaluation. AJR Am J Roentgenology 1984;143:1005–9.

247. Presti JC, Rao PH, Chen Q, et al. Histopathological, cytogenetic and molecular characterization of renal cortical tumors. Cancer Res 1991;1544–52.

248. Rainwater LM, Hosaka Y, Farrow GM, Lieber MM. Well differentiated clear cell renal carcinoma. Significance of nuclear deoxyribonucleic acid patterns studied by flow cytometry. J Urol 1987;137:15–20.

249. Reddy ER. Bilateral renal cell carcinoma — unusual occurrence in three members of one family. Br J Radiol 1981;54:8–11.

250. Ro JY, Ayala AG, Sella A, Samuels ML, Swanson DA. Sarcomatoid renal cell carcinoma: clinicopathologic. A study of 42 cases. Cancer 1987;59:516–26.

251. Robson CJ, Churchill BM, Anderson W. The results of radical nephrectomy for renal cell carcinoma. J Urol 1969;101:297–301.

252. Siminovitch JP, Montie JE, Straffon RA. Lymphadenectomy in renal adenocarcinoma. J Urol 1982;127:1090–1.

253. Solomon D, Schwartz A. Renal pathology in von Hippel-Lindau disease. Hum Pathol 1988;19:1072–9.

254. Störkel S, Steart PV, Drenckhahn D, Thoenes W. The human chromophobe cell renal carcinoma: its probable relation to intercalated cells of the collecting duct. Virchows Arch [Cell Pathol] 1989;56:237–45.

255. Syrjänen K, Hjelt L. Grading of human renal adenocarcinoma. Scand J Urol Nephrol 1978;12:49–55.

256. Thoenes W, Störkel S, Rumpelt HJ. Human chromophobe cell renal carcinoma. Virchows Arch [Cell Pathol] 1985;48:207–17.

257. _____, Störkel S, Rumpelt HJ, Moll R, Baum HP, Werner S. Chromophobe cell renal carcinoma and its variants—a report on 32 cases. J Pathol 1988;155:277–87.

258. Tomera KM, Farrow GM, Lieber MM. Sarcomatoid renal carcinoma. J Urol 1983;130:657–9.

259. Travis WD, Banks PM, Unni KK, Farrow GM. Sarcomatoid renal cell carcinoma: an immunohistochemical study of 15 cases (poster). Am Soc Clin Pathol, April 19-24, Washington, D.C., 1986.

260. Ulrich W, Horvat R, Krisch K. Lectin histochemistry of kidney tumours and its pathomorphological relevance. Histopathology 1985;9:1037–50.

261. Wenz W. Tumors of the kidney following retrograde pyelography with colloidal thorium dioxide. Ann NY Acad Sci 1967;145:806–10.

262. Wick MR, Cherwitz DL, Manivel JC, Sibley R. Immunohistochemical findings in tumors of the kidney. In: Eble JN, ed. Tumors and tumor-like conditions of the kidneys and ureters. New York: Churchill Livingstone, 1990:207–47.

263. Yoshida MA, Ohyashiki K, Ochi H, et al. Cytogenetic studies of tumor tissue from patients with nonfamilial renal cell carcinoma. Cancer Res 1986;46(4 Pt 2):2139–47.

264. Yoshida SO, Imam A, Olson CA, Taylor CR. Proximal renal tubular surface membrane antigens identified in primary and metastatic renal cell carcinomas. Arch Pathol Lab Med 1986;110:825–32.

265. Zbar B, Brauch H, Talmadge C, Linehan M. Loss of alleles of loci on the short arm of chromosome 3 in renal cell carcinoma. Nature 1987;327:721–4.

266. Zincke H, Swanson SK. Bilateral renal cell carcinoma: influence of synchronous and asynchronous occurrence on patient survival. J Urol 1982;128:913–5.

Oncocytoma

267. Akhtar M, Kott E. Oncocytoma of kidney. Urology 1979;14:397–400.

268. Alanen KA, Ekfors TO, Lipasti JA, Nurmi MJ. Renal oncocytoma: the incidence of 18 surgical and 12 autopsy cases. Histopathology 1984;8:731–7.

269. Ambos MA, Bosniak MA, Valensi QJ, Madayag MA, Lefleur RS. Angiographic patterns in renal oncocytomas. Radiology 1978;129:615–22.

270. Barnes CA, Beckman EN. Renal oncocytoma and its congeners. Am J Clin Pathol 1983;79:312–8.

271. Bennington JL, Mayall BH. DNA cytometry on four-micrometer sections of paraffin-embedded human renal adenocarcinomas and adenomas. Cytometry 1983;4:31–9.

272. Cohan RH, Dunnick NR, Degesys GF, Korobkin M. Computed tomography of renal oncocytoma. J Comp Assist Tomogr 1984;8:284–7.

273. Cohen C, McCue PA, Derose PB. Histogenesis of renal cell carcinoma and renal oncocytoma. An immunohistochemical study. Cancer 1988;62:1946–51.

274. Davis CJ, Mostofi FK, Sesterhenn IA, Ho CK. Renal oncocytoma. Clinicopathologic study of 166 patients. J Urogen Pathol 1991;112:805–8.

275. Eble JN, Hull MT. Morphologic features of renal oncocytoma: a light and electron microscopic study. Hum Pathol 1984;15:1054–61.

276. _____, Sledge G. Cellular deoxyribonucleic acid content of renal oncocytomas: flow cytometric analysis of paraffin-embedded tissues from eight tumors. J Urol 1986;136:522–4.

277. Hamperl H. Beitrage zur normalen and pathologischen histologie menschlicher speicheldrüsen. Z Mikrosk Anat Forsch 1931;27:1–55.

278. Jaffe RH. Adenolymphoma (onkocytoma) of the parotid gland. Am J Cancer 1932;16:1415–23.

279. Klein MJ, Valensi QJ. Proximal tubular adenomas of the kidney with so-called oncocytic features: a clinicopathologic study of 13 cases of a rarely reported neoplasm. Cancer 1976;38:906–14.

280. Kovacs G, Welter C, Wilkens L, Blin N, Deriese W. Renal oncocytoma. A phenotypic and genotypic entity of renal parenchymal tumors. Am J Pathol 1989;134:967–71.

281. Lewi HJ, Alexander CA, Fleming S. Renal oncocytoma. Br J Urol 1986;58:12–5.

282. Lieber MM, Hosaka Y, Tsukamato T. Renal oncocytoma. World J Urol 1987;5:71–9.

283. _____, Tomera KM, Farrow GM. Renal oncocytoma. J Urol 1981;125:481–5.

284. Moura AC, Nascimento AG. Renal oncocytoma: report of a case with unusual presentation. J Urol 1982;127:311–3.

285. Psihramis KE, Dal Cin P, Dretler SP, Prout GR Jr, Sandberg AA. Further evidence that renal oncocytoma has malignant potential. J Urol 1988;139:585–7.

286. Rainwater LM, Farrow GM, Lieber MM. Flow cytometry of renal oncocytoma: common occurrence of deoxyribonucleic acid polyploidy and aneuploidy. J Urol 1986;135:1167–71.

287. Rodriguez CA, Buskop A, Johnson J, Fromowitz F, Koss LG. Renal oncocytoma: preoperative diagnosis by aspiration biopsy. Acta Cytol 1980;24:355–9.

288. Syrjänen K, Hjelt L. Ultrastructural characteristics of human renal cell carcinoma in relation to the light microscopic grading. Scand J Urol Nephrol 1978;12:57–65.

289. Thoenes W, Störkel S, Rumpelt HJ, Moll R, Baum HP, Werner S. Chromophobe cell renal carcinoma and its variants—a report on 32 cases. J Pathol 1988;155:277–87.

290. Tremblay G. The oncocytes. Methods Achiev Exp Pathol 1969;4:121–40.

291. Walter TA, Pennington RD, Decker HJ, Sandberg AA. Translocation t(9;11)(p23;q12): a primary chromosomal change in renal oncocytoma. J Urol 1989;142:117–9.

292. Waters DJ, Holt SA, Andres DF. Unilateral simultaneous renal angiomyolipoma and oncocytoma. J Urol 1986;135:568–70.

293. Weiner SN, Bernstein RG. Renal oncocytoma: angiographic features of two cases. Radiology 1977; 125:633–5.

294. Woodard BH, Tannenbaum SI, Mossler JA. Multicentric renal oncocytoma. J Urol 1981;126:247–8.

295. Zippel L. Zur kenntnis der onkocyten. Virchows Arch Pathol Anat 1942;308:360–82.

Rare Tumors with Epithelial or Renal Parenchymal Differentiation

296. Aaronson IA, Sinclair-Smith C. Multiple cystic teratomas of the kidney [Letter]. Arch Pathol Lab Med 1980; 104:614.

297. Barajas L. The development and ultrastructure of the juxtaglomerular cell granule. J Ultrastruct Res 1966; 15:400–13.

298. Biava CG, West M. Fine structure of normal human juxtaglomerular cells. II. Specific and nonspecific cytoplasmic granules. Am J Pathol 1966;49:955–79.

299. Byrd RL, Evans AE, D'Angio GJ. Adult Wilms' tumor: effect of combined therapy on survival. J Urol 1982; 127:648–51.

300. Capella C, Eusebi V, Rosai J. Primary oat cell carcinoma of the kidney. Am J Surg Pathol 1984;8:855–61.

301. Castillo OA, Boyle ET Jr, Kramer SA. Multilocular cysts of the kidney: a study of 29 patients and a review of the literature. Urology 1991;37:156–62.

302. Davila RM, Kissane JM, Crouch EC. Multilocular renal cyst. Immunohistochemical and lectin-binding study. Am J Surg Pathol 1992;16:508–14.

303. Dunnick NR, Hartman DS, Ford KK, Davis CJ Jr, Amis ES Jr. The radiology of juxtaglomerular cell tumors. Radiology 1983;147:321–6.

304. Eble JN. Unusual renal tumors and tumor-like conditions. In: Eble JN, ed. Tumors and tumor-like conditions of the kidneys and ureters. New York: Churchill Livingstone, 1990:145–76.

305. Essenfeld H, Manivel JC, Benedetto P, Albores-Saavedra J. Small cell carcinoma of the renal pelvis: a clinicopathologic, morphologic and histochemical study of 2 cases. J Urol 1991;144:344–7.

306. Farrow GM, Harrison EG Jr, Utz DC. Sarcomas and sarcomatoid and mixed malignant tumors of the kidney in adults—Part III. Cancer 1968;22:556–63.

307. Fetissof F, Benatre A, DuBois MP, Lanson Y, Arbeille-Brassart B, Jobard P. Carcinoid tumor occurring in a teratoid malformation of the kidney: an immunohistochemical study. Cancer 1984;54:2305–8.

308. Gleeson MH, Bloom SR, Polak JM, Henry K, Dowling RH. Endocrine tumor in kidney affecting small bowel structure, motility, and absorptive function. Gut 1971;12:773–82.

309. Goldblum JR, Lloyd RV. Primary renal carcinoid. Case report and literature review. Arch Pathol Lab Med 1993;117:855–8.

310. Grignon DJ, Ro JY, Ayala AG. Mesenchymal tumors of the kidney. In: Eble JN, ed. Tumors and tumor-like conditions of the kidneys and ureters. New York: Churchill Livingstone, 1990:123–44.

311. Hamilton I, Reis L, Bilimoria S, Long RG. A renal lipoma. Br Med J 1980;281:1323–4.

312. Hannah J, Lippe B, Lai-Goldman M, Bhuta S. Oncocytic carcinoid tumor of the kidney associated with periodic Cushing's syndrome. Cancer 1988;61:2136–40.

313. Kilton L, Matthews MJ, Cohen MH. Adult Wilms' tumor: a report of prolonged survival and review of literature. J Urol 1980;124:1–5

314. Kojiro M, Ohishi H, Isobe H. Carcinoid tumor occurring in a cystic teratoma of the kidney: a case report. Cancer 1976;38:1636–40.

315. Madewell JE, Goldman SM, Davis CJ Jr, Hartman DS, Feigin DS, Lichtenstein JE. Multilocular cystic nephroma: a radiographic-pathologic correlation of 58 patients. Radiology 1983;146:309–21.

316. Mills SE, Weiss MA, Swanson PE, Wick MR. Small cell undifferentiated carcinoma of the renal pelvis. A light microscopic immunocytochemical and ultrastructural study. Am J Surg Pathol 1988;1:83–8.

317. Resnick ME, Unterberger H, McLoughlin PT. Renal carcinoid producing the carcinoid syndrome. Med Times 1966;94:895–6.

318. Robertson PW, Klidjian A, Harding LK, Walters G, Lee MR, Robb-Smith AH. Hypertension due to a renin-secreting renal tumor. Am J Med 1967;43:963–76.

319. Squires JP, Ulbright TM, DeSchryver-Kecskemeti K, Engleman W. Juxtaglomerular cell tumor of the kidney. Cancer 1984;53:516–23.

320. Têtu B, Ro JY, Ayala AG, Ordonez NG, Johnson DE. Small cell carcinoma of the kidney. A clinicopathologic, immunohistochemical and ultrastructural study. Cancer 1987;60:1809–14.

321. Unger PD, Russell A, Thung SN, Gordon RE. Primary renal carcinoid. Arch Pathol Lab Med 1990;114:68–71.

Medullary Fibroma (Renomedullary Interstitial Cell Tumor)

322. Glover SD, Buck AC. Renal medullary fibroma: a case report. J Urol 1982;127:758–60.

323. Lerman RJ, Pitcock JA, Stephenson P, Muirhead EE. Renomedullary interstitial cell tumor (formerly fibroma of the renal medulla). Hum Pathol 1972;3:559–68.

324. Mandal AK. The renal papilla and hypertension. An up-to-date review. Pathol Annu 1981;16(Pt 2):295–313.

325. Stuart R, Salyer WR, Salyer DC, Heptinstall RH. Renomedullary interstitial cell lesions and hypertension. Hum Pathol 1976;7:327–32.

326. Warfel KA, Eble JN. Renomedullary interstitial cell tumors [Abstract]. Am J Clin Pathol 1985;83:262.

Leiomyoma

327. Clinton-Thomas CL. A giant leiomyoma of the kidney. Br J Surg 1956;43:497–501.
328. Fisher KS, van Blerk PJ. Childhood leiomyoma of kidney. Urology 1983;21:74–5.
329. Petersen RO. Urologic pathology. Philadelphia: JB Lippincott, 1986:121.

Lipoma

330. Dineen MK, Venable DD, Misra RP. Pure intrarenal lipoma—report of a case and review of the literature. J Urol 1984;132:104–7.
331. Xipell JM. Incidence of benign renal nodules (a clinicopathologic study). J Urol 1971;106:503–6.

Hemangioma - Lymphangioma

332. Garcia MM, Tello DM, Junquera SR, Uria GV, Aguire FR, Fernandez de Retana JO. Multiple cavernous hemangiomas of the kidney. Eur Urol 1988;14:90–2.
333. Grignon DJ, Ro JY, Ayala AG. Mesenchymal tumors of the kidney. In: Eble JN, ed. Tumors and tumor-like conditions of the kidneys and ureters. New York: Churchill Livingstone, 1990:123–44.
334. Joost J, Schaefer R, Altwein JE. Renal lymphangioma. J Urol 1977;118(1 Pt 1):22–4.
335. Pickering SP, Fletcher BD, Bryan PJ, Abramowsky CR. Renal lymphangioma: a cause of neonatal nephromegaly. Pediatr Radiol 1984;14:445–8.
336. Schofield D, Zaatari GS, Gay BB. Klippel-Trenaunay and Sturge-Weber syndromes with renal hemangioma and double inferior vena cava. J Urol 1986;136:442–5.
337. Singer DR, Miller JD, Smith G. Lymphangioma of kidney. Scott Med J 1983;28:293–4.

Mesoblastic Nephroma in Adults

338. Bitter JJ, Harrison DA, Kaplan J, Irwin GA. Mesoblastic nephroma. J Comput Assist Tomogr 1982;6:180–3.
339. Block NL, Grabstald HG, Melamed MR. Congenital mesoblastic nephroma (leiomyomatous hamartoma): first adult case. J Urol 1973;110:380–3.
340. Durham JR, Bostwick DG, Farrow GM, Ohorodnik JM. Mesoblastic nephroma of adulthood. Report of three cases. Am J Surg Pathol 1993;10:1029–38.
341. Levin NP, Damjanov I, Depillis VJ. Mesoblastic nephroma in an adult patient. Recurrence 21 years after removal of the primary lesion. Cancer 1982;49:573–7.
342. Lopez JP, Redorta JP, Robles JM, Perez EM, Marcellan CR. Leiomyomatous renal hamartoma in an adult. Eur Urol 1988;14:80–2.
343. Trillo AA. Adult variant of congenital mesoblastic nephroma. Arch Pathol Lab Med 1990;114:533–5.
344. Van Velden DJ, Schneider JW, Allen FJ. A case of adult mesoblastic nephroma: ultrastructure and discussion of histogenesis. J Urol 1990;143:1216–9.

Sarcomas

345. Asa SL, Bedard YC, Buckspan MB, Klotz PG, Bain J, Steinhardt MI. Spontaneous hypoglycemia associated with hemangiopericytoma of the kidney. J Urol 1981;125:864–7.
346. Cano JY, D'Altorio RA. Renal liposarcoma: case report. J Urol 1976;115:747–9.
347. Cason JD, Waisman J, Plaine L. Angiosarcoma of kidney. Urology 1987;30:281–3.
348. Cavaliere A, Fratini D, Legittimo C, Tosi F, Lolli E. Renal fibrosarcoma: single case in a ten-year survey. Pathologica 1984;76:615–21.
349. Chatterjee D, Powell A. Renal hemangioendothelioma. Int Surg 1982;67:373–5.
350. Farrow GM, Harrison EG Jr, Utz DC, ReMine WH. Sarcomas and sarcomatoid and mixed malignant tumors of the kidney in adults—Part I. Cancer 1968;22:545–50.
351. Grignon DJ, Ro JY, Ayala AG. Mesenchymal tumors of the kidneys. In: Eble JN, ed. Tumors and tumor-like conditions of the kidneys and ureters. New York: Churchill-Livingstone, 1990:123–44.
352. Kollias G, Giannopoulos T. Primary malignant fibrous histiocytoma of the kidney: report of a case. J Urol 1987;138:400–1.
353. Mayes DC, Fechner RE, Gillenwater JY. Renal liposarcoma. Am J Surg Pathol 1990;14:268–73.
354. Mortensen PH. Primary osteogenic sarcoma of the kidney. Br J Urol 1989;63:101–2.
355. Siniluoto TM, Päivänsalo MJ, Hellström PA, Leinonen AS, Kyllonen AP. Hemangiopericytoma of the kidney: a case with preoperative ethanol embolization. J Urol 1988;140:137–8.
356. Srinivas V, Sogani PC, Hajdu SI, Whitmore WF Jr. Sarcomas of the kidney. J Urol 1984;132:13–6.
357. Takashi M, Murase T, Kato K, Koshikawa T, Mitsuya H. Malignant fibrous histiocytoma arising from the renal capsule: report of a case. Urol Int 1987;42:227–30.
358. Terris D, Plaine L, Steinfeld A. Renal angiosarcoma. Am J Kidney Dis 1986;8:131–3.
359. Tsukamoto T, Lieber MM. Sarcomas of the kidney, urinary bladder, prostate, spermatic cord, paratestis and testis in adults. In: Raaf JH, ed. Soft tissue sarcomas: diagnosis and treatment. St. Louis: Mosby Yearbook, 1992.

Angiomyolipoma

360. Bennington JL, Beckwith JB. Tumors of the kidney, renal pelvis and ureter. Atlas of Tumor Pathology, 2nd Series, Fascicle 12. Washington, D.C.: Armed Forces Institute of Pathology, 1975.
361. Blute ML, Malek RS, Segura JW. Angiomyolipoma: clinical metamorphosis and concepts for management. J Urol 1988;139:20–4.

362. Chen KT, Bauer V. Extra-renal angiomyolipoma. J Surg Oncol 1984;25:89–91.

363. Farrow GM, Harrison EG Jr, Utz DC, Jones DR. Renal angiomyolipoma. A clinicopathologic study of 32 cases. Cancer 1968;22:564–70.

364. Ferry JA, Malt RA, Young RH. Renal angiomyolipoma with sarcomatous transformation and pulmonary metastases. Am J Surg Pathol 1991;15:1083–8.

365. Glenthøj A, Partoft S. Ultrasound-guided percutaneous aspiration of renal angiomyolipoma: report of two cases diagnosed by cytology. Acta Cytol 1984;28:265–8.

366. Goodman ZD, Ishak KG. Angiomyolipomas of the liver. Am J Surg Pathol 1984;8:745–50.

367. Hulbert JC, Graf R. Involvement of the spleen by renal angiomyolipoma: metastasis or multicentricity? J Urol 1983;130:328–9.

368. Katz DA, Thom D, Bogard P, Dermer MS. Angiomyolipoma of the fallopian tube. Am J Obstet Gynecol 1984;148:341–3.

369. Klapproth HJ, Poutasse EF, Hazard JB. Renal angiomyolipomas—report of 4 cases. Arch Pathol 1959;67:400–41.

370. Kutcher R, Rosenblatt R, Mitsudo SM, Goldman M, Kogan S. Renal angiomyolipoma with sonographic demonstration of extension into the inferior vena cava. Radiology 1982;143:755–6.

371. Lynne CM, Carrion HM, Bakshandeh K, Nadji M, Russel E, Politano VA. Renal angiomyolipoma, polycystic kidney, and renal carcinoma in a patient with tuberous sclerosis. Urology 1979;14:174–6.

372. Perez-Atayde AR, Iwaya S, Lack EE. Angiomyolipomas and polycystic renal disease in tuberous sclerosis. Ultrastructural observations. Urology 1981;17:607–10.

373. Price EB, Mostofi FK. Symptomatic angiomyolipoma of the kidney. Cancer 1965;18:761–74.

374. Silpananta P, Michel RP, Oliver JA. Simultaneous occurrence of angiomyolipoma and renal cell carcinoma. Clinical and pathologic (including ultrastructural) features. Urology 1984;23:200–4.

375. Stapleton FB, Johnson D, Kaplan GW, Griswold W. The cystic renal lesion in tuberous sclerosis. J Pediatr 1980;97:574–9.

Lymphoid Tumors

376. Farrow GM, Harrison EG Jr, Utz DC. Sarcomas and sarcomatoid and mixed malignant tumors of the kidney in adults — Part III. Cancer 1968;22:556–63.

377. Lee SC, Roth LM, Brashear RE. Lymphomatoid granulomatosis. A clinicopathologic study of four cases. Cancer 1976;38:846–53.

378. Liebow AA, Carrington CR, Friedman PJ. Lymphomatoid granulomatosis. Hum Pathol 1972;3:457–558.

379. Lipford EH, Margolick JB, Longo DL, Fauci AS, Jaffe ES. Angiocentric immuno-proliferative lesions: a clinicopathologic spectrum of post-thymic T-cell proliferations. Blood 1988;72:1674–81.

380. Martinez-Maldonado M, Ramirez de Arellano GA. Renal involvement in malignant lymphomas. A survey of 49 cases. J Urol 1966;95:485–8.

381. Nicholas PW, Koss M, Levine AM, Lukes RJ. Lymphomatoid granulomatosis: a T-cell disorder? Am J Med 1982;72:467–71.

382. Osborne BM, Brenner M, Weitzner S, Butler JJ. Malignant lymphoma presenting as a renal mass: four cases. Am J Surg Pathol 1987;11:375–82.

383. Richmond J, Sherman RS, Diamond HD, Crauer LF. Renal lesions associated with malignant lymphomas. Am J Med 1962;32:184–207.

Metastatic Tumors to the Kidneys

384. Petersen RO. Kidney: metastatic neoplasms. In: Urologic pathology. Philadelphia: JB Lippincott, 1986:134–6.

Non-neoplastic Tumorous Conditions

385. Ask-Upmark E. Uber juvenile maligne nephrosclerose und ihr verhältnis zu störungen in der nierenentwicklung. Acta Pathol Microbiol Scan 1929;6:382–442.

386. Becker JA. Xanthogranulomatous pyelonephritis. A case report with angiographic findings. Acta Radiol [Diagn] (Stockh) 1966;4:139–44.

387. Ceccarelli FE Jr, Wurster JC, Chandor SB. Xanthogranulomatous pyelonephritis in an infant. J Urol 1970;104:755–7.

388. Flynn JT, Molland EA, Paris AM, Blandy JP. The underestimated hazards of xanthogranulomatous pyelonephritis. Br J Urol 1979;51:443–4.

389. Gerber WL, Catalona WJ, Fair WR. Michigan S, Melson L. Xanthogranulomatous pyelonephritis masquerading as occult malignancy. Urology 1978;11:466–71.

390. Goodman M, Curry T, Russel T. Xanthogranulomatous pyelonephritis (XGP): a local disease with systemic manifestations. Report of 23 patients and review of the literature. Medicine (Baltimore) 1979;58:171–81.

391. Grainger RG, Longstaff AJ, Parsons MA. Xanthogranulomatous pyelonephritis: a reappraisal. Lancet 1982;1:1398–401.

392. Ljungqvist A, Lagergre C. The Ask-Upmark kidney. Acta Pathol Microbiol Scand 1962;56:277–83.

393. Malek RS, Elder JS. Xanthogranulomatous pyelonephritis: a critical analysis of 26 cases and of the literature. J Urol 1978;119:589–93.

394. Noyes WE, Palubinskas AJ. Xanthogranulomatous pyelonephritis. J Urol 1969;101:132–6.

395. Royer P, Habib R, Broyer M, Nouaille Y. Segmental hypoplasia of the kidney in children. Adv Nephrol Necker Hosp 1971;1:145–59.

396. Rubenstein M, Meyer R, Bernstein J. Congenital anomalies of the urinary system. I. A post-mortem survey of developmental anomalies and acquired lesions in a children's hospital. J Pediatr 1961;58:356–66.

397. Schlagenhaufer F. Uber eigentimliche staphylomycosen der nieren und der pararenalen bindegewehes. Frankfurt Zeitschr Pathol 1916;19:139–48.

398. Tolia BM, Iloreta A, Freed SZ, Fruchtman B, Bennett B, Newman HR. Xanthogranulomatous pyelonephritis: detailed analysis of 29 cases and a brief discussion of atypical presentations. J Urol 1981;126:437–42.

399. Vinik M, Freed TA, Smellie WA, Weidner W. Xanthogranulomatous pyelonephritis: angiographic considerations. Radiology 1969;92:537–40.

2
TUMORS OF THE URINARY BLADDER

NORMAL ANATOMY

The urinary bladder forms during the first 12 weeks of gestation as the result of three events (6). First, the trigone (base) develops by dilatation, fusion, and eventual incorporation of portions of the mesonephric ducts into the urogenital sinus, forming a triangular area that receives the terminal portions of the future ureters. The müllerian ducts are close to this area but their influence, if any, on the formation of the trigone is not known. Second, the posterior walls, dome, and portions of the lateral walls arise from mesenchyme surrounding the urogenital sinus when that space is transected by the urorectal septum. Third, the anterior wall and portions of the lateral walls develop in conjunction with closure of the infraumbilical portion of the abdominal wall. The bulk of the resulting organ is derived from tissue at the rostral portion of the urogenital sinus. Despite the embryologic continuity of the urogenital sinus with the allantois and urachus, neither of these structures is involved in the formation of the urinary bladder. The allantois is an embryonic structure lined by entoderm that connects to the urachus. It is rudimentary in humans. The urachus is formed during the descent of the anterior abdominal wall, when the rostral portion of the urogenital sinus is attenuated into a tubular structure. This tube is torn apart as the embryo elongates, but remnants persist in the anterior abdominal wall and, occasionally, in the bladder wall of the fully developed human. These remnants may be lined by various types of epithelium, most often transitional. They rarely connect directly to the adult bladder lumen. The most embryologically complicated portion of the bladder is its base, a fact that might help to explain the propensity of all types of tumors to arise in this area.

The fully developed urinary bladder is designed to store and expel urine. Anchored deep in the pelvis, the organ consists of a meshwork of thick muscle bundles surrounding a highly vascular lamina propria lined by a stratified epithelium (fig. 2-1) (10). In usual histologic preparations, the muscles of the wall (detrusor muscles) exist in rounded bundles separated by an interstitium containing scant collagen. The lamina propria is a layer of loose connective tissue which normally contains a few lymphocytes and a network of thin-walled blood vessels. Some of these vessels are so closely applied to the epithelial lining that any process that denudes or ulcerates the mucosa results in abnormal numbers of red blood cells in the urine. In well-oriented specimens, the lamina propria can sometimes be divided into inner and outer zones by a discontinuous layer of thick-walled blood vessels and wispy muscle fibers, reminiscent of a muscularis mucosae. A well-developed muscularis mucosae occurs in less than 5 percent of human urinary bladders and the practical value of recognizing this potential division of the lamina propria remains to be demonstrated (5). In contrast to the well-defined, rounded muscle fascicles of the detrusor, muscle remnants in the lamina propria are smaller, irregularly occurring fibers with fewer discrete boundaries. Correct identification of these wispy fibers is important for the accurate pathologic staging of bladder neoplasms.

The bladder is lined by multiple layers of relatively flat cells, like squamous mucosa, in which the superficial elements are large and secrete small amounts of mucin, like glandular mucosa. Perhaps for this reason, the term "transitional cell" epithelium has become deeply entrenched in the medical lexicon. A more general and preferred term for this mucosa is urothelium. Several features of the urothelium are important to an understanding of bladder neoplasia (6). Invaginated nests of urothelial cells (Brunn nests) may occur throughout the urothelium but are most common at the bladder base. Their greater frequency in adults than in newborns and late stage fetuses suggests an acquired phenomenon, perhaps as a reaction to trauma or infection. The exact number of layers in the normal human bladder urothelium is unknown but varies between three and seven, depending on the degree of bladder distension. An increase in the number of cell layers is not in

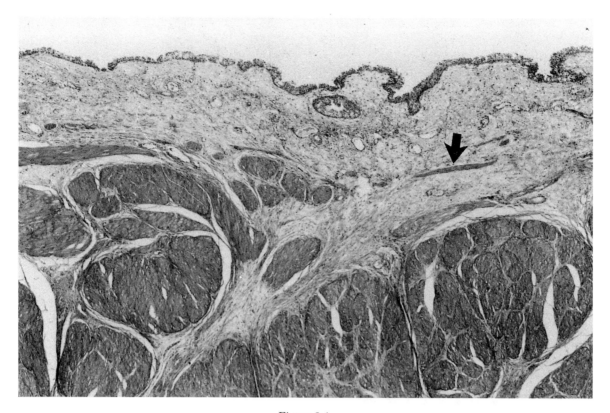

Figure 2-1
NORMAL URINARY BLADDER
Wisps of smooth muscle (arrow) occur in the lamina propria. Their configuration is different from the muscle bundles of the detrusor. A well-developed muscularis mucosae is not present in most human urinary bladders.

itself neoplastic but is considered abnormal, especially when the mucosal thickening occurs on a fibrovascular stalk. Urothelial cell proliferation is almost always accompanied by nuclear atypia so that a determination of neoplasia based solely on increased layering is rarely a problem.

Normal urothelial cells are of two distinctive types (fig. 2-2): cells of the superficial layer and the underlying intermediate and basal cells. The cells comprising all but the superficial layer are small and uniform, with well-defined borders and amphophilic cytoplasm rich in glycogen. The glycogen often dissolves in routine preparations, leaving cleared areas which have sometimes been erroneously described as vacuoles. These cells have sparse desmosomes, facilitating their ability to flatten and slide over one another during bladder distension (7). They also manifest blood group isoantigens and keratins (especially 7, 8, 18,19) of molecular weights ranging from 40 to 70 kilodaltons (2,11). Epidermal growth factor

receptors are on the surfaces of the deepest cells (9). In tissue sections, the nuclei of subsuperficial intermediate and basal cells are ovoid, with the long axis oriented at right angles to the surface. Nuclei are regularly arranged in the epithelium. They have evenly dispersed, very finely granular chromatin which accentuates the regularly contoured nuclear borders. Nucleoli are small and inapparent in tissue fixed in formalin. The normal urothelium has an estimated turnover time of approximately 1 year and it is unusual to see mitoses.

The superficial layer of urothelium is composed of a specialized group of cells that could be considered terminally differentiated. These cells are much larger than the underlying elements; this, plus their location, have suggested the term "umbrella" cells. Superficial cells tend to have acidophilic cytoplasm and store small amounts of neutral mucin but are primarily modified to maintain the integrity of the mucosa during expansion and contraction as well as to prevent

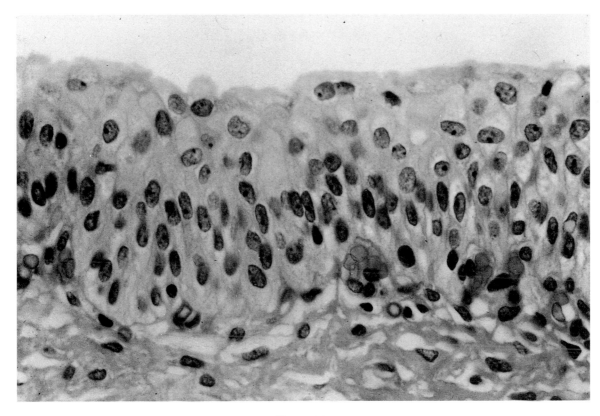

Figure 2-2
NORMAL UROTHELIUM
A single layer of large, occasionally binucleated superficial cells covers multiple layers of intermediate and basal cells. Note the even distribution and polarization of the nuclei. Fixation in Hollande solution (a picric acid–based fixative) tends to accentuate nucleoli, which would not be apparent in formalin-fixed preparations.

urine transport. These cells have a rigid surface membrane which maintains its shape after exfoliation (fig. 2-3). In young and early middle-aged individuals, the surface membrane is reinforced with plaques of asymmetric unit membrane alternating with sections of symmetric surface (7). This structure tends to break down with age and is lost early in carcinogenesis, but may reform after successful therapy. Superficial cells may manifest blood group antigens and cytokeratins but lack epidermal growth factor receptors. A few are binucleate. The nuclei are large even though the nuclear-cytoplasmic ratios are low. They have evenly dispersed chromatin, regularly contoured borders, and, often, detectable nucleoli, even in formalin-fixed specimens. As the first layer of epithelial defense, superficial cells are exposed to various noxious substances and often appear reactive. In such cases, their nuclei are enlarged and their chromatin more coarsely clumped. Nucleoli may be prominent. Mitoses are rare in superficial cells, even in situations of great stimulation. In general, the presence of superficial cells is a sign of normal maturation and differentiation. Neoplasms manifesting superficial cells are usually not aggressive.

Most current knowledge of normal urothelial cell structure and function has been gained through experimental studies using animals and tissue culture. It appears that urothelial cells incorporate certain glycoproteins into their cell membranes and communicate with their environment through surface receptors (11). Blood group antigens are the best characterized surface glycoproteins but others, such as epidermal growth factor receptors, have been documented (8,9). In some instances, the surface receptors are associated with gene products which serve as transducers. Most of these substances are glycoproteins of unknown function, recognized

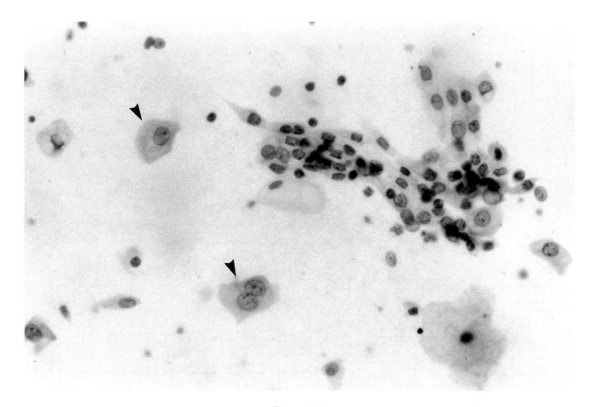

Figure 2-3
NORMAL UROTHELIAL CELLS
Superficial cells (arrows) retain their shape in urinary specimens. They are much larger and have larger nuclei than the intermediate and basal cells.

by their reactions to specific antibodies refined from extracts of tissue or urine (3). Many antigens occur in both normal and neoplastic cells. In general, the more anaplastic the cells, the more primitive is their antigenic expression. Thus, in a high-grade transitional cell carcinoma there are reduced receptors for antibodies to normal adult blood group antigens and increased expression of primitive precursors such as the Thomsen-Friedenreich antigen (1). Urine itself is rich in at least a few factors, such as epidermal growth factor, which might affect cell proliferation (4,9). These data strongly indicate that carcinogenesis in human bladders involves cellular machinery already in place.

CLASSIFICATION

The classification of urinary bladder tumors used in this atlas is presented in Table 2-1. Differences between this scheme and other formulations can be better understood in light of certain general principles. Classification systems are most profitably viewed as devices through which complex processes are separated into smaller units having commonly held characteristics. Among other goals, a classification scheme aims to lend stability and order to the study of disease and foster better communication by the use of a single set of terms. For most diseases, including bladder tumors, classification is expressed in pathologic terms based upon the morphology of tissues as viewed through the light microscope, after fixation in formalin and staining with hematoxylin and eosin (H&E). If the essential characteristics of each lesion in a classification scheme were known, the morphology remained constant over time, tumors in each category had a distinct behavior pattern, and each tumor reacted similarly to treatment, then any formulation could be readily accepted and used by all pathologists. So long as key tumor-related factors remain elusive and morphology alone cannot predict the behavior of every neoplasm in

Table 2-1
CLASSIFICATION OF URINARY BLADDER TUMORS

EPITHELIAL NEOPLASMS
    Transitional cell neoplasms
        Papilloma
            Inverted
            Exophytic
        Carcinoma
            Low grade
            High grade
        Carcinoma in situ
        Variants of transitional cell carcinoma
            Transitional cell carcinoma with gland-like
                lumina
            Transitional cell carcinoma, nested type
            Sarcomatoid carcinoma
    Squamous cell carcinoma
        Verrucous carcinoma
    Mixed carcinoma
    Adenocarcinoma
        Signet ring cell carcinoma
        Clear cell carcinoma
        Villous tumors
    Poorly differentiated carcinoma - small cell
        carcinoma
    Rare neoplasms
        Carcinosarcoma
        Carcinoid tumor
        Melanoma
        Lymphoepithelial carcinoma
        Plasmacytoid carcinoma
        Carcinoma with spindle cell stroma
        Giant cell carcinoma

NONEPITHELIAL NEOPLASMS
    Mesenchymal tumors
        Benign
        Malignant
    Pheochromocytoma (paraganglioma)
    Lymphoma
    Plasmacytoma
    Germ cell neoplasms

NON-NEOPLASTIC TUMOROUS CONDITIONS
    Condyloma acuminatum - squamous papilloma
    Metaplasia
        Squamous
        Intestinal
        Nephrogenic
    Inflammation
        Postoperative spindle cell nodule
        Inflammatory pseudotumor
            (pseudosarcomatous fibromyxoid tumor)
        Malakoplakia
        Xanthogranulomatous cystitis
        Granulomas
    "Cystitis"
        Glandularis et cystica
        Follicular
        Bullous
            Polypoid
            Fibroepithelial polyp
        Emphysematous
    Amyloidosis
    Rests, choristomas, hamartomas
        Cysts
        Endometriosis and endocervicosis
        Ectopic prostate
        Paraganglionic tissue
        Extramedullary hematopoiesis
        Hamartoma

every patient, pathologists must be prepared to alter their classifications as concepts change and to accept the fact that no system can be entirely complete.

Since bladder tumors must be at least partially removed for pathologic examination and almost all are subsequently excised completely, it is impossible to determine the natural history of large groups of lesions and classifications are devised that rely heavily upon concepts of neoplasia rather than actual observations. Thus, using the concept that disseminated carcinomas arise through an orderly sequence of increasing cellular anaplasia and recurrence is a sign of impending progression, papillary tumors of very low cytologic grade are classified according to their anticipated growth potential and called carcinomas. In contrast, using the concept that the growth potential of any particular urothelial neoplasm depends upon its degree of cellular anaplasia at the time of clinical recognition, and that recurrences per se are not a sign of impending progression, very low-grade papillary lesions are classified according to their morphology and called papillomas.

Considering the paucity of solid information, there is surprisingly little variation among classification systems for bladder neoplasms (12–19). An array of tumors are recognized, including some space-occupying, non-neoplastic lesions. With few exceptions, similar diagnostic terms are used. These terms were introduced or adapted for classification at various times, under differing theories, by different observers, with varying understanding of the language. As a result, pathologists might differ in their interpretation of the same lesion or use the same name for different tumors.

BLADDER NEOPLASIA

A detailed discussion of the historical development of terminology in bladder neoplasia is beyond the scope of this Fascicle but we can describe our concept of bladder carcinogenesis, indicate how this view affects our nomenclature, and define the use of certain terms. This might be especially important to individuals who have learned to recognize bladder tumors by names other than those used in this atlas.

The discussion is written with the view that bladder neoplasms arise through a complicated interaction between carcinogenic stimuli and host resistance; that the dynamic is continuous during the patient's life; and that the morphologic appearance of most neoplasms represents a relatively stable, though not necessarily static, relationship between opposing forces. Although exceptions may exist, neoplasms are generally characterized as lesions that do not respond normally to host mechanisms regulating their reproduction, maturation, and aging. They can be reliably recognized under the light microscope only when they acquire one or both of the following characteristics: a proliferation of cells that results in an abnormal configuration and does not spontaneously regress, and significant cellular anaplasia. Bladder neoplasms are malignant when their cells demonstrate the capacity to invade adjacent tissue or metastasize. Recognizing that neoplasia and malignancy are exceedingly difficult to define, these observations are offered as guidelines to facilitate the reader's understanding rather than as incontrovertible truths.

Bladder tumors differentiating toward normal urothelium are called transitional cell neoplasms, although terms such as epithelioma and epidermoid carcinoma have been used in the past. A significant percentage are benign in the sense that their cells have many features of normal urothelium and, once these tumors are removed, approximately 90 to 95 percent of affected patients do not develop higher grade neoplasms, invasion of the muscular wall, or metastases (31,32). Transitional cell carcinomas are divided into a small group with features of low cytologic grade and a larger group with features of high cytologic grade. Correlations among classification schemes identifying 3, 4, or 5 grades of transitional cell neoplasms are not exact (Table 2-2). In general, almost all papillomas in this atlas would be included among the grade I carcinomas in the World Health Organization (WHO) system (37). In contrast, approximately half of the high-grade tumors would be included among grade II lesions using the WHO system.

In organs lined by urothelium, only transitional cell neoplasms can be considered well differentiated. Bladder carcinomas recapitulating the epithelium of colon or skin are considered poorly differentiated regardless of how much they resemble the normal epithelium of these organs. The aggressive behavior of the majority of glandular and squamous carcinomas supports this view, although exceptions like villous adenoma and verrucous carcinoma exist. Therefore, grading of glandular and squamous cell neoplasms has not been widely accepted.

Intraepithelial lesions are not tumors in the classic sense of space-occupying masses, but many are neoplastic on clinical and cytologic grounds. The terms used for intraepithelial lesions are also influenced by the previously described concept of carcinogenesis. Carcinoma in situ (CIS) is defined as a flat, noninvasive urothelial lesion composed of cells with significant anaplasia. Such lesions include those with cellular maturation toward the surface, often termed

Table 2-2

GRADING SYSTEMS FOR TRANSITIONAL CELL NEOPLASMS*

		WHO	Bergkvist	Broders/Ash	Murphy
Papilloma	0	X	X	—	X
	1		X		
Carcinoma	1	X	–	X	
					X (low grade)
G	2	X	X	X	
R					X (high grade)
A	3	X	X	X	
D					
E	4	–	X	X	

*Histologic definitions for each grade apply within each scheme and designations of grade are not necessarily interchangeable among systems. This table is intended to provide approximate equivalents within the most common grading systems. For example, most tumors classed as carcinoma, grade I in the WHO system would be considered papillomas in Murphy and Bergkvist. In contrast, many tumors classed as grade II in WHO would be considered high grade in Murphy.

"severe dysplasia" in other systems. Intraepithelial cellular atypia of mild and moderate degrees, so-called "dysplasia" or "atypical hyperplasia," have been difficult to define in morphologic terms. Mild and moderate degrees of urothelial dysplasia may occur in bladders that never develop carcinoma and the biological nature of these lesions is highly controversial. They are probably not neoplasms according to the definition used here but no discussion of intraepithelial neoplasia would be complete without their inclusion. Intraepithelial carcinomas of squamous and glandular types have not been well defined in the urothelium and are not discussed.

A few names merely reflect common English usage. The term "metaplasia" ordinarily connotes the transition from one morphologically normal tissue to another and is not used in reference to malignant tumors (see Mixed Carcinoma). "Undifferentiated" is a somewhat misleading term when coupled with carcinoma, since the lesion in question must be differentiated to some degree or it could not be identified as a carcinoma. Malignancies classified into this category in other formulations are termed "poorly differentiated" in this atlas.

Superficial carcinoma is a term used by urologists to describe a urothelial neoplasm that has not invaded into the detrusor muscle. Used in this way, superficial carcinoma includes a variety of pathologic lesions ranging from cytologically benign transitional cell papillomas to high-grade cancers of any histologic type which have invaded the lamina propria. This designation has some clinical merit but does not describe a single pathologic entity and is not further discussed.

General Features. Bladder tumors comprise a heterogeneous group of lesions; however, since all arise in an organ of relatively simple structure and function, general statements concerning their characteristics are justified (38). Epithelial tumors comprise approximately 95 percent of all bladder neoplasms and 75 to 90 percent of these differentiate as transitional cell lesions. Among the remainder, squamous cell carcinomas comprise 2 to 15 percent; mixed carcinomas 4 to 6 percent; adenocarcinoma, less than 2 percent; and poorly differentiated carcinomas, less than 0.5 percent. Given these statistics, it is not surprising that the best studied bladder tumors are transitional cell neoplasms and most of our knowledge in this area applies to them.

The etiology of human bladder neoplasia is essentially unknown. The role of transmissible agents such as human papillomavirus is controversial (20,23). In its function as a reservoir for urine, the bladder is exposed to a complex array of chemicals, often in concentrated forms, and many experts believe that the majority of tumors result primarily from environmental factors (36). This theory is supported by increased frequency of bladder tumors in industrial areas, especially in areas associated with petrochemicals, and by the proven relationship between bladder carcinoma and exposure to both cigarette smoke and arylamines (24). Worldwide, the greatest concentration of bladder neoplasms occurs in areas infested with *Schistosoma hematobium* (30). Nitrosamines, metabolites of the nitrates commonly added to processed meats, are well-established carcinogens in laboratory rodents but their relationship to human cancer is unclear. Other environmental factors associated with an increased relative risk for human bladder tumors include benzidine, auramine, phenacetin, and cyclophosphamide (38). Certain other compounds, such as saccharin, might have a co-carcinogenic function.

Except for the arylamine class of chemicals and perhaps the calcified eggs of *S. hematobium*, a causal role for bladder cancer has not been proven for any environmental factor. Even in experimental situations, animals must be exposed to high doses over prolonged periods and the majority of resulting neoplasms do not metastasize. Current concepts of human carcinogenesis and the empirical observation that few individuals exposed to any suspected environmental factor actually develop bladder neoplasms strongly suggest that the human host has important mechanisms to defend against all phases of the process. It is likely that neoplasms in humans are not solely a function of environmental overdose but result from a combination of exposure to cancerous stimuli and defects in host resistance.

The histogenesis of epithelial neoplasia has been studied in both experimental animals and humans (38). Animal studies demonstrate that neoplasms can arise through a time-sequenced series of cellular changes of increasing degrees of anaplasia. The histologic type of tumor and its growth pattern depend upon both the species of animal and the type of chemical carcinogen, another indication of the importance of the host in the process. In contrast to humans, animals can be exposed to such large, continuous doses of chemicals that almost all develop carcinomas, a situation in which any host resistance has been artificially overcome. In experimental systems of chemical carcinogenesis, the initial epithelial changes consist of generalized hyperplasia with slight nuclear atypia (atypical hyperplasia). The epithelial cells develop in a disordered fashion which includes abnormalities of cellular arrangement and atypical nuclear changes (dysplasia) (39). The earliest point in this process at which cellular changes reflect the establishment of a neoplasm remains unknown.

Studies of bladder tumor histogenesis in humans have been largely limited to monitoring small populations exposed to chemicals in the workplace and histologic examination of the grossly normal urothelium of patients who already have neoplasms elsewhere in the bladder (28,34,35,40,41,44). Workers exposed to suspected carcinogens may develop overt bladder malignancies but have often remained free of neoplasms throughout the study period. Even those shedding malignant-looking cells into their urine may not develop clinical cancer. The cystoscopically "normal" mucosa in bladders containing papillary or nodular tumors is often abnormal when examined pathologically. This might mean that bladder neoplasms arise through a field change phenomenon wherein the entire epithelium is reactive to carcinogenic stimuli but in which lesions are developing at different rates. It is equally likely, however, that most areas of abnormal epithelium not overtly malignant at diagnosis either temporarily or permanently lack the capacity to develop into true carcinomas. Whatever thinking is correct, the evolution of bladder neoplasms from low grade and noninvasive to high grade and disseminated has been observed in only a small percentage of clinical cases.

Bladder tumors may arise via intravesical seeding of the normal mucosa by cells from an existing neoplasm. This theory is supported by laboratory studies documenting colonization of urothelium by highly anaplastic cultured tumor cells and observations in humans of an increased frequency of new tumors at the bladder dome after surgical resection (22,43). It is further substantiated by the finding of similar chromosomal aberrations in multiple coexistent bladder tumors from the same patients (42). Intravesical seeding does not account for the development of the initial neoplasm nor does it adequately explain the mechanism by which tumor cells might survive in urine with sufficient energy to invade normal epithelium and replicate. There is no convincing clinical evidence that procedures that might facilitate intravesical seeding, for example multiple surgical interventions, increase the frequency of new tumors in bladders harboring transitional cell neoplasms.

There is growing consensus that most transitional cell neoplasms can be separated into two fairly well-defined categories based upon cytologic grade (31–34). Low-grade lesions must be papillary to be recognized as neoplastic. Flat lesions of this cytologic grade have been difficult to define and nodular tumors composed entirely of low-grade neoplastic cells are essentially nonexistent. Almost all low-grade transitional cell neoplasms are DNA diploid and manifest other features of normal differentiation. They are associated with an excellent long-term prognosis. In contrast, high-grade tumors are usually nodular, but both papillary and flat lesions are easily defined and recognized. DNA aneuploidy occurs in 80 to 95 percent and most tumors lack cells with normal differentiation. Essentially all deaths related to transitional cell neoplasia occur among patients with high-grade tumors.

Bladder tumors are most reliably detected and monitored using some combination of cystoscopy, histology, and cytology (38). Measurements of total nuclear DNA using flow cytometry or image analysis are widely applied but not yet standard; they are discussed in the section, Special Techniques. All methods have limitations and none can detect the presence of bladder tumors at every point in time. They are best used in combination.

Cystoscopy is particularly beneficial for localizing bladder tumors and detecting very low-grade papillary lesions. Certain areas of the bladder mucosa are difficult to visualize and some tumors may be too small to see. Intraepithelial lesions, like CIS, cannot be reliably identified cystoscopically, and evaluation of the urothelium for cancer after topical chemotherapy is not completely reliable. Determination of

the depth of invasion and tumor grade represent further limitations to this method.

Since bladder tumors are defined in histologic terms, histology is the most accurate procedure for documenting the presence of a neoplasm during initial and follow-up examinations. Using this method, tumor type, grade, and level of invasion can be established. In addition to pitfalls associated with tissue processing and the diagnostic discrepancies attendant upon observer variation, histology is primarily limited by sampling. Cystoscopically visible tumors may not be adequately sampled and, more often, important lesions that are small, intraepithelial, or otherwise inaccessible to direct visualization may not be represented in random or selected-site biopsies.

Urinary cytology should be integrated into every detection and monitoring program (38). Randomly voided specimens without prior patient preparation are adequate, although saline lavage should be performed if the bladder is to be instrumented for other reasons. Samples can be preserved in the cold (not frozen) or in dilute alcohol solutions. Best results for evaluation of fine nuclear details are obtained with membrane filtration or cytocentrifugation with subsequent Papanicolaou staining. Using adequate preparations, almost all true bladder carcinomas, many benign papillomas, and nonepithelial neoplasms can be detected. The method is especially useful for monitoring patients after treatment with topical drugs and in cases of CIS. It also has prognostic value, since patients with positive cytology following topical therapy are at high risk for an adverse outcome. Very low-grade tumors are difficult to detect cytologically because their cells lack many of the features of malignancy. Ordinarily, urinary cytology is not useful in localizing lesions nor is it reliable for determining the depth of invasion. The disaggregated cells in urinary samples do not always accurately reflect tumor grade as observed in histologic sections (38).

Clinical Features. The clinical features of bladder tumors vary considerably in different parts of the world (45). In countries where *S. hematobium* is endemic and the most prevalent histologic type is squamous carcinoma, patients present with hematuria and symptoms of chronic irritation. Bladder carcinoma is a leading cause of cancer-related deaths (27,30). In other locations, different frequencies and environmental relationships exist. Many of the clinical characteristics discussed here can be generally applied but one should be aware that they are drawn primarily from studies in the United States. In the United States, urinary tract tumors comprise 4 to 10 percent of all cancers. Men are affected more often than women (2.7 to 1) and whites more often than blacks (2 to 1) (38). A familial predisposition has not been well documented. According to statistics from the Surveillance, Epidemiology, and End Results (SEER) databank, the incidence has been rising steadily over the last two decades and more than 50,000 new cases/year are expected (21). In contrast, the death rate has remained constant at approximately 10,000/year during this period. No racial bias has been established for survival once cancer has been documented. Urinary tract tumors account for 3 to 5 percent of cancer-related deaths in the United States. Bladder neoplasia is primarily encountered in men aged 50 to 70 years (median and mean, 64 to 68 years). With the exception of certain myosarcomas, bladder tumors are rare in children and adults less than 40 years of age. When epithelial neoplasms occur in the young, they are predominantly low-grade, noninvasive transitional cell tumors (29).

The signs and symptoms of bladder neoplasia are nonspecific (26). Patients with epithelial tumors usually experience gross or microscopic hematuria. Those with intraepithelial lesions often complain of dysuria, frequency, and suprapubic pain. Mass lesions, with or without a feeling of pelvic fullness, are associated primarily with sarcomas. The majority of bladder tumors, whether neoplastic or non-neoplastic, benign or malignant, occur at the base (trigone), a region that includes the ureteral orifices and extends into the bladder neck. At least 60 percent of primary neoplasms occur as single lesions and 72 percent of all tumors are localized to the bladder at clinical diagnosis. Based on cystoscopic estimates, over half are less than 2.5 cm in diameter (25). Fewer than 10 percent of patients present with metastases. In contrast to the location of primary tumors, so-called "recurrent" bladder neoplasms commonly occur at other sites, such as the dome (22). Most lesions arising subsequent to resection of a primary neoplasm do not occupy the exact same site and are therefore actually new occurrences.

Since almost all bladder tumors are treated soon after diagnosis, the natural history of these lesions cannot be studied. Observations of treated patients document a relationship between prognosis and histologic type. In general, nontransitional cell carcinomas tend to be progressive and are often associated with an adverse outcome. This is also true for transitional cell cancers of high cytologic grade and mixed tumors containing high-grade transitional cell components. In contrast, adverse patient outcome is unusual if the initial lesion is a transitional cell tumor of low cytologic grade, despite the tendency of these lesions to recur.

TRANSITIONAL CELL NEOPLASMS

Transitional Cell Papilloma. Transitional cell papillomas may be inverted or exophytic.

Inverted Papilloma. This is a benign tumor comprising less than 1 percent of transitional cell neoplasms (116,133). It is distinctive both grossly and microscopically (fig. 2-4). Cystoscopically, these tumors appear as solitary, raised, pedunculated or polypoid lesions with a smooth surface. Most are under 3 cm in greatest dimension but rare lesions have grown to as large as 8 cm. Histologically, cords of transitional cells appear as if a papillary lesion had invaginated into the lamina propria (69). The central portions of the cords contain maturing transitional cells and the surrounding tissue is stroma, exactly the opposite of an exophytic papilloma, where the central stroma is surrounded by the epithelial cells. Inverted papillomas grow as expansile masses and do not infiltrate the muscular wall. They rarely coexist with carcinomas. Conversely, carcinomas occasionally have intertwining invasive papillae which resemble an inverted papilloma. Cystic areas and foci of squamous metaplasia are common in inverted papillomas. Neuroendocrine differentiation has been reported (154). Occasionally, inverted papillomas exist in association with florid proliferations of Brunn nests (102). Both histologic patterns may represent host reactions to similar stimuli but their exact histogenetic relationship is unclear.

Cellular atypia is common in inverted papillomas but true anaplasia is rare. Atypical nuclear changes might result from compression of cells within tightly packed trabeculae. This theory is

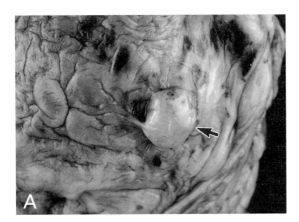

Figure 2-4
INVERTED TRANSITIONAL
CELL PAPILLOMA

A: The tumor appears grossly as a small submucosal nodule (arrow). (Courtesy of Dr. George M. Farrow, Rochester, MN.)

B: Inverted transitional cell papilloma.

C: In contrast to exophytic papilloma, the epithelial cells are oriented toward the central portions of the trabeculae, as if the fingers of a glove had been invaginated into its hand.

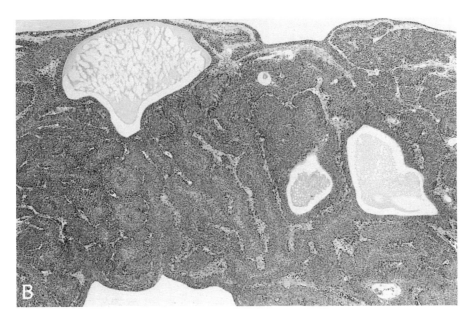

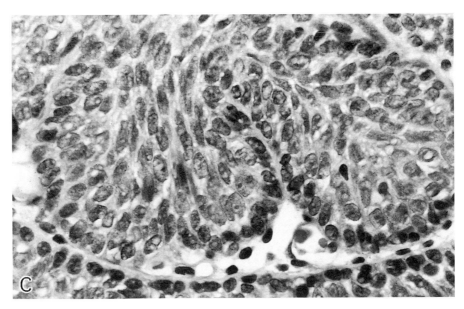

supported by cytologic studies in which features of malignancy have not been recognized among disaggregated transitional cells from bladders harboring inverted papillomas (62). The ultrastructure, antigenic composition, and DNA content of inverted papilloma cells have been noncontributory to the diagnosis and prognosis in the few evaluated cases (46).

If the diagnosis of inverted papilloma is confined to the prototype lesion discussed here, these tumors are benign. Recurrent lesions have been observed in less than 5 percent of reported cases and progression from pure inverted papilloma to carcinoma has not been documented. The temptation to expand the definition of inverted papilloma to include all polypoid lesions with predominantly subsurface growth patterns, such as florid proliferations of Brunn nests, should be resisted.

Exophytic Papilloma. This is a benign neoplasm composed of transitional cells arranged on a delicate fibrovascular stalk. Although well differentiated, the cells of these tumors are rarely completely normal in either arrangement or morphology. As defined here, exophytic papillomas comprise as much as 25 percent of transitional cell neoplasms (92). Most such tumors are classified as carcinoma in the WHO and Broders/Ash terminology but exact extrapolations among classification systems cannot be achieved and pathologists using these schemes may recognize occasional lesions as grade 1 carcinomas when they do not qualify as papillomas (Table 2-2) (51,58,114,116). In this atlas, papillomas conform closely to lesions classified as grade 0 and grade 1 tumors in the Bergkvist system (55).

Exophytic transitional cell papillomas are distinctive primarily because their cells resemble normal urothelium (106,117). Almost all have structurally normal chromosomes and diploid DNA (116,118). Normal blood group ABH antigen expression occurs in over 80 percent. Proliferative activity, as measured by mitotic and labeling indices, is in the normal range as is the expression of genes such as c-Ha-*ras* and gene products such as epidermal growth factor receptor. Papilloma cells lack significant anaplasia and are difficult to recognize in urinary samples. As defined here, they do not invade the detrusor muscle or metastasize. These tumors are considered neoplastic primarily because of their pro-

pensity to recur and their relationship to a spectrum of cellular features, the most severe of which occur in aggressive cancers.

In histologic preparations, exophytic transitional cell papillomas are composed of multiple layers of cells which retain their superficial cell layer and cover delicate fibrovascular stalks (figs. 2-5–2-7). Neoplastic cells often extend onto flat areas of urothelium adjacent to the bases of the stalks. The number of cell layers is not an important diagnostic feature, but since the tumor cells lack significant anaplasia and may rarely be completely normal by light microscopy, the characteristics of the stalk are essential for recognition of this neoplasm. The stalks of transitional cell papillomas may have dilated blood vessels, edema, or even foamy macrophages but structures with broad stalks rich in connective tissue are not papillomas.

The cells of exophytic transitional cell papillomas tend to be evenly distributed on the stalks. They have moderately distinct borders and homogeneous, amphophilic to acidophilic cytoplasm (Table 2-3). Cytoplasmic clearing is almost always reduced when compared to normal cells from the same case (fig. 2-8). Nuclei may be round or elongated and maintain their normal perpendicular orientation to the surface and basal lamina (fig. 2-9). Irregularities of nuclear borders are common and best appreciated in cytologic samples. Chromatin is evenly dispersed and finely granular. Nucleoli are small or absent. Mitoses may occur, especially in tissue fixed in picric acid–based solutions, but are not numerous.

When separated from the stalk and either exfoliated or washed into cytologic samples, the cells of transitional cell papillomas cannot always be distinguished from normal elements. The unequivocal diagnosis of neoplasia cannot usually be made and the cells have been recognized as abnormal in only 24 to 60 percent of cases (116, 137,167). In many specimens, abundant cells are the principal clue to the presence of a papilloma (fig. 2-10). Detection of these elements is best achieved with Papanicolaou preparations (Table 2-4). Recognizable neoplastic cells are larger than the normal basal and intermediate cells essentially always present in the same specimen. They may be isolated or aggregated. Tight papillary clusters occur but are not an important diagnostic feature. Cytoplasmic vacuolization is not a

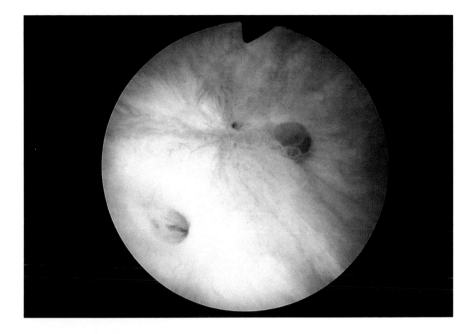

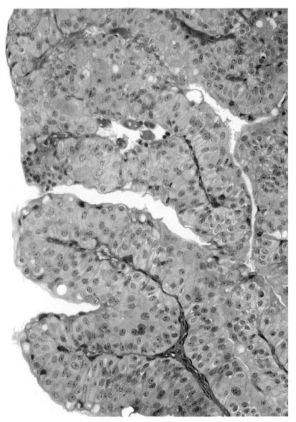 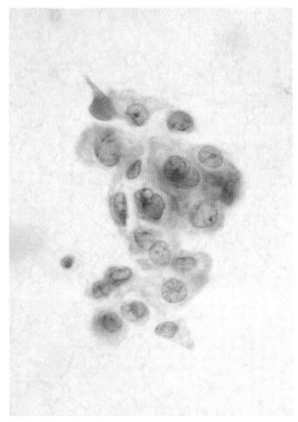

Figure 2-5
EXOPHYTIC TRANSITIONAL CELL PAPILLOMA
A: Cystoscopic photograph. (Courtesy of Dr. Mark S. Soloway, Miami, FL.)
B: Exophytic transitional cell papilloma.
C: Cytology of exophytic papilloma. The cells have large, eccentric nuclei and irregular nuclear borders. The variation in nuclear size and shape is particularly prominent in this illustration.

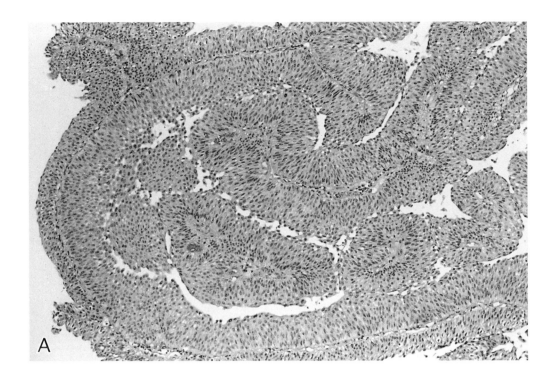

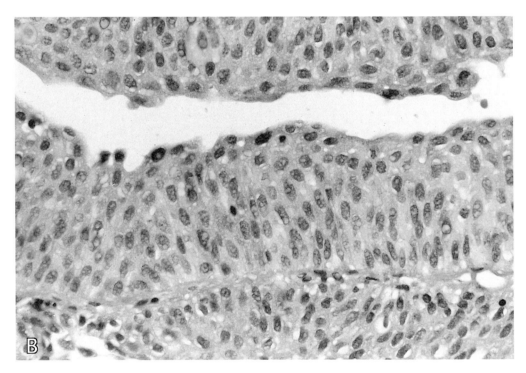

Figure 2-6
EXOPHYTIC TRANSITIONAL CELL PAPILLOMA

A: Well-oriented, uniform transitional cells arranged on delicate fibrovascular stalks. The tissue was fixed in formalin.

B: The nuclei are oriented with their long axis perpendicular to the surface and base. There is degeneration in the superficial cell layer.

C: Cells from an exophytic papilloma. Although not normal, these cells lack significant anaplastic features. This is an important clue to the nature of the neoplastic process in this patient's bladder.

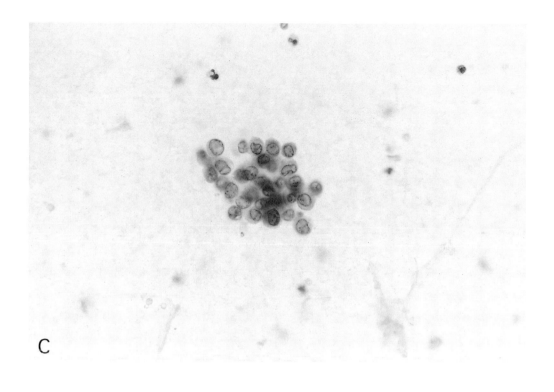

C

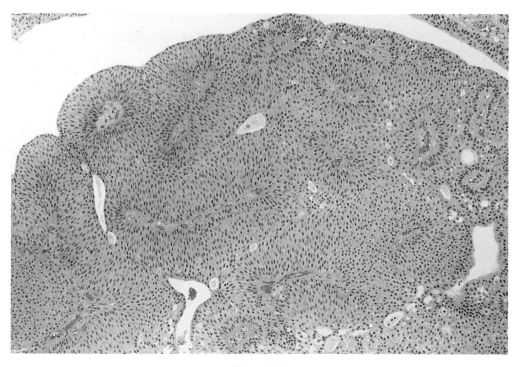

Figure 2-7
EXOPHYTIC TRANSITIONAL CELL PAPILLOMA
Short, branching papillae in this lesion give it a more nodular appearance than the tumor in figure 2-6.

Table 2-3

GUIDELINES FOR EVALUATING TRANSITIONAL CELL NEOPLASMS*

| | Configuration | | Cell Distribution | | Pleomor-phism | Nuclear Features | | |
	Papillary	Nodular	Even	Clustered		Chromatin Fine	Chromatin Coarse	Large Nucleoli
Papilloma	+++**	0	+++	0	+	+++	0	±
Carcinoma								
low grade	++	+	+++	0	+	++	±	+
high grade	+	+++	0	+++	+++	+	+++	++

*Table 4.2 from Murphy WM. Urothelial neoplasia. In: Weinstein RS, Gardner WA Jr, eds. Pathology and pathobiology of the urinary bladder and prostate. Baltimore: Williams & Wilkins, 1992:77–111.

**Key to features: 0 - absent; + - may occur sporadically; ± - occurs in some tumors but not constant; ++ - occurs in most tumors; +++ - characteristic feature which occurs in all or almost all cases.

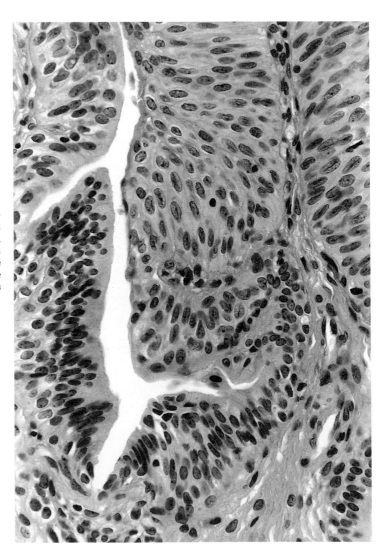

Figure 2-8
NORMAL VERSUS
NEOPLASTIC UROTHELIUM

This photograph depicts the base of a papilloma. The papilloma cells (right) are larger than the normal cells (left and base) and have larger, more irregular nuclei. Note the marked reduction in cytoplasmic clearing in the neoplastic cells. The differences in nuclear morphology illustrated here also appear in cytologic preparations. Tissue was fixed in Hollande solution.

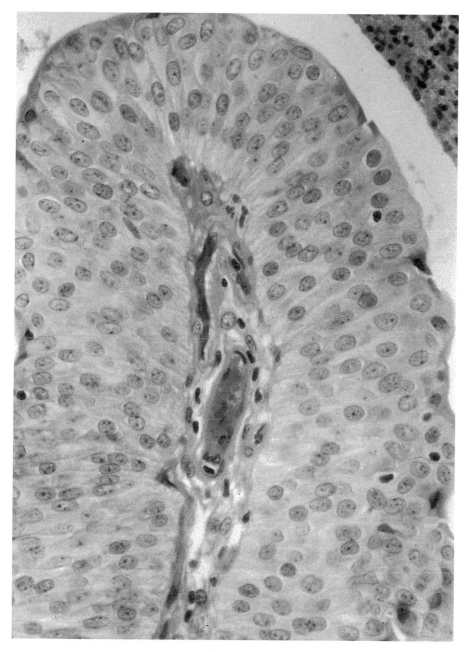

Figure 2-9
EXOPHYTIC TRANSITIONAL CELL PAPILLOMA

feature of low-grade neoplastic cells although cytoplasmic degeneration may occur. Nuclear-cytoplasmic ratios are greater than 1 to 2 and the nuclei often occupy an extremely eccentric position in the cells. Many nuclei have irregular borders. These most commonly appear as shallow depressions, notches, or creases and correlate with morphometrically calculated abnormalities expressed as the nuclear shape index. Nucleoli are inconspicuous or absent in papilloma cells. Although most often indicative of a papilloma, cells with these characteristics may occasionally be exfoliated or washed from the surfaces of low-grade carcinomas or dysplastic lesions.

Table 2-4

CELLULAR FEATURES OF UROTHELIAL NEOPLASIA*

		Low Grade	High Grade
Cells	Arrangement	Papillary and loose clusters	Isolated and loose clusters
	Size	Increased, uniform	Increased, pleomorphic
	Number	Often numerous	Variable
Cytoplasm		Homogeneous	Variable
N:C ratio**		Increased	Increased
Nuclei	Position	Eccentric	Eccentric
	Size	Enlarged	Variable
	Morphology	Variable within aggregates	Variable
	Borders	Irregular notches (creases)	Irregular
	Chromatin	Fine, even	Coarse, uneven
Nucleoli		Small, absent	Variable

*Table 2 from Murphy WM, Soloway MS, Jukkola AF, Crabtree WN, Ford KS. Urinary cytology and bladder cancer. Cancer 1984;53:1555–65.
**N:C ratio = nuclear:cytoplasmic ratio.

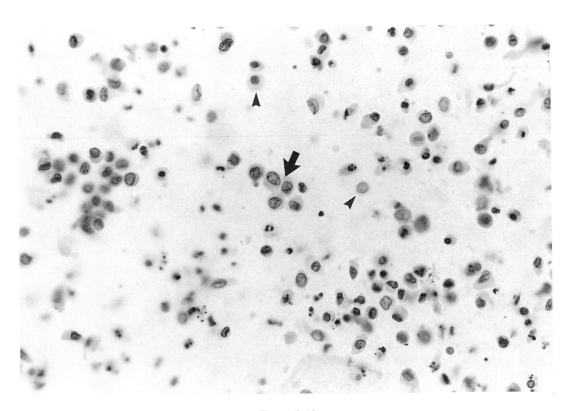

Figure 2-10

PAPILLOMA CELLS IN URINARY CYTOLOGY

Numerous atypical cells are present (arrow). They can be distinguished from cells with normal morphology (arrow heads).

Electron microscopy and immunohistochemistry have not contributed significantly to the diagnosis or prognosis of exophytic transitional cell papillomas. Antibodies that identify low-grade neoplasms are not in general use and are discussed in the section, Special Techniques.

Transitional Cell Carcinoma, Low Grade. This is a well-differentiated malignant neoplasm composed of relatively small, uniform cells arranged on a delicate fibrovascular stalk. As defined here, these tumors comprise 13 to 30 percent of transitional cell neoplasms (Table 2-2). These lesions are recognized as carcinoma in other classification schemes, some designated as grade 1 and others as grade 2a or A (51,61,114). A few have been called "atypical papilloma." They are distinctive in having a well-ordered growth pattern and cell differentiation associated with the capacity for deep invasion (92). This lesion has only recently been defined in morphologic terms and remains to be completely characterized. Data accumulated to date indicate that only 20 percent have DNA aneuploidy and 8 to 12 percent are lethal. Cells from these lesions have easily identifiable neoplastic features in cytologic preparations (61,92,118).

Histologically, all low-grade transitional cell carcinomas are predominantly papillary, but invasive components may exist. Most often, the superficial cell layer is partially preserved. Rarely, small foci of glandular and squamous differentiation occur, although these patterns are more common in high-grade transitional cell tumors. Low-grade transitional cell carcinomas have a characteristic light microscopic appearance at low magnification (figs. 2-11–2-13) (Table 2-3). The cells are uniform in size and evenly distributed but densely packed. They have indistinct borders and little or no cytoplasmic clearing. Nuclei often retain a semblance of normal orientation but are rounded and slightly pleomorphic. Nuclear borders are irregular and, as in papillomas, are more easily appreciated in cytologic preparations. Chromatin is evenly dispersed and finely granular. Large nucleoli may occupy some nuclei but are not a prominent feature of low-grade tumors. Mitoses may be numerous, especially in preparations fixed in picric acid–based solutions. They are often scattered throughout the tumor rather than concentrated in basal areas.

Neoplastic cells from low-grade transitional cell carcinomas are readily recognized by experienced observers in cytologic preparations (Table 2-4) (98,115,137). Most occur in loose clusters and have the high nuclear-cytoplasmic ratios, markedly eccentric nuclei, irregular nuclear borders, and chromatin pattern characteristic of low-grade neoplasms (figs. 2-12C, 2-13B). These features are accentuated in carcinoma cells as compared to papilloma cells, but differ more in degree than in kind. Therefore, papillomas and low-grade carcinomas cannot always be distinguished in cytologic samples. It is not uncommon for a few cells disaggregated from a low-grade carcinoma to have the coarse chromatin and large nucleoli of a high-grade neoplasm. Ultrastructural and immunohistochemical studies of low-grade transitional cell carcinomas have not yet contributed significantly to their diagnosis and prognosis.

Transitional Cell Carcinoma, High Grade. This is a moderately to poorly differentiated malignant neoplasm composed of pleomorphic cells most often arranged in nodules (fig. 2-14). In contrast to papillomas and low-grade transitional cell carcinomas, these lesions are more often multifocal and associated with separate foci of carcinoma in situ. As defined here, high-grade transitional cell carcinomas account for 50 to 60 percent of all transitional cell neoplasms and approximately 60 to 80 percent of true carcinomas (Table 2-2) (61,116). These tumors are also considered malignant in other classification systems. In the WHO terminology, they include all grade III and most of the aneuploid grade II cancers (114). In the Broders/Ash system, they encompass some grade 4 tumors (51,58). Transitional cell carcinoma, high grade is distinguished primarily by its cytologic anaplasia (116). Almost all tumors have aneuploid DNA; blood group antigen expression is absent or abnormal in approximately 90 percent; and cytologic recognition is readily achieved in most cases by even inexperienced observers.

In histologic preparations, high-grade transitional cell carcinomas are usually infiltrating neoplasms whose cells are arranged in sheets, nests, and broad cords (figs. 2-15–2-17). Papillary and flat components are common but do not usually predominate. Rarely, small portions of a low-grade papillary neoplasm are composed of high-grade carcinoma; at low magnification the

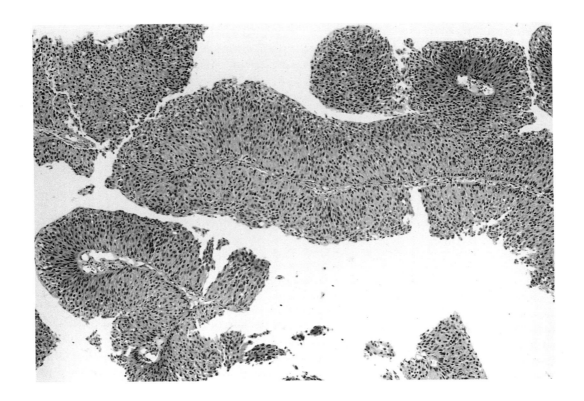

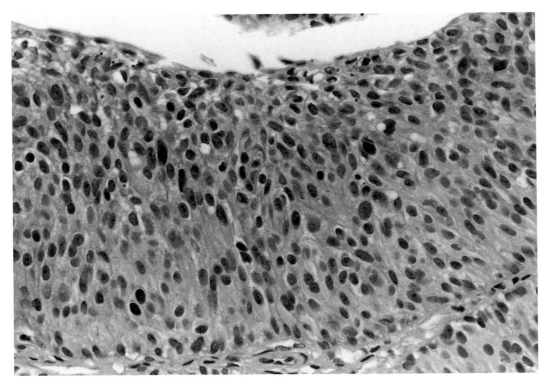

Figure 2-11
TRANSITIONAL CELL CARCINOMA, LOW GRADE
Top: These tumors are characteristically papillary. Nuclei are uniformly distributed but densely packed.
Bottom: The nuclei of this case are more irregularly shaped than those of most low-grade transitional cell carcinomas.

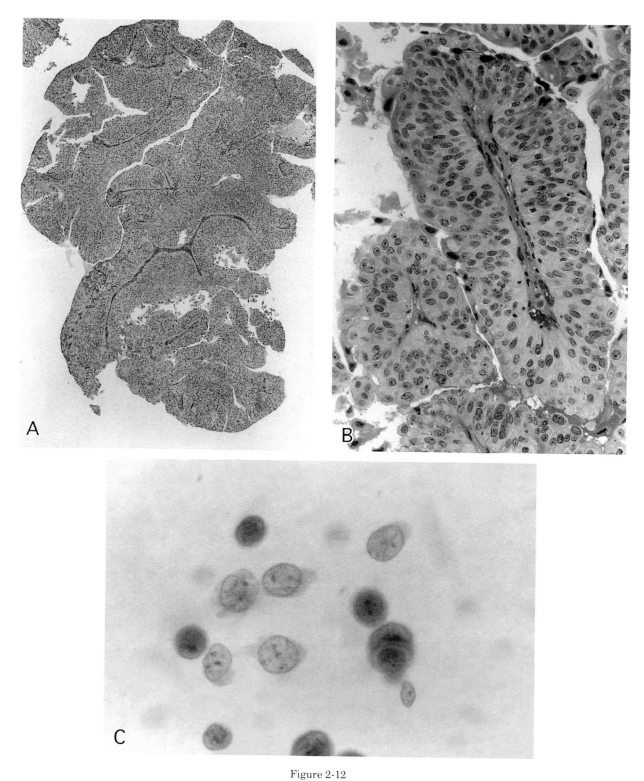

Figure 2-12
TRANSITIONAL CELL CARCINOMA, LOW GRADE
A: At low magnification, the densely packed but evenly distributed nuclei are characteristic.
B: Higher magnification of A.
C: Urinary cytology reveals neoplastic cells with high nuclear-cytoplasmic ratios and marked nuclear eccentricity as well as a characteristic chromatin pattern and irregular nuclear borders.

213

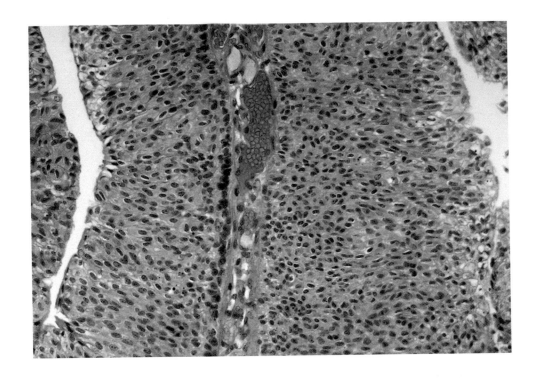

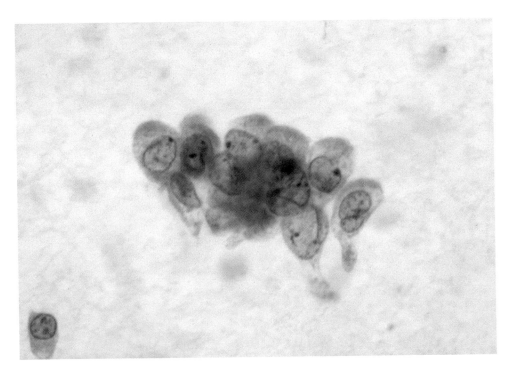

Figure 2-13
TRANSITIONAL CELL CARCINOMA, LOW GRADE
Top: Densely packed but uniformly distributed cells with small nuclei and high nuclear-cytoplasmic ratios are characteristic.
Bottom: Urinary specimen shows tumor cells in the center and a normal cell at the lower left.

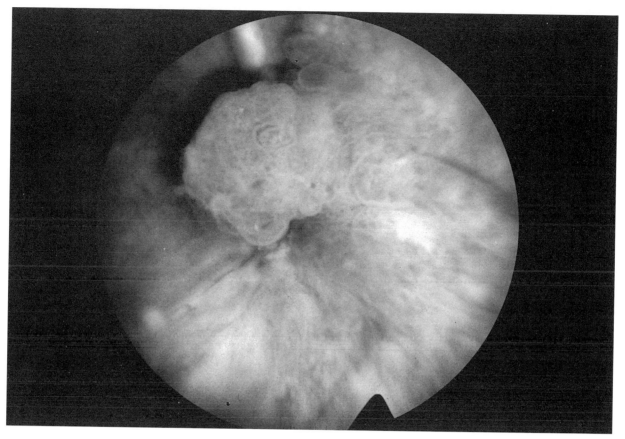

Figure 2-14
TRANSITIONAL CELL CARCINOMA, HIGH GRADE
(Courtesy of Dr. Mark S. Soloway, Miami, FL.)

lesion may seem to be a low-grade neoplasm or even a papilloma (fig. 2-18).

The cells of high-grade transitional cell carcinoma tend to cluster in histologic preparations. Their borders may be sharply defined or indistinct. Cytoplasm is usually homogeneous but vacuolization is common. Nuclei are markedly pleomorphic in shape. Significant variation in size is usually not a prominent feature. Chromatin is irregularly dispersed and coarsely granular, a feature more easily appreciated in formalin-fixed than picric acid–fixed tissues. Large nucleoli appear in many but not all nuclei. Mitoses are common and may be abnormal.

Transitional cell carcinomas of high cytologic grade may manifest heterologous elements of both epithelial and stromal origin (74,171). Small foci of glandular and squamous differentiation occur, especially in large tumors (fig. 2-19).

Calcification and areas of histologically benign osseous and cartilaginous tissue have been described (fig. 2-20). Giant cells of both stromal and epithelial origin may develop (174). In some cases, a few giant cells may contain human chorionic gonadotropin (HCG).

HCG has been detected in serum of 10 to 30 percent of bladder cancer patients and in more than 50 percent of individuals with disseminated disease (60,90). Tissue localization is much less frequent, probably because the hormone is not stored in secretory granules but released soon after production. Since the free beta subunit has no endocrine function, signs and symptoms related to hormonal abnormalities are rare. The almost exclusive association of increased HCG levels with transitional cell differentiation (not choriocarcinoma) and the production of this hormone by normal urothelial cells in culture suggest a

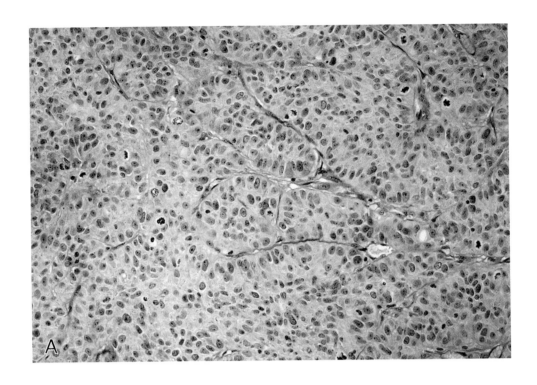

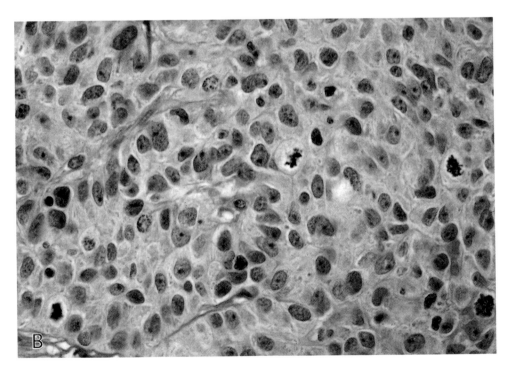

Figure 2-15
TRANSITIONAL CELL CARCINOMA, HIGH GRADE

A: Transitional cell carcinoma, high grade at low magnification.

B: At high magnification, nuclear pleomorphism is the most characteristic feature.

C: Urinary cytology obtained during follow-up.

D: Flow cytometric histogram obtained during follow-up. In the top histogram, 24 percent of the cells examined fell outside the normal G1G0 range. The bottom histogram was created from the same specimen as in C.

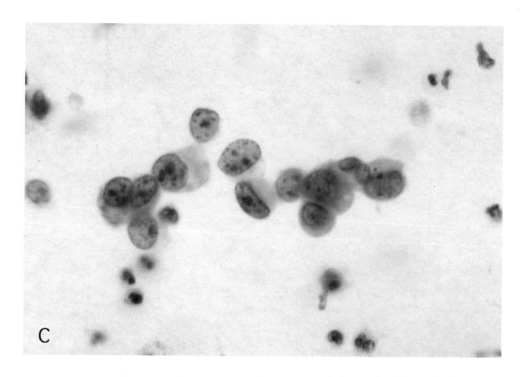

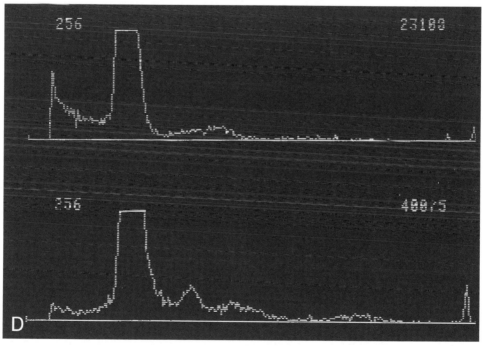

relationship at the genetic transcriptional level. It is tempting to consider transitional cell carcinomas that produce HCG as a distinctive variant. The distinction is lost at the histologic level, however, where tumors associated with increased serum HCG cannot be reliably distinguished from those lacking the hormone (fig. 2-21). The value of HCG in identifying a subgroup of patients with a poor prognosis has been disputed, undoubtedly because most patients with elevated hormone levels already have advanced disease (60,90).

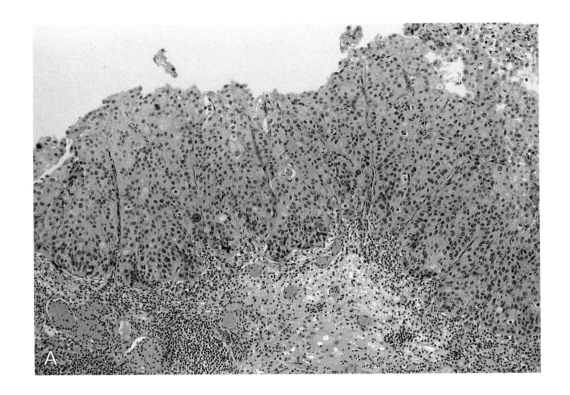

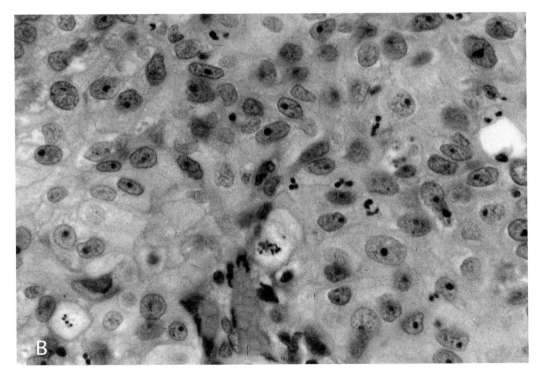

Figure 2-16
TRANSITIONAL CELL CARCINOMA, HIGH GRADE

A: A predominantly papillary neoplasm with minimal infiltration of the lamina propria (right).

B: At higher magnification, the nuclear pleomorphism, coarsely granular chromatin, and prominent nucleoli can be appreciated.

C: Urinary cytology.

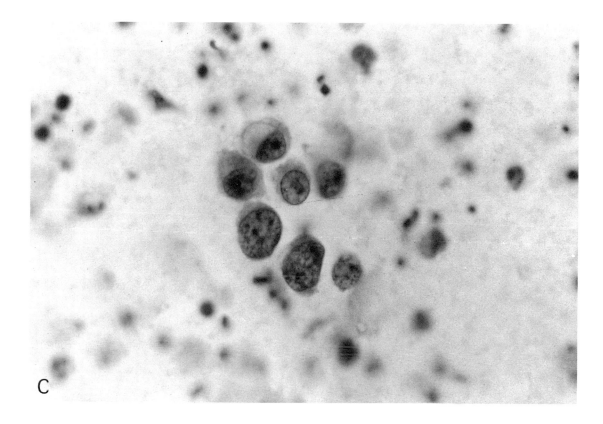

C

Cytologic samples from bladders harboring high-grade transitional cell carcinomas almost always contain readily recognizable anaplastic cells (figs. 2-15–2-17) (97,115,137). Neoplastic elements are isolated or loosely clustered. They may be associated with a background of degenerating blood, cellular debris, and inflammation but this so-called "tumor diathesis" is not a reliable diagnostic feature. High-grade neoplastic cells characteristically have moderate to high nuclear-cytoplasmic ratios. Malignant cells with very low nuclear-cytoplasmic ratios may be difficult to distinguish from superficial cells affected by topical therapy and should not form the sole basis for diagnostic interpretation. Cytoplasmic degeneration and vacuolization are common in high-grade neoplastic cells. As in histologic preparations, nuclear pleomorphism is the most reliable diagnostic feature. Chromatin is coarsely granular and nearly always irregularly dispersed. Large nucleoli occur in some high-grade neoplastic cells. In usual cytologic preparations, high-grade transitional cells cannot always be distinguished from other types of high-grade lesions, such as adenocarcinomas.

In contrast to papillomas and low-grade transitional cell carcinomas, high-grade transitional cell carcinomas have more cellular heterogeneity. The characterization of various neoplastic clones may provide important clues to the more aggressive behavior of these cancers. Electron microscopy has not been particularly useful in this regard but immunochemistry might play a more significant role (see Special Techniques).

Carcinoma in Situ. This is a flat, noninvasive, transitional cell neoplasm composed of cells of high cytologic grade (117). Squamous and glandular variants are not well characterized. Anaplastic cells appear in all layers but do not always replace the full thickness of the urothelium. Similar lesions have been called moderate and severe dysplasia in other formulations. Although these neoplasms may vary in their degree of cytologic anaplasia, grading has not been widely accepted.

The clinical features of urothelial carcinoma in situ (CIS) differ from those of other transitional cell neoplasms. Primary lesions are rare, occurring in less than 1 percent of individuals with urinary symptoms (76). In contrast, foci of CIS

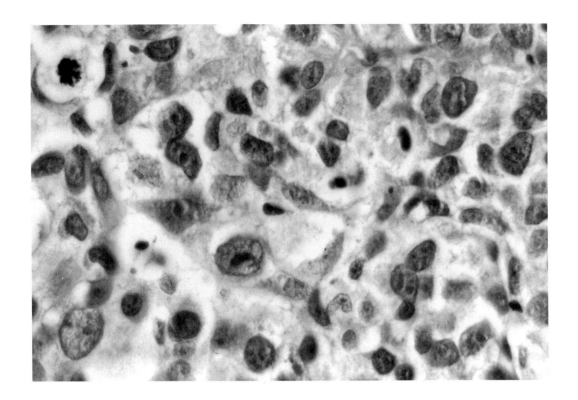

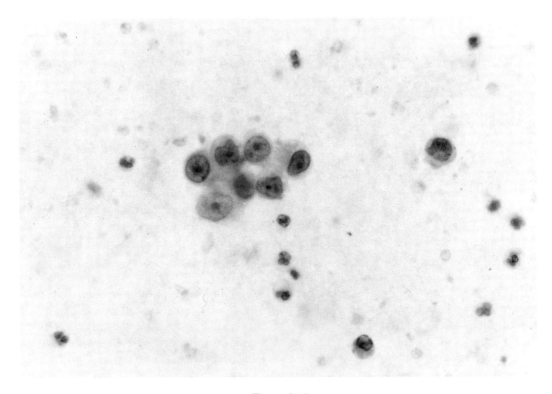

Figure 2-17
TRANSITIONAL CELL CARCINOMA, HIGH GRADE
Top: Marked nuclear pleomorphism and clustering are characteristic of high-grade transitional cell carcinoma.
Bottom: Urinary sample corresponding to top figure.

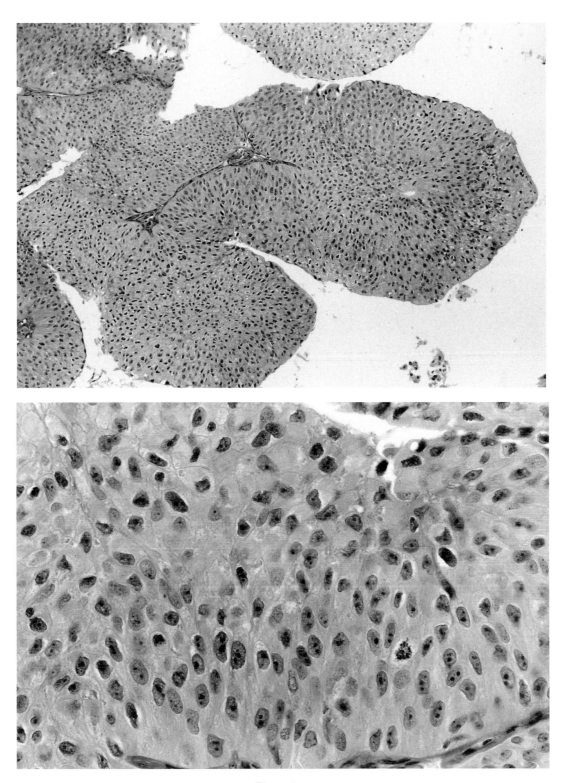

Figure 2-18
TRANSITIONAL CELL CARCINOMA, HIGH GRADE

Top: At low magnification, this predominantly papillary tumor might be mistaken for a papilloma. Similar lesions have been labeled "atypical papilloma" in the past.

Bottom: At high magnification, the nuclear anaplasia is apparent.

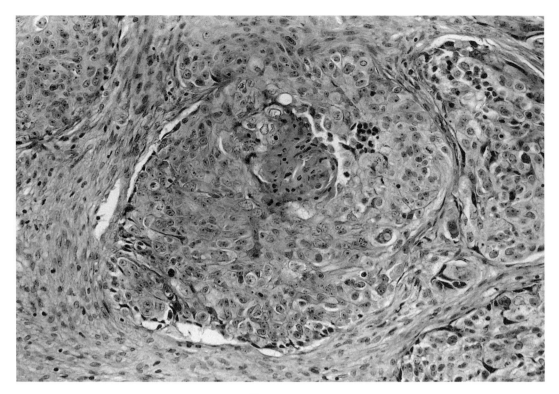

Figure 2-19
TRANSITIONAL CELL CARCINOMA, HIGH GRADE WITH SQUAMOUS DIFFERENTIATION

Figure 2-20
TRANSITIONAL CELL CARCINOMA
WITH OSSIFICATION
Photomicrograph of ossification in a carcinoma of the bladder
from a 68-year-old man. (Fig. 28 from Fascicle 31a, 1st Series.)

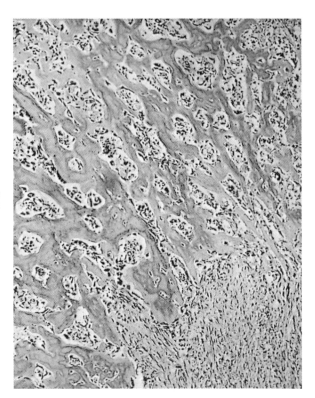

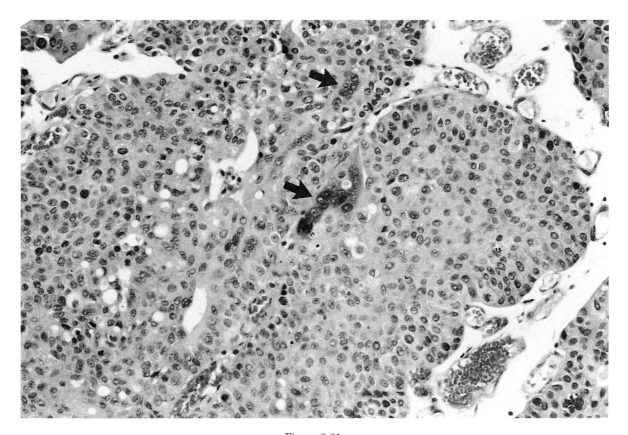

Figure 2-21
TRANSITIONAL CELL CARCINOMA WITH SYNCYTIOTROPHOBLASTIC GIANT CELLS
The giant cells in this photograph (arrows) reacted positively with antibodies to human chorionic gonadotropin (HCG). In our experience, HCG-containing cells are not always multinucleated and many cannot be distinguished from other anaplastic elements without immunohistochemistry. (Courtesy of Dr. Jonathan I. Epstein, Baltimore, MD.)

have been identified in nearly every bladder removed for invasive carcinoma (99). The tendency for patients to have symptoms for years prior to diagnosis and for lesions to persist without invasion for years after detection is frequently observed (76,111). CIS is usually multifocal, often involving urothelium in areas other than the bladder base. Signs and symptoms of primary CIS are more suggestive of an infection than a neoplasm. Their severity tends to parallel the extent of the lesion. Hematuria is common but patients are more concerned with dysuria, frequency, and suprapubic pain. At cystoscopy, CIS may appear as either erythematous or normal mucosa.

The pathologic features of urothelial CIS are also distinctive. Lesions are almost always observed in association with previous or coincident high-grade transitional cell carcinomas; they rarely coexist with papillomas. Despite their

morphologic resemblance to high-grade transitional cell carcinoma, the cells of CIS seem to prefer an intraepithelial environment. They expand by undermining the adjacent mucosa and do not usually invade stromal tissue even under favorable conditions, as when biopsies have created large mucosal defects (fig. 2-22).

The biologic potential of CIS is related to its mode of presentation. Lesions appearing as the initial urothelial neoplasm are associated with a low frequency of invasion and an even lower rate of patient death (75,132). In contrast, an adverse outcome is likely when CIS occurs in association with papillary or invasive carcinoma (136). Whereas CIS is a constant finding in advanced carcinomas, it is less common among patients with small or superficial tumors (99,121). The data suggest that most lesions of urothelial CIS recognized pathologically and treated clinically

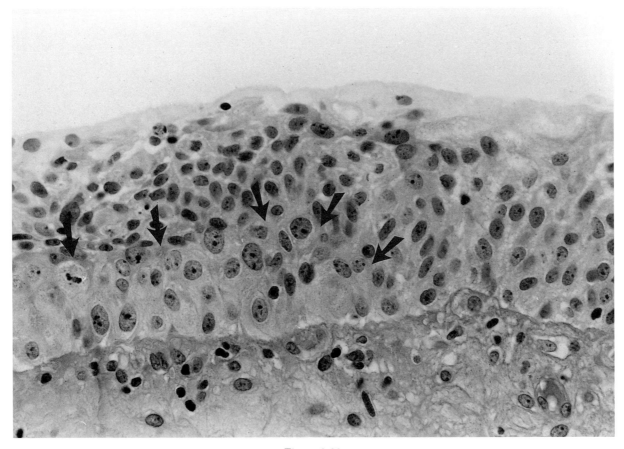

Figure 2-22
CARCINOMA IN SITU UNDERMINING ADJACENT UROTHELIUM
The interface between neoplastic and normal urothelium is indicated by the arrows.

do not evolve into invasive transitional cell carcinoma but are stunted growths which lack the capacity to invade and only acquire adverse prognostic attributes in cases of advanced disease. Nevertheless, urothelial CIS is a serious disease associated with a significant risk of aggressive behavior in some patients.

Histologically, CIS may exist in several patterns (99,116). Most often, cells with high nuclear-cytoplasmic ratios, amphophilic cytoplasm, and indistinct borders are irregularly arranged over discrete areas of urothelium (figs. 2-23, 2-24). The demarcation between CIS and adjacent mucosa is nearly always sharp, even when coexistent epithelial atypicalities are present. Hyperplasia, i.e, more than seven cell layers, is unusual. Slight maturation may occur as cells progress toward the epithelial surface and remnants of the superficial cell layer may be preserved. Nuclear pleomorphism is prominent. Nuclei have coarsely granular, irregularly dispersed chromatin. Many have large nucleoli. Mitoses are variable and occasionally abnormal. Rarely, cells with nuclear characteristics similar to those of the common lesion may be very small and densely aggregated, a pattern that has sometimes been called the *small cell variant of CIS* (fig. 2-25). In approximately 10 percent of cases, CIS comprises large cells with relatively low nuclear-cytoplasmic ratios, fairly well-defined borders, and slightly acidophilic cytoplasm (fig. 2-26) (132). When seen en face, this lesion resembles extramammary Paget disease and has been called the *pagetoid variant*. Pagetoid CIS is rarely, if ever, the primary lesion and usually comprises only small foci in a CIS of the usual pattern. All histologic variants of CIS may be associated with marked inflammation of the

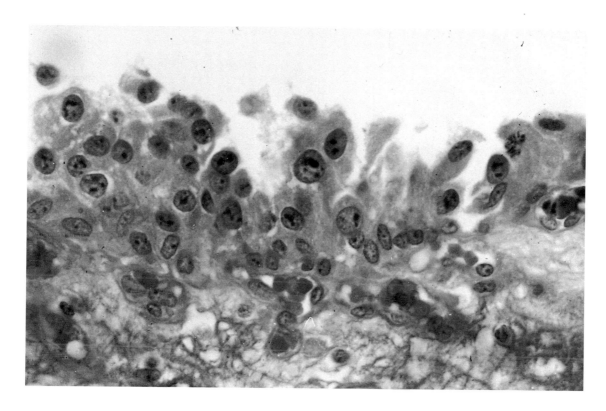

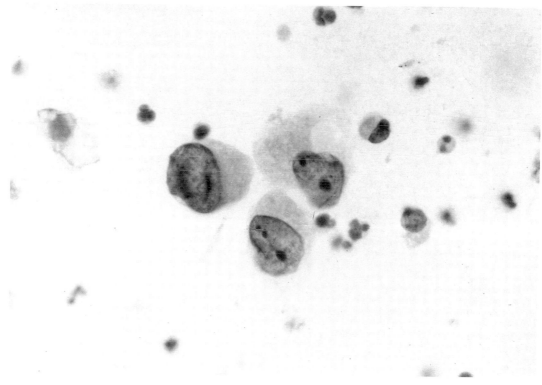

Figure 2-23
CARCINOMA IN SITU
Top: Partial denudation is characteristic of these lesions.
Bottom: High-grade malignant tumor cells are readily identified in most cytologic specimens.

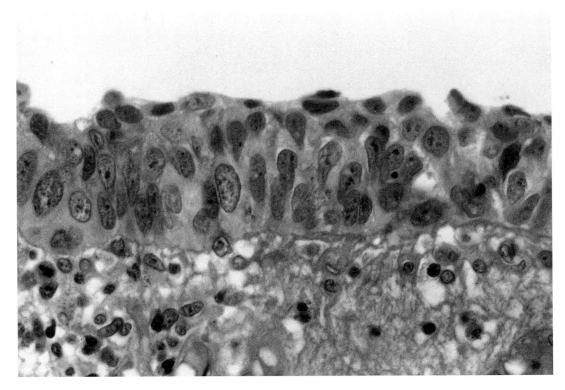

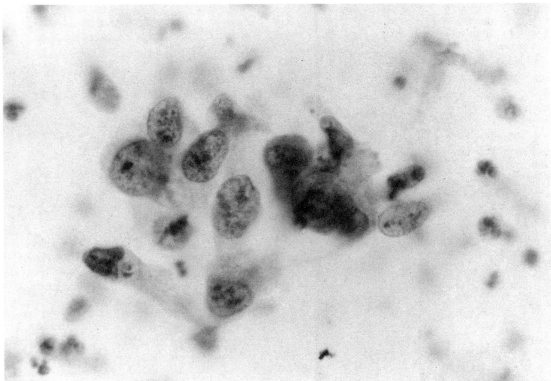

Figure 2-24
CARCINOMA IN SITU
Top: In this example, the superficial cell layer is partially preserved.
Bottom: High-grade tumor cells in the urinary cytology.

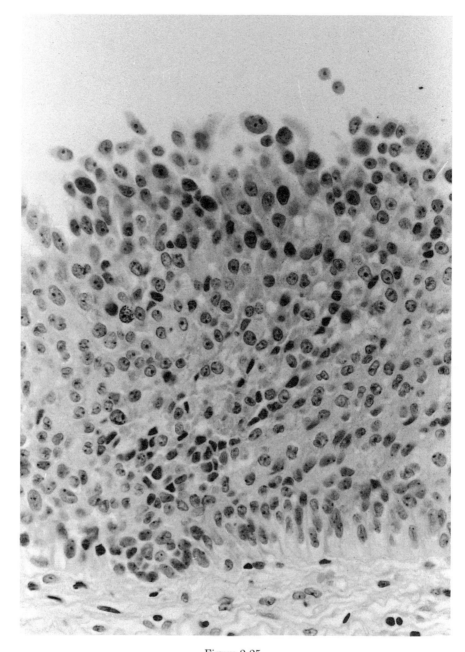

Figure 2-25
CARCINOMA IN SITU, SMALL CELL VARIANT

lamina propria. The relationship of the inflammation to the neoplasm is unclear.

A common feature of urothelial CIS is lack of intercellular cohesion, resulting in extensive denudation of the epithelium in tissue sections. In such cases, the pathologist should resist the temptation to interpret the material as "negative," as if no abnormality were present. Clues to the nature of

the process can be obtained by examining remnant epithelial cells for cytologic anaplasia and a urinary specimen for exfoliated cells.

Cytologic samples from untreated urothelial CIS often contain numerous neoplastic cells. With few exceptions, these cells have features of any high-grade bladder neoplasm. In our experience, in situ lesions cannot be reliably distinguished

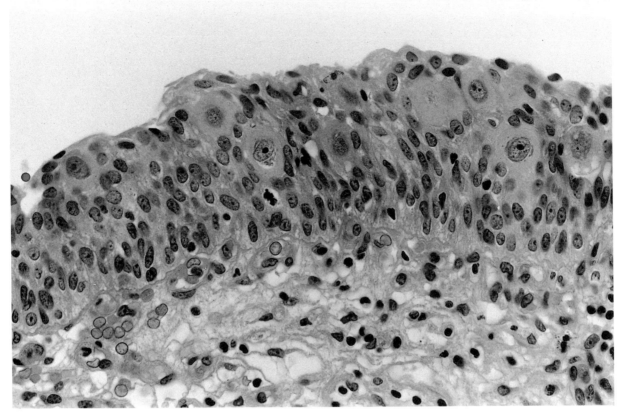

Figure 2-26
CARCINOMA IN SITU, PAGETOID VARIANT

from invasive tumors using urinary cytology alone. Malignant tumor cells are readily identified in urinary samples and despite an inability to determine location or depth of invasion, cytology is currently the most reliable method for detection of both primary and recurrent/persistent cancer in this group of patients.

Abnormalities in DNA ploidy and blood group antigen expression may be even more prominent in areas of CIS than in areas of invasive transitional cell carcinoma (64,116,158). These changes further document the extreme cellular derangement of CIS and suggest that invasion and metastasis require more than anaplasia alone.

Dysplastic Intraepithelial Lesions. *Dysplasia* and *atypical hyperplasia* are the most commonly used terms to describe a group of urothelial changes that resemble lesions of similar names in other organs. This terminology is a highly controversial subject but essential to any discussion of urothelial neoplasms, since these lesions tend to define the limits of the qualitative light microscopic approach to the subject. The concept that all carcinomas arise from preexisting epithelium is widely accepted, but the processes by which intraepithelial neoplasms develop in humans are largely unknown. Until the carcinogenic process is better understood, controversy concerning epithelial changes of lesser morphologic severity than CIS is inevitable. No single term seems to encompass all facets of the problem and various designations have been proposed: dysplasia, CIS grade 1, atypical hyperplasia, atypia, simple hyperplasia, and urothelial intraepithelial neoplasia. As defined here, urothelial dysplasia describes a spectrum of histologic changes occurring in flat, noninvasive urothelium. These changes may arise from a variety of stimuli, including neoplastic and non-neoplastic, but can be distinguished morphologically from other lesions recognized as either reactive, regenerative, or CIS (Table 2-5).

Table 2-5

COMPARISON OF DYSPLASIA TO
CARCINOMA IN SITU AND REACTIVE UROTHELIUM*

	CIS**	Dysplasia	Reactive
Cell layers	Variable	Variable	Variable
Mucosal infiltrate	Absent	Absent	Variable
Polarization	Abnormal	Slightly abnormal	Slightly abnormal
Cytoplasm	Homogeneous	Homogeneous	Vacuolated
N:C ratio†	Increased	Slightly increased	Normal, slightly increased
Nuclei Position	Eccentric	Eccentric	Normal
Borders	Pleomorphic	Notches, creases	Regular, smooth
Chromatin	Coarse	Fine	Fine, dusty
Distribution	Uneven	Even	Even
Nucleoli	Large	Large	Small, absent
Mitoses	Variable	Variable	Variable

*Table 2-10 from Murphy WM. Diseases of the urinary bladder, urethra, ureters, and renal pelves. In: Urological pathology. Philadelphia: WB Saunders, 1989:96.
**CIS = Carcinoma in situ.
†N:C ratio = Nuclear:cytoplasmic ratio.

The clinical features associated with dysplastic urothelial abnormalities are poorly characterized. Almost all cases have been uncovered in bladders that have already developed carcinomas (76,99). The incidence of dysplastic lesions in the general population is unknown; the frequency among bladder cancer patients varies from 20 to 86 percent (76,99,121). Lesions are more easily documented and probably much more common in association with advanced disease. Experiences in clinic and hospital populations, where patients were only partially selected because of known bladder neoplasia, suggest that the frequency of dysplastic changes among noncancer patients is less than 5 percent (116). The lack of visible cystoscopic abnormalities, obvious cytologic changes, and serum markers make early detection of this lesion a sporadic, serendipitous event.

Concern about the importance of dysplastic urothelial lesions centers upon the following observations: dysplastic lesions are often observed in bladders harboring carcinomas; the cells in dysplastic lesions bear a morphologic resemblance to those in low-grade papillary tumors; experimental animals exposed to large doses of chemical carcinogens develop carcinomas through a series of intraepithelial changes of increasing cytologic severity; the ultrastructural and antigenic composition of dysplastic lesions more closely resemble CIS than normal urothelium; and the appearance of urothelial dysplasia in patients with a history of bladder cancer may increase the risk for an adverse outcome (47,88, 121,122). This information is somewhat tempered by the following: dysplastic lesions are uncommon in noncancer patients; the frequency and severity of dysplasia seems to parallel rather than precede advanced neoplastic disease; few studies have documented an increased risk for adverse outcome among patients with mildly dysplastic lesions; and only 10 percent of patients with dysplasia in the best-documented series died from bladder cancer over a 10-year period (83,116,121,140).

Current information indicates that urothelial abnormalities described as dysplasia are risk factors for an adverse outcome, especially among patients with previous or coincident neoplasms. The degree of risk is apparently small. Until methods to identify these lesions in patients without bladder neoplasms can be developed, their clinical significance remains obscure.

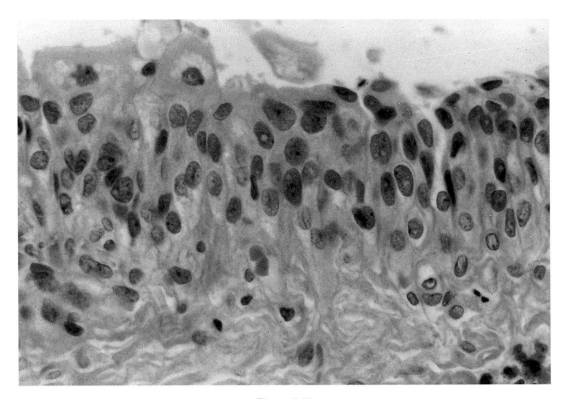

Figure 2-27
UROTHELIAL ATYPIA (DYSPLASIA, ATYPICAL HYPERPLASIA, SIMPLE HYPERPLASIA)
Note the nuclear clustering and irregularities of shape and orientation. Not all cells in this photograph are atypical, a common situation in dysplastic lesions which tends to confound accurate interpretation.

Dysplastic lesions can be recognized in histologic preparations by the disorientation and clustering of their nuclei (fig. 2-27) (116,122). When compared to normal cells in other areas of the specimen, dysplastic cells have a more homogeneous cytoplasm and larger nuclei. Nuclei tend to crowd together and overlap. The notches, creases, and shallow depressions of nuclear borders seen in papillomas are present but less pronounced. Chromatin is finely granular and evenly dispersed. Nucleoli are absent or small. Mitoses are rare.

Dysplastic cells can also be seen in urinary samples. Not surprisingly, they resemble the changes previously described for papillomas. They are more difficult to identify than neoplastic cells, even by experienced observers.

Variants of Transitional Cell Carcinoma. These tumors can be defined as transitional cell neoplasms having unexpected histologic patterns or cellular products (Table 2-1). The unexpected element, whether a gland-like lumen, cell nest, or focus of spindle cells, may occur as a

minor component in many transitional cell neoplasms. It becomes noteworthy only when florid. Anecdotal reports, such as transitional cell carcinoma with rhabdoid features, appear sporadically in the literature (84). Well-characterized variants are described in the following section.

Carcinoma with Gland-like Lumina. This is an uncommon tumor characterized by the presence of small clusters of intercellular or intracellular lumina surrounded by neoplastic transitional or squamous cells (figs. 2-28, 2-29) (68,71,171,173). Lumina may occur in all grades of transitional cell carcinoma but seem more noticeable in high-grade tumors. They are usually small but may reach cystic proportions. Most appear empty in usual histologic preparations but some contain granular acidophilic material or necrotic tumor cells. Appropriate histochemical reactions reveal small amounts of predominantly acid mucins in almost all cases. Ultrastructural studies have confirmed the light microscopic findings. In most instances, these gland-like structures probably

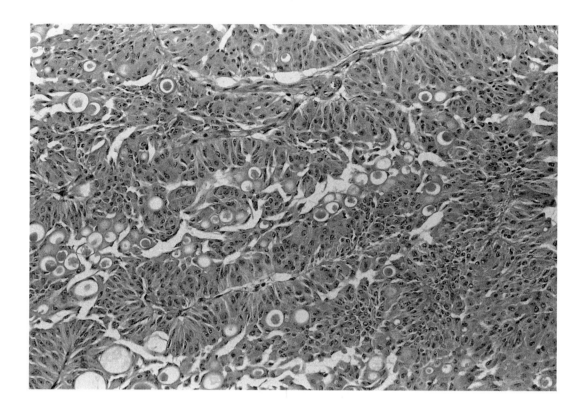

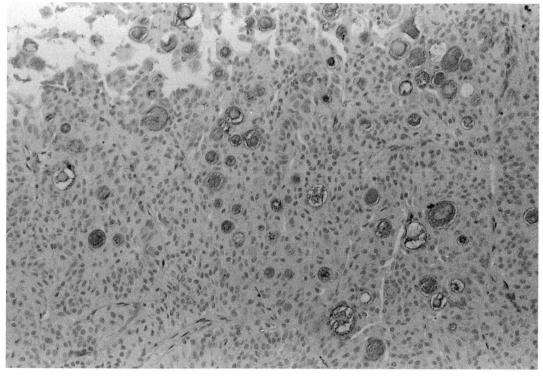

Figure 2-28
TRANSITIONAL CELL CARCINOMA WITH GLAND-LIKE LUMINA
Top: Transitional cell carcinoma with gland-like lumina.
Bottom: Transitional cell carcinoma with gland-like lumina. (Alcian blue stain)

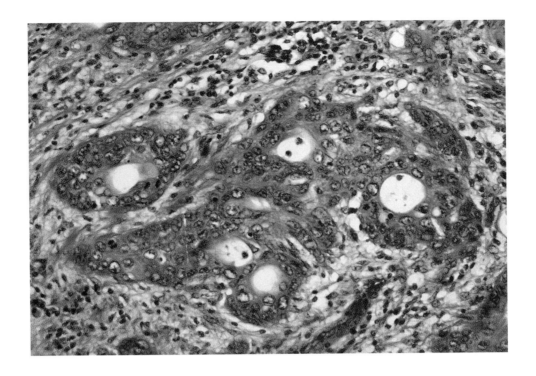

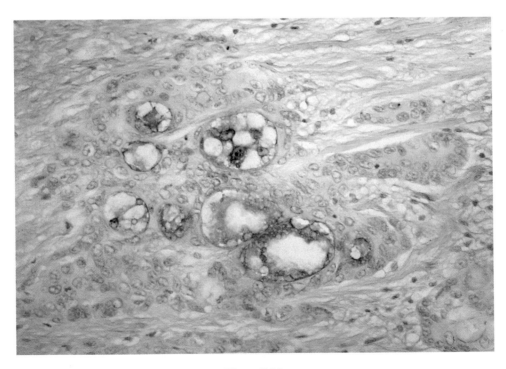

Figure 2-29
TRANSITIONAL CELL CARCINOMA WITH GLAND-LIKE LUMINA
Top: Transitional cell differentiation is seen in the cells surrounding the gland-like spaces of this deeply invasive tumor.
Bottom: Same tumor stained with mucicarmine.

reflect a genetically programmed ability of transitional cells to form and line spaces (like bladders). The glandular debris and necrotic cells found in a few lumina suggest a degenerative etiology in some cases. The presence of gland-like spaces has no known prognostic significance. Differentiation of transitional cell carcinomas with gland-like lumina from mixed transitional cell-adenocarcinomas is somewhat arbitrary but important when the transitional cell neoplasm is of low cytologic grade. In the bladder, we concentrate on the lining cells rather than the secretory products and define glands as those structures differentiating toward colonic epithelium.

Transitional Cell Carcinoma, Nested Type. This is a rare bladder tumor in which neoplastic transitional cells are arranged in structures resembling florid proliferations of Brunn nests (fig. 2-30) (119,156). Reported cases have occurred in males aged 53 to 97 years who presented with hematuria, urgency, or signs of ureteral obstruction. Lesions have usually been small, multifocal, and localized to ureteral orifices. Their distinctive feature is the arrangement of tumor cells in nests and abortive tubules suggestive of cystitis glandularis et cystica. Many of the neoplastic cells are only slightly atypical but some markedly anaplastic elements occur in every case. The pathology is deceptive in that these tumors tend to be highly aggressive. Transitional cell carcinoma, nested type can be differentiated from prostatic carcinoma by its location, histology, and negative reactions for prostate-specific antigen and prostatic acid phosphatase. A lack of colonic differentiation distinguishes it from adenocarcinoma. These tumors differ from proliferations of Brunn nests by their invasive growth pattern and nuclear anaplasia.

Sarcomatoid Carcinoma. This unusual tumor is composed predominantly of spindle cells surrounding isolated islands of pure or mixed transitional cell carcinoma (fig. 2-31) (138,171,172). In contrast to transitional cell carcinoma with spindle cell stroma, these spindle cells are malignant and manifest various amounts of both vimentin and cytokeratins. Many such tumors have been called spindle cell carcinoma or even carcinosarcoma in previous reports (100,165). Clinical features do not differ significantly from those of patients with high-grade transitional cell carcinomas. Microscopically, the tumors resemble malignant fibrous histiocytomas and multiple sections may be necessary to uncover the islands of epithelial differentiation. Positive reactions of at least some of the spindle cells to cytokeratin antibodies is confirmatory. Most sarcomatoid carcinomas are high stage at diagnosis and 5-year survival has been less than 30 percent. Individuals with low-stage disease have a more favorable outlook.

Special Techniques. A great deal of information concerning normal and neoplastic urothelium is available from techniques other than routine light microscopy. Flow cytometry, digitizing image analysis, immunohistochemistry, in situ hybridization, in situ and in vitro tissue labeling, silver impregnation, direct chromosomal analyses, polymerase chain reactions, and gel chromatography are used to examine tissues and cells for their antigenic composition, nuclear morphometry, DNA ploidy, chromosomal structure, genes and gene products, and growth kinetics.

Antigenic Composition. The antigenic composition of normal and neoplastic urothelium has been characterized primarily through the study of blood group–related antigens, carcinoembryonic antigens, cytokeratins, and antibodies to poorly characterized glycoproteins of various molecular weights. Substances specific for urothelium have yet to be discovered and many antibodies react to normal as well as neoplastic cells.

The best-characterized blood group–related antigens are ABH, Lewis a,b, and X, and Thomsen-Friedenreich (T) (65,93,129,130,143, 170). ABH and Lewis a and b are expressed on normal cell membranes whereas the Lewis X and T antigens are primarily found in neoplastic epithelium. Expression of ABH and Lewis antigens is influenced by a gene product first found in saliva and carried by almost 80 percent of the population (so-called "secretors"). In general, normal expression of blood group–related antigens is lost in transitional cell neoplasms. Even low-grade tumors may lack ABH antigens or express Lewis X. High-grade cancers often express T antigens. Biochemical changes in the membranes of neoplastic cells are complex and vary even among cells of one tumor. Blood group–related antigens are easily altered during processing and consistent results have been difficult to obtain in nonresearch settings.

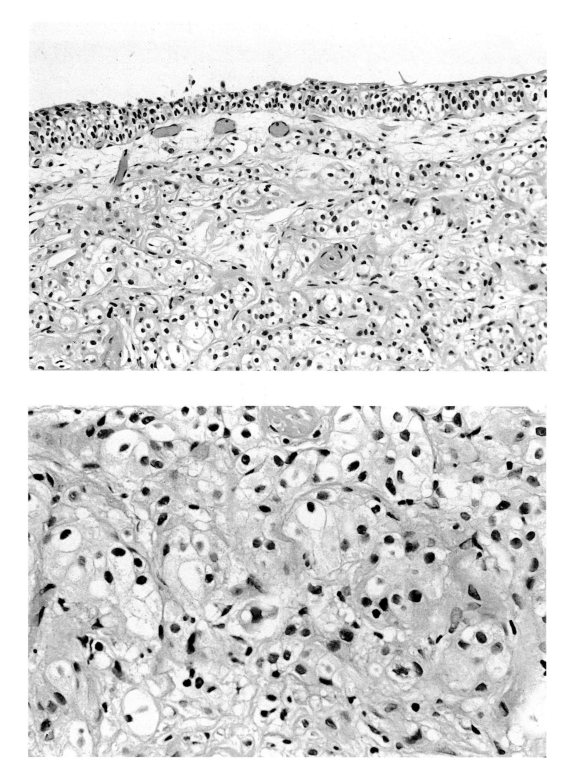

Figure 2-30
TRANSITIONAL CELL CARCINOMA, NESTED TYPE

Top: The tumor characteristically presents as multiple, deceptively benign-appearing nests in the lamina propria. In contrast to cystitis glandularis, the nests lack cellular organization around lumina and seem to infiltrate rather than cluster.

Bottom: At higher magnification, the cellular disorganization and atypia are easily appreciated. (Both figures courtesy of Dr. Daniel M. Lundblad, Parkersburg, WV.)

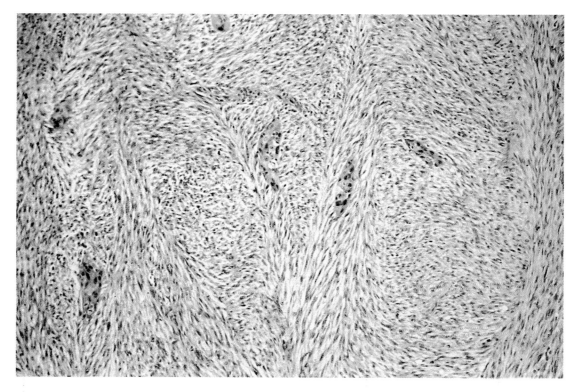

Figure 2-31
SARCOMATOID CARCINOMA
The neoplasm comprises islands of epithelial cells surrounded by spindle cells reactive for cytokeratins and vimentin.

Carcinoembryonic antigens are a group of gly-coproteins produced by cells of endodermal derivation (125,145,163). These substances are produced in the highest amounts by immature, reactive, and neoplastic cells but have been observed in normal urothelium. Their concentration in urine is increased in several conditions, most notably urinary tract infection. Like blood group–related substances, carcinoembryonic antigen expression is dynamic and too variable for routine clinical use.

Antibodies to cytokeratins detect epithelial cells and are particularly useful for identifying small foci of invasive carcinoma in poorly preserved tissue. Antibodies to a variety of poorly characterized urothelial proteins have been produced (54,63,79). Application of these antibodies to urinary specimens has increased the ability to detect neoplastic cells and differentiate cytologic grades (96,110). Assessment of the antigenic composition of transitional cell neoplasms may have practical value in increasing the diagnostic yield and degree of prognostic certainty in selected cases.

Morphometry. The size, quantity, variation, and disposition of any particulate cellular component can be quantitated with morphometry. The most versatile methods employ computer-based digitizing systems which can record actual measurements and calculate a vast array of means, coefficients, and indices on individual cells while integrating the information to create a quantitative profile of the tissue itself (70,162). Morphometry can deliver information on features such as nuclear shape and chromatin texture, which cannot be obtained by visual assessment using light microscopy. The best results are achieved from disaggregated cells, a requirement for which urinary specimens are especially well suited (143).

Studies exploring the practical value of morphometry as applied to bladder neoplasms have been primarily concerned with correlating quantitative features with grade and prognosis (57, 109, 151,161). Since computer-based systems for quantitation are usually used in an interactive mode, the significance of these correlations depends

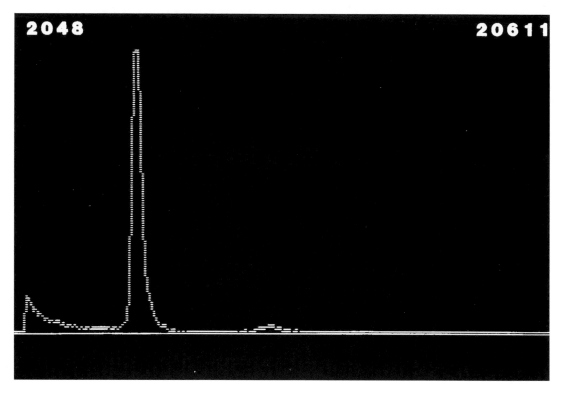

Figure 2-32
FLOW CYTOMETRY: NORMAL HISTOGRAM

upon the selection criteria of the observer. In general, quantitative measurements and calculations document a direct correlation between nuclear size and tumor grade. They seem to support the thesis that most transitional cell neoplasms can be separated into low-grade lesions with a good prognosis and high-grade cancers with an unfavorable outlook. In addition to potential value in diagnosis and prognosis, morphometric techniques deliver a level of precision that can be of practical value in quality assurance.

DNA Ploidy. DNA ploidy can be determined by measuring the optical density of nuclei stained stoichiometrically with dyes like Feulgen or by measuring the light scattered from nuclei exposed to laser beams after being reacted with immunofluorescent substances (153,157, 158). The most popular instruments are image analyzers and flow cytometers. Image analyzers process material relatively slowly compared to flow cytometers but offer the advantages of operator interaction and image storage. Flow cytometers can assess large numbers of nuclei in

seconds but generally destroy the specimen in the process. Neither method can detect every neoplasm nor can measurements of DNA alone accurately predict the course of the disease. The methodology requires a great deal of operator discretion; it is inaccurate to consider quantitation of DNA content as a totally objective test.

Terminology for expressing DNA ploidy has not been standardized. In general, normal histograms are called diploid or euploid whereas abnormal histograms are labeled aneuploid (figs. 2-32, 2-33) (157). Aneuploid histograms are often further subdivided as tetraploid or hypertetraploid when an abnormal amount of DNA is recorded in the 4C position. Histograms with a sloping right shoulder to the G1G0 peak are labeled hyperdiploid (fig. 2-34) (122). Current terminology in this area can lead to misconceptions. Even though results are expressed in terms of ploidy, the method actually measures total DNA rather than the number of normal chromosomes. Chromosomal abnormalities that do not alter the total amount of DNA cannot be

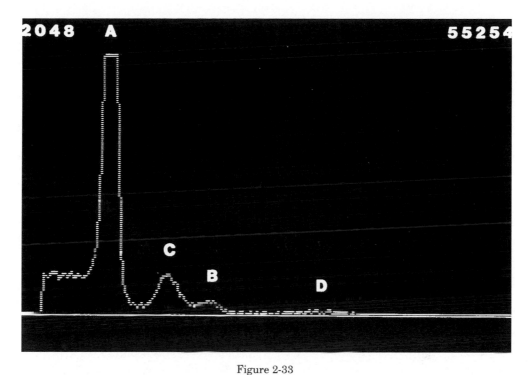

Figure 2-33
FLOW CYTOMETRY: ANEUPLOID HISTOGRAM
A and B mark the normal G1G0 peak and the normal G2M peak. C and D represent the aneuploid peak and its G2M peak.

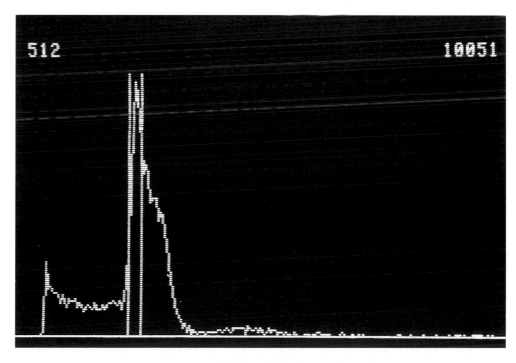

Figure 2-34
FLOW CYTOMETRY: HYPERDIPLOID HISTOGRAM
The significance of this type of histogram is controversial. In this case, 62 percent of the cells examined fell outside the normal G1G0 peak and the patient had transitional cell carcinoma of the bladder.

detected in usual preparations. When multiple abnormal peaks occur in DNA histograms, they are often described as different cell lines, although similarities in total DNA can hardly be construed as evidence for genetic lineage.

Used in conjunction with light microscopy, measurements of DNA ploidy can be important in clinical practice (126,157). Essentially all bladder lesions containing aneuploid cells are neoplastic and almost all are malignant. Depending upon the classification system, this may be an important factor in separating transitional cell neoplasms into groups with different prognoses (77). Using the WHO classification, for example, the majority of grade II transitional cell carcinomas with DNA aneuploidy behave like grade III cancers whereas similarly classified neoplasms with DNA diploidy act more like grade I tumors. DNA ploidy has been of value in detecting transitional cell neoplasms in cytologic specimens (53, 101,120). Coupled with monoclonal antibodies for epithelial differentiation, DNA ploidy methodology can detect malignant elements in specimens having few tumor cells or tumor cells masked by inflammatory debris (78). Knowledge of DNA ploidy may influence the type and extent of treatment and serve as a predictive factor for patient outcome (Table 2-6) (89). The precision of available instrumentation is an important factor in quality assurance. The increased level of certainty that a positive histogram brings to a light microscopic interpretation should not be minimized, especially since pathologists cannot be expert microscopists in every facet of the field.

Chromosomal Structure. The chromosomal structure of urothelial tumors has been studied with increasingly sophisticated techniques for more than two decades (103,148,155). Established methods can reveal chromosomal aberrations that do not affect the total amount of nuclear DNA and are therefore not detectable using flow cytometry or digitizing image analysis (150). Changes may occur in the modal number, the physical structure, or the gene placement of one or many chromosomes. To date, no abnormalities have been specific for urothelial neoplasms. The information available from chromosomal analysis can be briefly summarized as follows: some chromosomal aberrations can be found in almost all transitional cell neoplasms; these aberrations are often constant among multiple coexistent tumors and re-

Table 2-6

CLINICAL VALUE OF DNA PLOIDY IN UROTHELIAL NEOPLASIA

Detect neoplastic cells

Subdivide intermediate grade tumors

Confirm light microscopic diagnosis

Increase level of diagnostic certainty

Avoid "bad day" errors

Allay skepticism of clinicians

Improve quality assurance

Establish database

current low-grade tumors from the same patient but differ from patient to patient; chromosomal changes in low-grade transitional cell neoplasms are rarely as numerous or varied as in high-grade neoplasms; genetic changes in the chromosomes of low-grade neoplasms are often not observed in high-grade tumors; at present, abnormalities of gene placement tend to be more predictive of recurrence than progression; and prognosis is currently best correlated with the total number of different abnormalities or, more accurately for the majority of studies, tumors that have already progressed have more chromosomal abnormalities than those that have not yet progressed at the time of evaluation (52,82,128,134,159).

Chromosomal analysis has developed into a highly specialized field not easily understood by the novice. Results are expressed in a standardized but complicated terminology. For example, an unbalanced translocation involving the short arms of chromosomes 3 and 5 would be written as follows: -5,+der(5)t(3;5)(p14;p14) (52). Practical application is further hindered by the difficulty of interpreting the complex array of chromosomal changes found in urothelial neoplasms in terms of diagnosis and prognosis.

Genes and Gene Products. Information on the function of genes and gene products in the development of neoplasms in general and bladder tumors in particular is rapidly accumulating and only the most general statements can be made at this time (59,139,146). The data strongly indicate that cellular proliferation is regulated by a group of genes acting on different parts of the cell cycle. The term "oncogene" is misleading in that these genes are normal constituents of chromosomes and only become involved in oncogenesis under abnormal circumstances. Genes regulating proliferation (oncogenes) are themselves modulated by suppressor genes (97). Neoplasms may be initiated when mutations or overexpression of oncogenes allow cells to escape from the effects of suppressor genes or when abnormalities or deletions occur in the suppressors themselves (135,149). The process may involve factors produced by adjacent nonproliferating cells as well as alterations in the surface membrane receptors, transducers, nuclear transcription factors, and DNA repair enzymes of the proliferating cells. It may also have a quantitative aspect in that a critical mass of cells is required to produce sufficient substances, such as growth factors, to sustain independent growth.

From the genetic point of view, multiple alterations are required to produce a disseminated cancer (146). These alterations are not necessarily interdependent and one genetic change may not predispose to another. Mutations occur constantly in normal cells and their probability increases with increases in the growth fraction of any population so long as the proliferating tissue is not completely exfoliated. The process seems to involve a combination of normal and altered biochemical pathways. All steps in human carcinogenesis seem to be modulated in individual patients, perhaps related to inherited susceptibilities. Considering that the average human will have an estimated 10^{16} cell divisions in his lifetime and that the majority never develop a malignant neoplasm, one might conclude that the right combination of genetic aberrations to produce a cancer is a rare event and that it is difficult for humans to develop cancer.

Only a few genes and gene products have been associated with human bladder tumors at this time. The most constant abnormalities have been in overexpression of the *ras* family and in mutations of p53 and Rb (67,135,149). In contrast to the almost universal appearance of chromosomal aberrations in transitional cell neoplasms, most bladder tumors do not manifest nonrandom abnormalities in gene expression. Although the appropriate technology is readily available and increasingly applied in research and educational centers, widespread use of genetic testing in clinical bladder cancer settings must await further understanding of the significance of these changes.

Cell Kinetics. The study of cell kinetics offers information on the growth rate of tumors which might be valuable in determining their behavior. The various parts of the proliferating cell cycle can be assessed with available techniques (50,108,113, 164,169). Mitoses can be directly observed in usual histologic preparations. Synthesis rate can be estimated using flow cytometry and digitizing image analysis or quantitated after labeling with tritiated thymidine or bromodeoxyuridine. Cells in all parts of the cycle, including G1 and G2 phases, can be assessed using antibodies to Ki-67 and proliferating cell nuclear antigen (PCNA) or by counting nucleolar organizer regions after silver impregnation. Apoptosis, the orderly cell death programmed into G1, is less easily evaluated at this time.

Information on the cell kinetics of urothelial neoplasms is scanty (107,108,125,127,160). In general, the growth fraction is directly proportional to the degree of cellular anaplasia, so that high-grade tumors have a larger proportion of cycling cells than low-grade neoplasms. Cycling cells are apparently not uniformly distributed in neoplastic tissue nor is the number of synthesizing cells constant for any particular grade of carcinoma. Although all studies agree that the percentage of proliferating cells is relatively low even in high-grade bladder tumors, actual measurements have varied widely in published reports, regardless of the similarity in methods used (107,125,127,160). Most studies suggest a correlation between growth fraction and prognosis but the relationship is not yet particularly strong and has been disputed.

Differential Diagnosis. The differential diagnosis of *inverted papilloma* includes florid proliferations of Brunn nests and transitional cell carcinomas with anastomosing infiltrating papillae. Occasionally, florid proliferations of Brunn nests have a configuration so similar to inverted papilloma that they suggest a subtype of the tumor rather than a separate lesion (see section, Non-Neoplastic Tumorous Conditions). A well-demarcated polypoid pattern is usually not present and gland-like lumina, rather than microcysts, are common. Cells tend to form nests rather than cords and do not resemble invaginated papillae. Since both types of lesions are benign, this distinction has little practical importance. Any disruption of the normal growth pattern of transitional cells can be considered a risk factor for subsequent neoplasia, but the risk for proliferations of Brunn nests and inverted papilloma is very low. Transitional cell carcinomas differ from inverted papillomas in many ways: a completely smooth outer surface is rare; anastomotic papillae lack normal maturation toward the center; and neoplastic cells usually manifest significant anaplasia, as confirmed with urinary cytology.

Exophytic transitional cell papilloma must be differentiated from inverted papilloma, polypoid cystitis, nephrogenic metaplasia, and low-grade transitional cell carcinoma. Features distinguishing inverted papilloma from exophytic papilloma have already been described. Polypoid cystitis is a lesion with a broad-based, rather than delicate, papillary core which contains connective tissue identical to that in the lamina propria. The papillary core is almost always covered by normal or reactive urothelium. Nephrogenic metaplasia is distinguished by a lining composed of a single layer of cuboidal cells, almost always lacking significant cellular atypia. Most lesions also have a tubular component. Low-grade transitional cell carcinoma differs from exophytic papilloma primarily by a more dense concentration of cells and slight alterations in nuclear features. Mitoses are more randomly distributed and not concentrated in basal areas. In addition, the cells of low-grade carcinomas are characteristically smaller than those of papillomas and their nuclei are often disoriented in the tissue. These differences are best appreciated in histologic preparations at low magnification. In cytologic samples, where superior fixation accentuates differences in nuclear shape and chromatin granularity, the nuclei of low-grade carcinomas are more pleomorphic, with more granular chromatin.

Transitional cell carcinoma, low grade must be differentiated from papilloma and transitional cell carcinoma, high grade. These tumors are not confused with non-neoplastic conditions by knowledgeable observers. Features distinguishing papillomas from low-grade carcinomas have already been described. Low-grade carcinomas differ from high-grade tumors by having a more orderly growth pattern lacking prominent cell clustering; less pleomorphism of nuclei; evenly dispersed, finely granular chromatin; and few or no large nucleoli.

Transitional cell carcinoma, high grade must be distinguished from low-grade transitional cell carcinoma, mixed carcinoma, and poorly differentiated prostatic cancer. Features distinguishing high-grade from low-grade transitional cell carcinoma have already been discussed. The most important are the nuclear clustering and pleomorphism which characterize high-grade tumors. Mixed carcinomas usually contain large areas of high-grade transitional cell carcinoma and the most appropriate diagnostic term for tumors having glandular or squamous foci is somewhat arbitrary. Lacking specific guidelines, we distinguish mixed carcinomas from transitional cell carcinomas with squamous, glandular, or other types of differentiation by the degree of differentiation and the proportion of the heterogeneous elements in the histologic sections. Given that nonkeratinizing squamous cell differentiation cannot be distinguished from high-grade transitional cell differentiation by light microscopy, squamous change is recognized when some degree of keratinization of the cytoplasm occurs. If this occurs as very small foci, especially if they are localized to the surface of the tumor and lack keratin pearls, we label the lesion high-grade transitional cell carcinoma with squamous differentiation. Small areas of glandular differentiation with only slight luminal mucin are treated similarly for diagnostic purposes. Except for documenting extreme heterogeneity, the category of mixed carcinoma is probably unimportant. Poorly differentiated prostatic cancers occasionally present at the bladder base and their differentiation from high-grade transitional cell tumors is very important. The best method is through immunohistochemical reactions for prostatic antigens, since there are no known cellular substances specific for transitional cells. In contrast to high-grade transitional cell carcinomas, poorly differentiated prostatic carcinomas have prominent nucleoli in almost every nucleus; small, uniform nuclei; and finely granular, evenly dispersed chromatin.

The differential diagnosis of *carcinoma in situ* includes reactive/regenerative epithelium, drug effects on normal urothelium, and intraepithelial lesions of lesser degrees of cellular atypia (dysplasia/atypical hyperplasia). CIS is distinguished from reactive/regenerative urothelium by irregular distribution of nuclei, nuclear pleomorphism, coarsely granular chromatin, and large nucleoli. Both lesions may have mitoses. CIS differs from drug affected urothelium in that abnormal nuclei are distributed throughout the urothelial thickness rather than only in the superficial cell layer. Differentiation of CIS from other intraepithelial abnormalities is discussed in the following section. Briefly, intraepithelial lesions composed of anaplastic cells, whether or not full thickness or hyperplastic, are considered CIS. Intraepithelial abnormalities that lack significant nuclear anaplasia are not considered carcinoma even though they may be important in identifying bladders at increased risk for future cancer.

Dysplastic lesions must be differentiated from reactive/regenerative epithelium and CIS. Dysplastic changes are best distinguished from reactive/regenerative epithelium at low magnification. Nuclear clustering is the hallmark of dysplastic change in contrast to the even distribution of nuclei in reactive/regenerative states. The nuclei of reactive/regenerative cells commonly manifest large nucleoli, often in almost every nucleus; tend to be round; and the chromatin often appears washed out due to nuclear swelling. Large nucleoli are not a feature of dysplastic epithelium. Nuclear features suggestive of dysplasia can be artifactually produced by epithelial compression. Dysplastic lesions are distinguished from CIS by lack of cellular anaplasia. Anaplastic cells have larger, more pleomorphic nuclei with more coarsely granular chromatin and, occasionally, very large nucleoli. Abnormal mitoses aid in differential diagnosis but are not usually present.

Mode of Dissemination. Since all clinically recognized transitional cell neoplasms are treated, information concerning their mode of dissemination must be gathered from two sources: the stage of disease at initial diagnosis and the progression of disease among patients with an unfavorable response to therapy. Empirical observations indicate that papillomas lack the capacity to disseminate. They appear to grow slowly into the bladder lumen or, in the case of inverted papilloma, into the lamina propria, but do not infiltrate the muscular wall. Complex infoldings of papillary fronds may look like invasion. The vessel-like spaces often observed surrounding small nests at the stromal surfaces of papillomas and other transitional cell neoplasms are apparently artifacts (fig. 2-35)

(105). The occasional appearance of anaplastic foci in a field of papilloma cells suggests that some papillomas progress through the development of high-grade clones (fig. 2-36).

Transitional cell carcinomas ordinarily progress via invasion of the muscular wall. Factors essential to this process are unknown but the correlation between cellular anaplasia and invasion suggests that a certain amount of cellular heterogeneity is important. Transitional cell carcinomas commonly involve the prostatic urethra and distal ureters. Spread to prostatic ducts has been documented in as much as 40 percent of cases and is often associated with CIS (fig. 2-37) (168). Metastases are usually associated with muscular wall invasion but have been observed in the regional lymph nodes of 14 percent of patients with superficial neoplasms (166). Metastases tend to follow lymphatics or blood vessels, and in order of declining frequency affect lymph nodes, lungs, liver, and bones (80,116).

CIS spreads by undermining the adjacent urothelium (see fig. 2-22). These lesions seem to prefer an intramucosal environment and do not invade even when surgical procedures have created large defects in the basal lamina. Since many high-grade transitional cell carcinomas are associated with CIS, intramucosal spread may be a significant method of bladder cancer dissemination, especially into the prostate gland and seminal vesicles. The possibility that progression of transitional cell carcinomas might occur through intravesical seeding is a controversial issue (see section, General Features).

Staging. Staging schemes, like grading systems, are designed to predict future activity by categorizing neoplasms on the basis of their behavior prior to clinical recognition (48,72,86, 116). Simple systems with few categories are the easiest to learn and use but convey the least information. Complex systems provide the most data but may be difficult to implement in nonresearch settings. Although intended to promote communication by establishing a stable basis for the study of cancer, staging schemes require periodic alterations as new information becomes available. A comparison of staging systems for bladder cancer is summarized in Table 2-7 (116). The formulation of the American Joint Cancer Committee and the International Union Against Cancer (AJCC-UICC) is recommended (48,86).

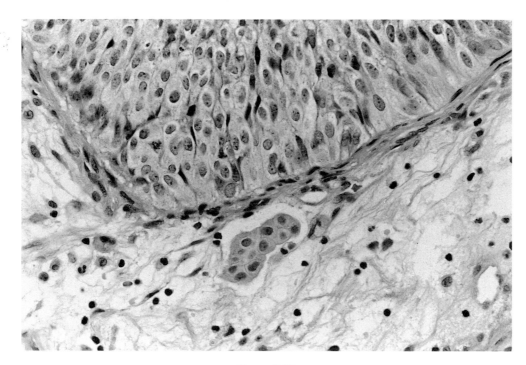

Figure 2-35
TRANSITIONAL CELL CARCINOMA, LOW GRADE
Artifactual space in lamina propria mimicking vascular invasion.

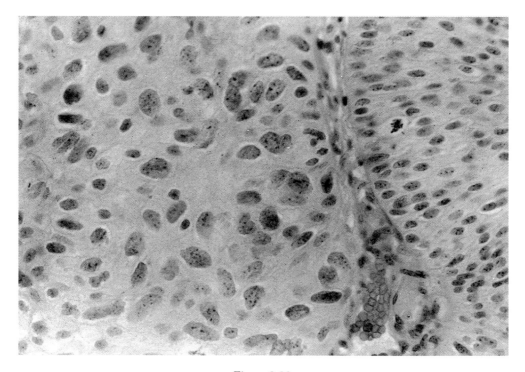

Figure 2-36
TRANSITIONAL CELL CARCINOMA, HIGH GRADE
When anaplastic areas occur in a low-grade papillary neoplasm, the tumor is best classified according to the higher grade focus.

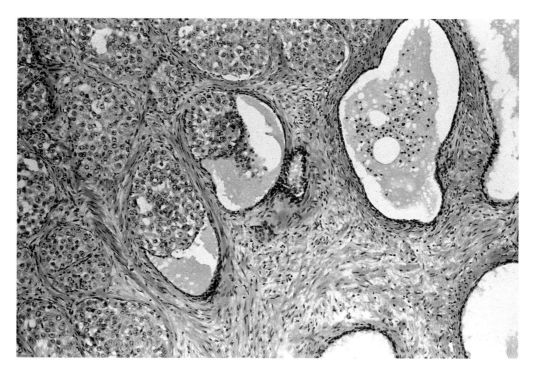

Figure 2-37
TRANSITIONAL CELL CARCINOMA INVOLVING PROSTATIC DUCTS

Table 2-7

STAGING SYSTEMS OF BLADDER CANCER*

Jewett 1946	Jewett 1952	Marshall 1952		Bladder Cancer Staging (Clinical-Pathological)	American Joint Cancer Committee UICC—1992**	
					Clinical	Pathological
		0	⌈ No tumor in specimen		T0	pT0
			⌊ No invasion	– carcinoma in situ	Tis	pTis
A	A			– papillary tumor	Ta	pTa
		A	Invasion	– lamina propria	T1	pT1
B	B1	B1		– superficial muscle	T2	pT2
	B2	B2		– deep muscle	T3a	pT3a
C	C	C		– paravesical tissue	T3b	pT3b
		D1	⌈	– contiguous organs or tissues	T4	pT4
			⌊ Metastases	– regional lymph nodes	N1-3 (<2cm, 2-5 cm, >5 cm)	pN1-3
		D2		– distant sites	M1	pM1

*Modified from Table 2-9 from Murphy WM. Diseases of the urinary bladder, urethra, ureters, and renal pelves. In: Murphy WM, ed. Urological pathology. Philadelphia: WB Saunders, 1989:85.
**UICC: International Union Against Cancer. The UICC and the AJCC also use the following codes: TX, NX, MX meaning items cannot be assessed and N0, M0 meaning no metastases to lymph nodes or distant sites.

Pathologic Effects of Treatment. The urinary bladder may be affected by a variety of therapeutic procedures (116). This is especially important to the pathologist, who must determine whether changes in treated urothelium represent residual or recurrent neoplasia, or alterations in normal cells caused by the therapy. The literature offers only a little help. Although abundant, it is usually not focused on the tissue and cellular manifestations of treated bladders. Assessment of treatment effects is often further hindered by incomplete information regarding the health of the patient prior to therapy, the extent of the disease, and the duration of exposure to the regimen. Established treatment modalities can be considered in four categories: surgery, chemotherapy, topical bacillus Calmette-Guérin, and X-ray therapy.

Surgical procedures disrupt the normal anatomy of the bladder and trigger nonspecific inflammatory responses that might confound the interpretation of subsequent tissue samples. These include granulomatous reactions suggestive of infectious disease and florid stromal proliferations (postoperative spindle cell nodules) suggestive of soft tissue neoplasms. Epithelial nests trapped in inflammatory tissue may suggest an invasive tumor. Regenerative epithelium can be confused with CIS, especially if it exhibits hyperdiploidy on flow cytometric histograms (120).

Chemotherapeutic drugs affecting the urinary bladder can be divided into two groups: systemic agents administered primarily for nonurological disease but concentrated in urine and topical chemicals used for prophylaxis or treatment of bladder neoplasms. Among systemic agents, the best studied is cyclophosphamide (Cytoxan). This is an alkylating agent most often given in multidrug cocktails for the treatment of leukemia and lymphoma. It has caused hemorrhagic cystitis characterized by denudation of epithelium with consequent irritative voiding symptoms and gross hematuria (152), and bladder cancers, although this is rare. Almost all bladder tumors have been carcinomas of high cytologic grade (142). They have no histologic or cytologic features that distinguish them from neoplasms occurring in patients not exposed to the drug.

Among the topical chemicals instilled for prophylaxis or treatment of bladder tumors, the most effective are alkylating agents (85,116).

Pathologic changes are thoroughly documented for triethylene thiophosphoramide (TTP) and mitomycin C (MMC) (123). Both are activated alkylating agents administered directly into the bladder, where they are in contact with urothelium for only a few hours. Pathologic changes associated with these drugs include exfoliation of both normal and abnormal urothelial cells with denudation of the bladder, degeneration, multinucleation, and bizarre reactive nuclear changes in superficial cells (fig. 2-38). Although characteristic, none of these alterations are specific for alkylating drugs in general or TTP and MMC in particular. They should not be confounding factors to the accurate interpretation of carcinoma for experienced observers (fig. 2-39). Exfoliation often results in a marked reduction in neoplastic cells in cytologic specimens, a situation that might decrease the effectiveness of flow cytometry as a monitoring technique (120). TTP and MMC have an abrasive effect on papillary tumors, destroying the tips of papillae and truncating the lesions to the point that they appear flattened or stubby in histologic preparations (fig. 2-40). It is important to differentiate stubby papillae from irregular areas of CIS or dysplasia in treated patients since this may constitute the difference between treatment failure (persistent tumor) and success (downgrading).

Topical bacillus Calmette-Guérin (BCG), like TTP and MMC, is instilled directly into the bladder for the prophylaxis and treatment of superficial bladder neoplasms (81,87,104,112). Few systemic complications have been documented even though the instillate consists of attenuated tubercle bacilli. The mechanism of action is unclear but the pathologic response is essentially identical to that observed in tuberculous cystitis (fig. 2-41). There is focal denudation of epithelium with an underlying granulomatous inflammation localized to the lamina propria and sparing the muscular wall. The granulomatous reaction indicates therapeutic activity of BCG and should be reported. Tubercle bacilli are not easily identified in these lesions; their presence does not affect future treatment.

Bladder tumors have been successfully downstaged by X-ray therapy, delivered either by intralesional implantation or external beam (49,145). The mechanism of action is unknown but may depend primarily on damage to blood

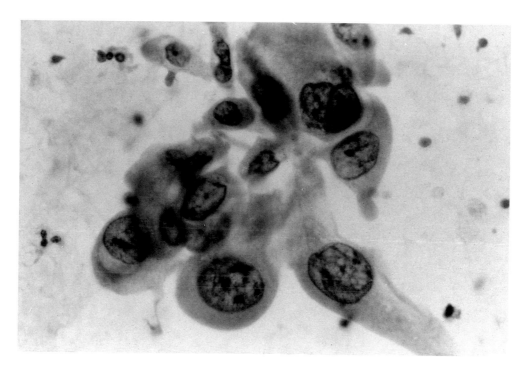

Figure 2-38
DRUG EFFECT
This is a characteristic but not pathognomonic reaction of superficial cells when exposed to alkylating agents like TTP/MMC.

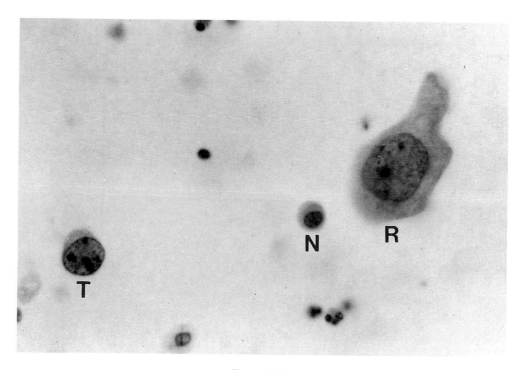

Figure 2-39
URINARY CYTOLOGY AFTER MITOMYCIN C THERAPY
The tumor cell (T) can be easily distinguished from the normal (N) and reactive superficial (R) cells.

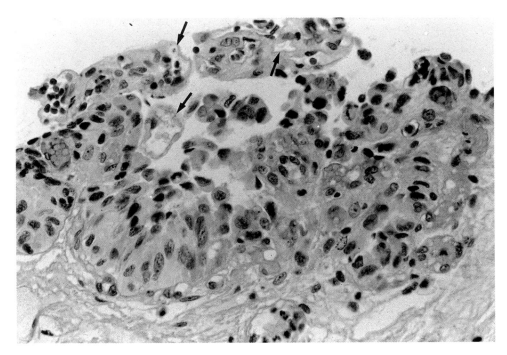

Figure 2-40
TRUNCATED PAPILLARY TUMOR AFTER MITOMYCIN C THERAPY
The denuded papillary cores can be recognized by their residual capillary lumina (arrows). (Fig. 2-58 from Murphy WM. Diseases of the urinary bladder, urethra, ureters, and renal pelves. In: Murphy WM, ed. Urological pathology. Philadelphia: WB Saunders, 1989:34–146.)

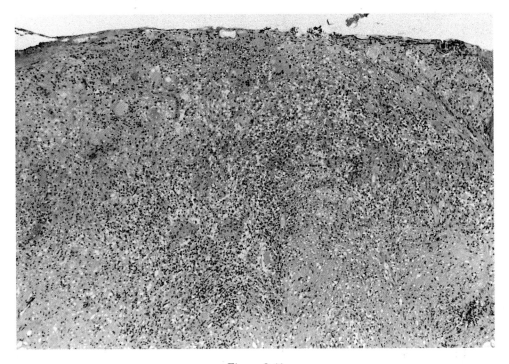

Figure 2-41
BLADDER EXPOSED TO TOPICAL BCG
There is denudation of the urothelium and a chronic inflammation with poorly formed granulomas in the lamina propria.

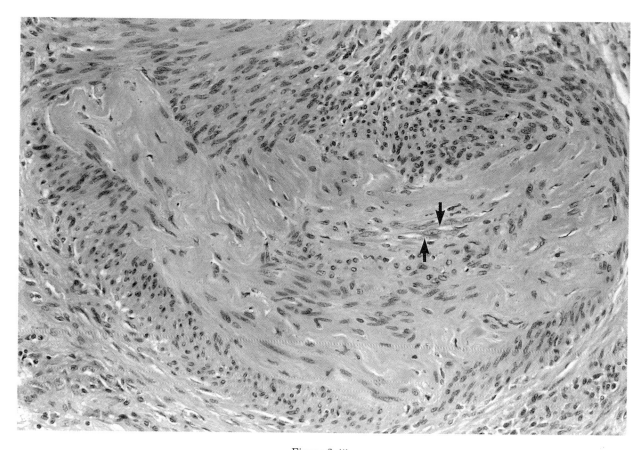

Figure 2-42
BLOOD VESSEL AFTER X-RAY THERAPY
Note the markedly narrow lumen (arrows) and thickened intima.

vessels. Endothelial swelling and necrosis are commonly observed soon after exposure of tissue to therapeutic doses of X rays. Marked mural thickening and hyalinization with luminal narrowing of blood vessels are late events (fig. 2-42). These changes are ordinarily accompanied by smoldering inflammation, nonhealing ulcers, lamina proprial edema, and interstitial fibrosis. So-called "radiation fibroblasts" are characteristic but not diagnostic of X-ray therapy. The bladder may be injured by X rays directed toward other pelvic organs (116,141). Atypical nuclear changes occurring in urothelial cells as well as several cases of both epithelial and stromal neoplasms have been recorded.

Urinary cytology is essential for the accurate monitoring of patients after treatment (73,116). Residual tumor is often undetectable endoscopi-cally, even when it occurs in areas accessible to the cystoscope. Biopsies sample only small portions of urothelium and are often denuded of diagnostic cells. Involvement of Brunn nests, prostatic ducts, distal ureters, and urethra are common and best evaluated by cytology. The appearance of malignant cells after an adequate course of therapy identifies patients at high risk for progressive disease.

Prognosis. The optimal approach to assessing the future course of a patient with a transitional cell neoplasm has not been established. There is general agreement that stage is the single most important factor, but accurate staging information is often available only in retrospect. Tumor configuration, multiplicity, size, DNA ploidy, growth fraction, marker chromosomes, and even overexpression of genes and gene products may have prognostic significance in certain situations (56,66,113,116,139,155,157, 160). The prognosis of patients with superficial transitional cell neoplasia is most profitably discussed in terms of the pathologic grade of the initial tumor (91,92,94).

Papillomas are benign by definition. Recurrences (actually new occurrences) of exophytic tumors appear in approximately 50 percent of cases but are usually of the same histologic grade as the primary lesion. The probability of progression is not directly related to either the frequency or total number of recurrences, although the overall frequency of progression among patients with recurrent papillomas is approximately 20 percent. Progression to high-grade transitional cell carcinoma has been recorded in fewer than 10 percent of patients presenting with papillomas (92,106). These patients then have the prognosis associated with the high-grade tumor. Death from bladder cancer has been observed in less than 5 percent of papilloma patients. It usually occurs more than 10 years after the initial diagnosis. Life-threatening events related to papillomas are rare and usually involve hemorrhage and infection resulting from neglected tumors. Papillomas respond favorably to almost any treatment. Successfully treated patients have a normal life expectancy.

The expected prognosis of patients with transitional cell carcinomas is greatly influenced by the classification system used. According to the guidelines in Table 2-3, low-grade carcinomas are predominantly papillary, noninvasive neoplasms associated with a 10- to 20-year actuarial survival of greater than 80 percent (92). Most deaths occur after 10 years of observation. In contrast, high-grade carcinomas are associated with a 10- to 20-year actuarial survival of 40 to 60 percent. When grade and stage have been specifically investigated, over 80 percent of all patients dying of transitional cell neoplasms have had high-grade tumors at the time of initial clinical recognition (92,95). Most of these patients had deeply invasive cancers but prognosis is unfavorable even among patients whose initial tumor is papillary and noninvasive.

Various treatments have been used for high-grade transitional cell carcinomas. The most popular are topical therapy for tumors localized to the epithelium or lamina propria and cystec- tomy for lesions involving the bladder wall or prostate gland. Statistical calculations indicate that life expectancy among all patients with transitional cell carcinoma is not normal even if the tumors are successfully treated (92).

Empirical observations of patients with CIS have produced contradictory results but much evidence suggests that primary CIS is a rather indolent neoplasm which does not spontaneously regress but invades sporadically and late (75,131). Cancer-related deaths at 10 years in the best studied populations have been less than 20 percent. As in all transitional cell neoplasms, prognosis is influenced by therapy (76,112). It is also directly related to the degree of bladder involvement at diagnosis. The prognosis of patients having CIS in association with other transitional cell neoplasms is generally unfavorable but the influence of the in situ cancer on the process is difficult to assess.

The course of patients with transitional cell neoplasms is influenced by a complex interaction of host- and tumor-related factors. The most accurate assessment is obtained by direct observation of patient outcome but this requires many years of monitoring during which diagnostic and treatment methods are constantly changing. Patients would benefit more if accurate predictions could be made at diagnosis and based upon the latest advances, but evaluation of the importance of new data requires time.

The current information indicates that: 1) the essential factors determining the growth and differentiation of a transitional cell neoplasm in any individual patient are established during the 25 to 30 cell generations required to produce a clinically recognizable tumor; 2) once established, these factors tend to remain constant in any individual, allowing prediction of future activity based upon previous behavior; 3) factors known to affect prognosis (stage, grade, multiplicity, DNA ploidy) are observed in combination rather than in sequence; 4) some prognostic factors are more predictive of future clinical course than others and most parameters are interrelated rather than independent; 5) the risk of progression is apparently not constant but decreases over time; and 6) the course of many patients with transitional cell neoplasms can be significantly modulated by medical intervention and prognosis can be expected to change as therapy becomes more effective.

SQUAMOUS CELL CARCINOMA

Definition. Squamous cell carcinomas comprise a group of urothelial neoplasms with histologic patterns and cytologic features of epidermis. As currently defined, these tumors must be sufficiently differentiated to have some combination of individual cell keratinization, keratin pearls, and intercellular bridges. Nonkeratinizing areas cannot be differentiated from high-grade transitional cell carcinomas and the distinction between mixed transitional cell–squamous cell carcinoma and pure squamous cell carcinoma in any particular case may be arbitrary. Despite the histologic definition of these tumors, the term "epidermoid" is not preferred, perhaps because it has been applied to transitional cell neoplasms in the past.

General Features. The etiology and pathogenesis of squamous cell carcinoma are best understood if cases are divided into those occurring de novo and those associated with long-term irritation of the bladder mucosa. More than 80 percent of cases occurring outside endemic areas of *S. hematobium* have arisen de novo (180,191, 194). Except for a high frequency of bacteriuria and symptoms suggesting mucosal irritation at diagnosis, there are no known predisposing factors among these patients. Concomitant or previous squamous metaplasia is uncommon and proliferative squamous lesions such as condyloma acuminatum or specific infections such as human papillomavirus are rare (184,195).

The frequency of squamous cell carcinoma among patients with long-term irritation of the bladder mucosa is sufficiently high to suggest that chronic irritation is a major etiologic factor. In regions endemic for *S. hematobium*, patients often develop chronically inflamed bladders loaded with calcified parasitic ova (178). Bladder cancer is a leading cause of death and approximately 75 percent of cases are of the squamous cell type. Increased frequencies of squamous carcinomas have been recorded among patients with nonfunctioning bladders requiring chronic indwelling catheterization, chronically infected diverticula, and bladder stones (175,187). Keratinizing squamous metaplasia (leukoplakia to the cystoscopist) is often present in the adjacent mucosa of patients with squamous cell carcinoma associated with long-term irritation. The lack of

squamous metaplasia in many such cases, the low frequency of squamous cancers among patients followed for squamous metaplasia, and the absence of significant cellular atypia in metaplastic lesions suggest that in most cases both the metaplasia and the carcinoma result from a common stimulus (176,189).

Most squamous cell carcinomas, even those arising in patients under medical surveillance for nonfunctioning bladders, are not detected until patients complain of hematuria or irritative bladder symptoms. By this time, the tumors tend to be large and deeply invasive. Urinary cytology is a potentially valuable method for monitoring high-risk patients but the literature contains few references to the efficacy of this technique (187).

Clinical Features. Squamous cell carcinomas comprise less than 5 percent of all urothelial neoplasms in most series but frequencies of 10 to 15 percent have been reported (180,181,191, 192). Compared to transitional cell neoplasms, squamous cell cancers are relatively more common in women: the male to female ratio in most series is less than 2 to 1. The disease may occur over a wide age range. Cases arising de novo are most common in patients aged 60 to 70 years; those occurring in association with chronic mucosal irritation appear somewhat earlier. Gross hematuria results in the detection of 70 percent of cases but at least one third of patients complain of dysuria, nocturia, frequency, or pain. Bacteriuria occurs in almost 50 percent of patients. Cystoscopy reveals nodular or plaque-like lesions with a shaggy white surface. In contrast to transitional cell neoplasms, squamous cell carcinomas are often widespread and involve areas other than the bladder base (177,191).

Pathologic Findings. Light microscopically, squamous cell carcinomas arise in the urothelium and infiltrate the underlying tissue in sheets, nests, and islands (figs. 2-43–2-46). Within each tissue configuration, the component cells tend to differentiate toward squamous epithelium reminiscent of epidermis, so that the periphery is composed of rather uniform basal cells which become keratinized as they progress toward the center or the surface. Keratinization of cells at the leading edge of a squamous cell neoplasm is a sign of invasion and can be an important feature in certain cases. Squamous cell carcinomas

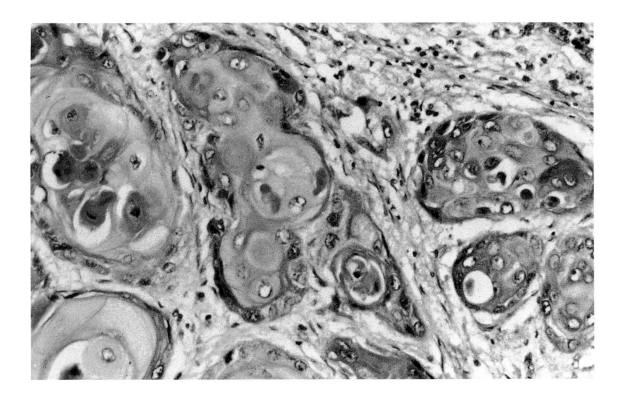

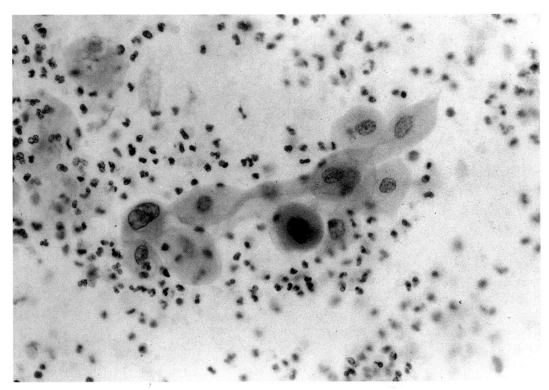

Figure 2-43
SQUAMOUS CELL CARCINOMA
Top: Nests of tumor cells with keratin pearl formation.
Bottom: Cytologic specimen with metaplastic squamous cells intermixed with neoplastic elements.

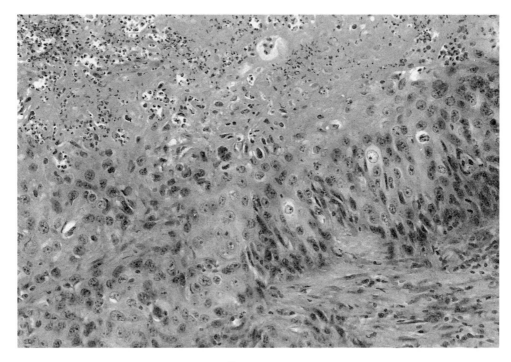

Figure 2-44
SQUAMOUS CELL CARCINOMA ARISING IN A BLADDER DIVERTICULUM
This is a poorly differentiated tumor with prominent necrosis.

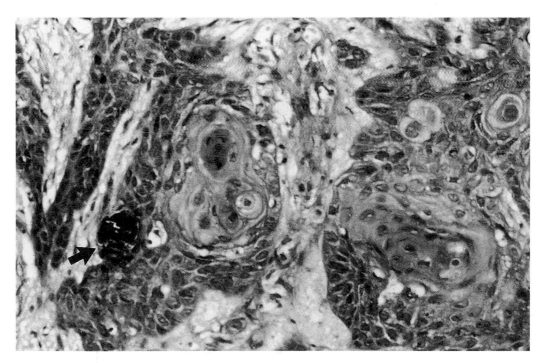

Figure 2-45
SQUAMOUS CELL CARCINOMA
This neoplasm is in a patient infested with *S. hematobium*. A calcified ovum (arrow) is present. (Courtesy of Dr. Samir N. Mina, Tanta, Egypt.)

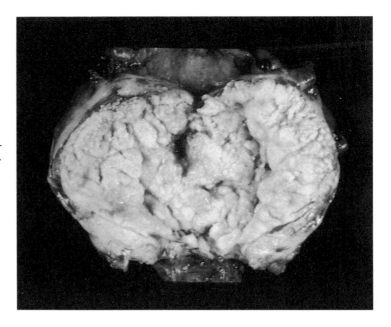

Figure 2-46
VERRUCOUS CARCINOMA OF BLADDER
In this gross specimen, the tumor nearly replaces the entire urothelium. (Courtesy of Dr. George M. Farrow, Rochester, MN.)

must be composed of some combination of well-defined intercellular bridges, individual cell keratinization, and keratin pearls or they are not pure squamous tumors. This requirement excludes very poorly differentiated cancers and may be a factor influencing the correlation between grade and prognosis.

The cells of squamous cell carcinoma are polygonal, with well-defined borders and amphophilic to acidophilic cytoplasm. Their nuclei are pleomorphic and occasionally bizarre, with irregularly distributed chromatin which may be either finely or coarsely granular. Prominent nucleoli and mitoses are common. Degenerated cells (dyskeratosis) are characteristic of squamous cell carcinoma.

Grading is based upon degree of keratinization and most schemes recognize three categories: well-, moderately, and poorly differentiated tumors (180,185,191,194). The value of this classification is confounded by several factors: most squamous cell carcinomas are large and deeply invasive at diagnosis; the most poorly differentiated cancers lack features of squamous differentiation; and tumors that closely resemble epidermis differ greatly from normal bladder mucosa and cannot be considered well differentiated if the host organ is used as the baseline. These factors probably account for the relatively low predictive value of grading and explain its indifferent acceptance among pathologists.

Squamous carcinoma cells appearing in urinary samples vary considerably in their morphology (186,190). The most characteristic elements are polygonal, fiber-like, or tadpole shaped. They have well-defined cellular borders and amphophilic to acidophilic, occasionally vacuolated cytoplasm (fig. 2-43). Nuclei are enlarged and slightly pleomorphic with irregularly distributed chromatin; often, they bulge into the adjacent cytoplasm instead of conforming to its elongated configuration. Nucleoli may be prominent but do not occur in most cells and are often obscured. More poorly differentiated cancers exfoliate cells indistinguishable from those of any high-grade neoplasm. Many neoplastic cells from squamous carcinomas are so well differentiated that they cannot be distinguished from squamous metaplasia, but almost all squamous cancers have some diagnostic cells in urinary samples. Degenerative changes are very common in these cells and many contain cytoplasmic vacuoles or pyknotic nuclei with condensed chromatin.

Special Techniques. A large number of squamous cell carcinomas have been examined for DNA ploidy using flow cytometry (193,196). Diploid DNA histograms have been recorded in 30 to 40 percent of cases. Most nondiploid tumors have distinct aneuploid peaks. Aneuploid cancers often have increased synthesizing fractions (S-phase). As expected, both ploidy and S-phase correlate with degree of nuclear anaplasia. Correlations with stage have been less clear. Chromosomal evaluation in at least one case revealed multiple aberrations, including abnormalities common in high-grade transitional cell carcinomas (188).

Variants of Squamous Cell Carcinoma. Squamous cell carcinoma may manifest heterogeneous patterns but the only histologically and clinically distinctive variant is *verrucous carcinoma*. This lesion is almost exclusively associated with *S. hematobium* infection, comprising approximately 3 percent of the bladder cancers arising in this group of patients (178,179). Rare examples unassociated with schistosomiasis have been recorded in single reports from patients with a condyloma acuminatum, diverticulum, and chronic infection (183,195). Like verrucous carcinomas at other sites, these tumors are indolent growths which spread by direct extension and do not metastasize. Histologically, verrucous carcinomas of the bladder resemble similar neoplasms at other sites (fig. 2-47). Acanthosis with rounded, "pushing" margins is characteristic. Slight cellular atypia may appear at the base or when the lesion is chronically inflamed but cellular anaplasia is not a feature. Mitoses are rare.

Differential Diagnosis. Squamous cell carcinomas must be differentiated from squamous metaplasia, condyloma acuminatum with nuclear atypia, mixed carcinomas with squamous components, and the verrucous variant. The presence of invasive nests and islands distinguishes squamous carcinoma from benign lesions with nuclear atypia and verrucous carcinoma. Diagnosis in the absence of clear-cut invasion depends primarily on the degree of cellular anaplasia since in situ squamous neoplasms have not been well defined in morphologic terms. Cases presenting diagnostic dilemmas in this regard are rare. More common is the problem of distinguishing pure squamous carcinomas from mixed lesions with squamous components (see differential diagnosis of high-grade transitional cell carcinoma). The diagnosis depends primarily on the proportion of tumor occupied by the questionable area. Pure squamous cell carcinoma must be composed almost entirely of neoplastic tissue differentiated toward keratinizing epithelium. As a practical matter, tumors presenting diagnostic difficulties are usually high stage and have similar prognoses and treatments regardless of the name appended to them.

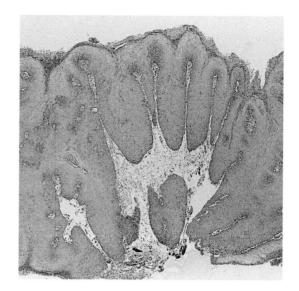

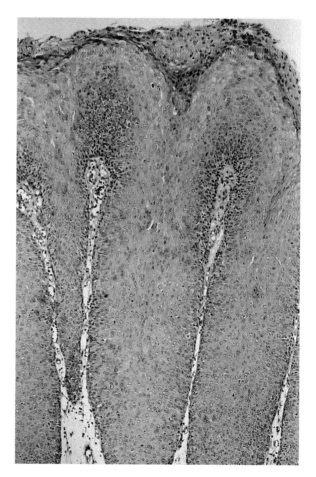

Figure 2-47
VERRUCOUS CARCINOMA
Top: The neoplasm is best appreciated at low magnification.
Bottom: Acanthosis and atypical parakeratosis without significant anaplasia or koilocytosis are characteristic.

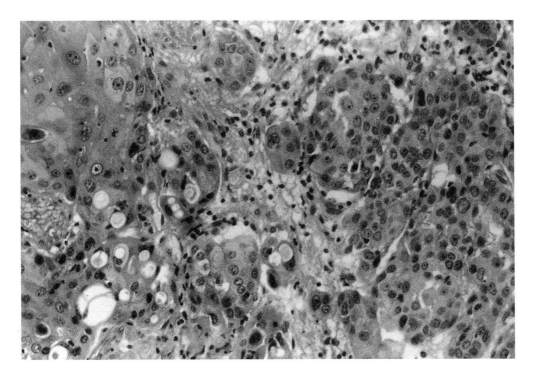

Figure 2-48
MIXED TRANSITIONAL CELL-SQUAMOUS CELL CARCINOMA
The transitional cell components of these lesions (right) are usually high grade and can be distinguished from the squamous components (left) by lack of the glassy acidophilic staining conferred by keratinization in the cytoplasm. (Fig. 84 from Murphy WM. Atlas of bladder carcinoma. Chicago: American Society of Clinical Pathologists Press, 1986:67.)

Mode of Dissemination. Most squamous cell carcinomas described in the literature have been large lesions at the time of detection (180,191,194). Invasion of the muscular wall was recorded in more than 80 percent. Prognosis has been poor although metastases are documented in only approximately 10 percent of cases. If these observations are accurate, it seems that squamous carcinomas grow locally, primarily as nodular lesions which invade the adjacent tissue rather than extending into the bladder lumen. Metastases are late events.

Staging. Squamous cell carcinomas have been staged according to a variety of methods (Table 2-7). The formulation of the AJCC-UICC is preferred (182).

Prognosis. Data on these patients, most of whom are older and present with bulky tumors often associated with chronic infections, are difficult to obtain. Most studies report crude 5-year survival rates of under 25 percent (180,191,194). At least one report cites a significant survival advantage for patients with diploid tumors (196).

MIXED CARCINOMA

Mixed carcinomas are urothelial neoplasms composed of two or more histologically distinctive components (197,198). These tumors comprise 4 to 6 percent of urothelial carcinomas. There are no characteristic general or clinical features. The most common lesions are composed of high-grade transitional cell and squamous cell carcinomas but any combination of glandular, poorly differentiated, squamous, and transitional cell carcinomas may occur (fig. 2-48). Mixed carcinomas tend to be large and deeply invasive at diagnosis. Cytology is useful for detection and monitoring, although each histologic component cannot always be discerned in urinary samples. The criteria for distinguishing mixed carcinomas from transitional cell carcinomas with small foci of squamous or glandular differentiation are not well defined (see differential diagnosis of high-grade transitional cell carcinoma). Prognosis depends primarily on stage at detection but may be influenced by the grade of the transitional cell component or the presence of poorly differentiated elements.

ADENOCARCINOMA

Definition. Adenocarcinomas are malignant glandular neoplasms histologically indistinguishable from similar tumors arising in the colon.

General Features. The etiology and pathogenesis of urothelial adenocarcinoma are unknown. Recognizing the close embryologic relationship of the bladder to the hindgut, the absence of intestinal differentiation in normal urothelium, the frequency of chronic mucosal irritation in association with adenocarcinoma, and the common occurrence of intestinal metaplasia in cancerous bladders, many experts accept the proposition that adenocarcinomas arise through a process of intestinal metaplasia stimulated by chronic irritation (217,218). This theory must be mitigated by the following factors: 1) some adenocarcinomas arise de novo without associated chronic irritation or intestinal metaplasia; 2) adenocarcinomas occurring in patients followed for intestinal metaplasia are rare and not all cancers arising in bladders with intestinal metaplasia are adenocarcinomas; 3) small amounts of intestinal metaplasia, such as occur in cystitis glandularis, have not been proven risk factors for subsequent malignancies; and 4) significant cellular atypia is uncommon in intestinal metaplasia, even in lesions adjacent to adenocarcinomas (199,200,206). Like squamous cell carcinomas, many adenocarcinomas probably arise as host reactions to long-term mucosal irritation and intestinal metaplasia is a commonly associated phenomenon. Whether metaplastic changes represent required precursors or concomitant lesions in glandular carcinogenesis is controversial. Most studies suggest that the risk of subsequent carcinoma is related to the degree of urothelial disturbance as reflected in the amount and distribution of intestinal metaplasia (200,211).

Among other factors associated with urothelial adenocarcinoma, exstrophy and persistent urachal remnants are most common. Exstrophy occurs when the cloacal membrane fails to properly differentiate, leaving the anterior abdominal wall, and thus the anterior bladder wall, undeveloped (211). Despite a markedly abnormal environment and widespread intestinal metaplasia, adenocarcinoma in exstrophied bladders is uncommon: it has been found in less than 10 percent of cases (204,211). Bladder cancers tend to occur late and are not confined to unrepaired defects, suggesting that carcinogenesis may be aborted and that even successful cancerous processes require time to develop and are not totally influenced by changing the mucosal environment to a more normal state.

In contrast to exstrophy, persistence of urachal remnants is a relatively normal condition and adenocarcinomas arising in such remnants, like similar tumors arising at the bladder base, are rare. Among urachal neoplasms, more than 80 percent are adenocarcinomas (202,206,211). Intestinal metaplasia is not a frequent associated finding although a few cases have arisen in association with cysts and villous adenomas. Adenocarcinomas arising in areas of urachal remnants differ clinically from those occurring at the bladder base, but these neoplasms are so similar in their pathology and behavior that they probably do not represent separate entities but a single group of cancers arising at different sites (206,211).

Adenocarcinomas, like most other bladder tumors, are usually not detected until patients recognize blood in their urine. Urinary cytology might be an important method for earlier detection but has received little attention in the literature.

Clinical Features. Adenocarcinomas comprise less than 2 percent of urothelial neoplasms (206,211,217). The majority (58 to 67 percent) arise at the bladder base, and almost all of the remainder occur in association with urachal remnants. Many clinical features vary with the primary site of the tumor (206). The male to female ratio of nonurachal neoplasms approaches 3 to 1 in contrast to almost 1 to 1 for urachal tumors. Adenocarcinomas may occur in young adults but most patients are middle-aged (mean approximately 62 years for nonurachal cases; 51 years for urachal cancers). Hematuria is the most common presenting sign, occurring in about 90 percent of patients regardless of the primary site of the tumor. Almost half of the patients with urachal neoplasms complain of irritative bladder symptoms (dysuria, nocturia, frequency, pain) whereas fewer than 15 percent with nonurachal neoplasms have these symptoms. Mucusuria is uncommon. Cystoscopically,

255

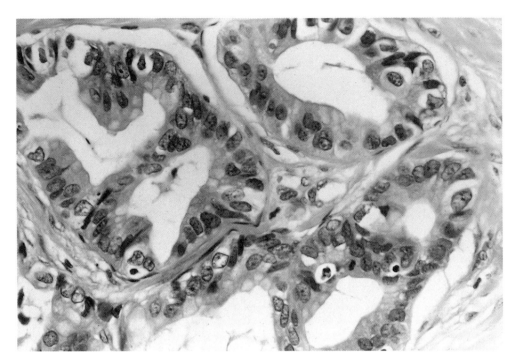

Figure 2-49
ADENOCARCINOMA ARISING IN THE URACHUS

adenocarcinomas ordinarily appear as single, nodular tumors which cannot be reliably distinguished from transitional cell neoplasms.

Pathologic Findings. Urothelial adenocarcinomas are histologically similar regardless of their primary site. Most are single lesions arising from the bladder mucosa but rare cases have extensively infiltrated the bladder wall with very little mucosal involvement. Urothelial adenocarcinomas cannot be distinguished from similar tumors of the colon and any histologic subtype common to the colon may occur in the bladder (figs. 2-49–2-51) (206,212). Most lesions have no distinctive histologic features and histologic subtyping has little significance to the patient so long as the signet ring pattern is considered an example of poor differentiation rather than a separate histologic entity.

Many authors classify the signet ring variant as a distinctive subtype of adenocarcinoma (205). When pure, these cancers are often diffusely infiltrating and high stage. Abnormalities in the urothelium are often difficult to find unless multiple sections are examined. Tumor cells with a characteristic signet ring appearance usually, but not always, react positively for mucins. As high-stage, usually unresectable malignancies, the signet ring type of bladder adenocarcinoma is associated with a particularly poor prognosis.

Adenocarcinomas produce colonic-type mucins in various amounts. Paneth cells and argentaffin cells have been identified in a few cases (211,214). Tumors react to antibodies directed to carcinoembryonic antigens and cytokeratins (206); rare cells react positively when exposed to antibodies to prostatic acid phosphatase (PAP) (203). Bladder adenocarcinomas have not contained cells reactive for both PAP and PSA.

Grading of urothelial adenocarcinomas has not been well accepted by pathologists, perhaps because only tumors with a significant number of signet ring cells have a distinctly different prognosis and almost all bladder adenocarcinomas are high stage at the time of clinical diagnosis. Like all nontransitional cell neoplasms, the normal standard for differentiation in adenocarcinomas is difficult to establish since the more a cancer resembles colon, the less differentiated it is if normal bladder is used as a baseline.

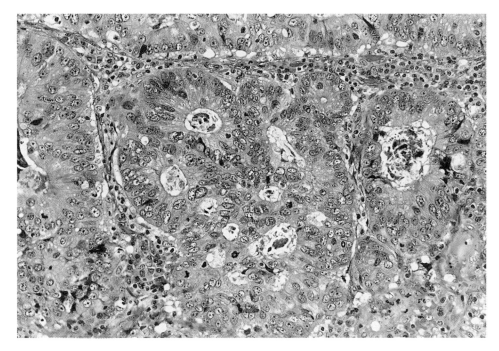

Figure 2-50
ADENOCARCINOMA ARISING IN THE BLADDER BASE

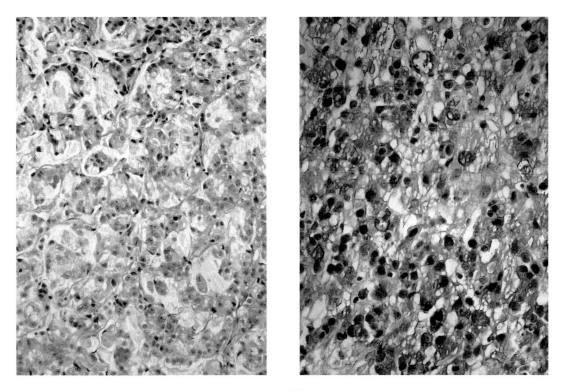

Figure 2-51
ADENOCARCINOMA

Left: Adenocarcinoma, mucinous type
Right: Adenocarcinoma stained with mucicarmine.

With few exceptions, the cells of bladder adenocarcinoma can be readily detected in urinary samples (208,210). Cancer cells are ordinarily of high cytologic grade but often lack features characteristic of glandular differentiation. Occasionally, adenocarcinomas may be so well differentiated that their disaggregated cells cannot be recognized as malignant in cytologic specimens.

Intraepithelial lesions with glandular differentiation are not well characterized. There are rare case reports, but the in situ lesions have been papillary rather than flat and are best considered villous variants (201,213). CIS associated with adenocarcinoma is rare and more often of transitional, rather than glandular, differentiation (206). Cystitis cystica and cystitis glandularis occur in approximately 50 percent of cases of adenocarcinoma located at the bladder base but are uncommon in association with urachal neoplasms. Significant cellular atypia in these areas of cystitis is uncommon.

Variants of Adenocarcinoma. Anecdotal reports, such as adenocarcinoma with hepatoid features, occur sporadically in the literature (215). If signet ring cancers are classified as poorly differentiated adenocarcinomas, the only well-characterized pathologic variants are clear cell carcinoma and villous tumors. Clear cell carcinoma is more common in the urethra and is discussed in that section.

Villous tumors are glandular neoplasms histologically indistinguishable from villous and tubulovillous adenomas and carcinomas of the colon (fig. 2-52) (201,202,209,213). These neoplasms are difficult to classify but can be considered particularly well-differentiated forms of adenocarcinoma. Almost all reports cite well-circumscribed tumors arising at the bladder dome; most are associated with histologically identifiable urachal remnants or cysts. Many tumors are larger than 4 cm in greatest dimension and some are locally invasive. A few lesions are associated with exstrophy, cystitis glandularis, chronic mucosal irritation, or even previous transitional cell neoplasms. Patients range in age from 18 days to 87 years, with most 40 to 60 years old. The male to female ratio is 2 to 1. Hematuria and mucusuria are the most common presenting signs. Follow-up information is incomplete in most reports, although complete surgical resection was achieved in almost all cases.

Special Techniques. DNA ploidy has been studied in a few bladder adenocarcinomas using flow cytometry (216). Diploid tumors accounted for 26 percent of cases, 21 percent were tetraploid, and 53 percent were aneuploid. There was no correlation with grade. Prognosis among patients with DNA diploid cancers was significantly better than for those with nondiploid lesions even though almost all cases were high stage.

Differential Diagnosis. Adenocarcinomas are characteristic neoplasms which present few differential diagnostic problems. Distinction from invasive colonic cancers or metastases with colonic differentiation cannot be achieved without appropriate clinical information. In rare cases, lesions resembling intestinal metaplasia may infiltrate the lamina propria or even the bladder wall. Despite their innocuous appearance, such lesions are best considered adenocarcinomas. In contrast, nodular areas of cystitis glandularis rich in goblet cells should be considered benign even if the nodules extend into the lamina propria. Adenocarcinomas must be distinguished from transitional cell neoplasms with glandular lumina. This distinction is somewhat arbitrary but not usually difficult if adenocarcinoma is defined as a malignant tumor differentiating toward colonic mucosa. Both types of lesions contain intracellular and luminal mucin, however, mucin is not abundant in the transitional cell lesion and goblet cell formation is not prominent. The "glands" of a transitional cell tumor with lumen formation are surrounded by cells with the pseudostratified appearance and superficial cell differentiation of transitional epithelium.

Mode of Dissemination. Long-term follow-up is not available for most reported cases of bladder adenocarcinoma. The available literature suggests that these lesions grow locally, primarily into the bladder wall rather than into the lumen. Intramucosal spread is uncommon (206). Well-documented metastases are infrequently cited even though most patient deaths are considered cancer related.

Staging. Almost all adenocarcinomas have invaded into the muscle wall at the time of diagnosis. Most previous reports have used some variation of the staging system of Marshall but the formulation of the AJCC-UICC is currently preferred (Table 2-7) (207).

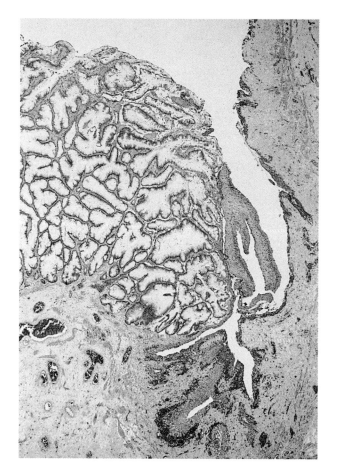 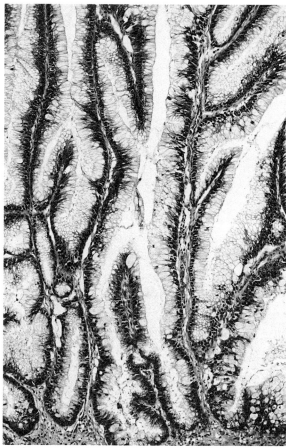

Figure 2-52
POLYPOID AND VILLOUS ADENOMA ARISING AT BLADDER DOME
Left: Low magnification of lesion.
Right: A predominantly villous area. (Both figures courtesy of Dr. Winfield Morgan, Morgantown, WV.)

Prognosis. Most reports cite a survival rate for bladder adenocarcinomas of 20 to 40 percent at 5 years but much of the literature on this subject is dated and the outlook for most current cases may not be so grim (206,211,217). Prognosis varies with stage, with survival approaching 75 to 100 percent among patients whose tumors are confined to the urinary bladder. Unfortunately, low-stage cancers account for fewer than 30 percent of reported cases. Except for the poor prognosis of signet ring cell tumors, correlation of prognosis with histologic type and grade has not been strong. Patients with urachal tumors tend to have a better short-term survival than those with nonurachal cancers, but the overall survival rate at 5 and 10 years is not significantly different (206).

POORLY DIFFERENTIATED CARCINOMA, SMALL CELL CARCINOMA

Definition. Poorly differentiated carcinomas are a group of malignant neoplasms that differentiate toward epithelium but lack well-formed epithelial structures. The best characterized poorly differentiated carcinoma is histologically similar to small cell carcinoma of the lung. Isolated case reports describing other lesions are listed under Rare Neoplasms.

General Features. The etiology and pathogenesis of small cell carcinoma of the urinary bladder are unknown. Pure small cell carcinomas are rare; almost half of reported cases describe mixed tumors with small cell components.

The rarity of the lesion and its relatively frequent occurrence in mixed carcinomas suggests an origin from a primitive precursor cell or aberrant differentiation of a transitional cell carcinoma in a patient with a marked deficiency in antitumor defense mechanisms. Although most lesions manifest some evidence of neuroendocrine differentiation and neuroendocrine cells may occur in normal bladders, histogenesis from a relatively mature neuroendocrine cell is not well accepted nor have small cell carcinomas been strongly associated with carcinoid tumors of the bladder (224). Cytologic detection of malignant tumor cells is readily achieved, although accurate typing is not always possible.

Clinical Features. Small cell carcinomas comprise less than 0.5 percent of all bladder neoplasms (219–221,224). Their clinical features do not differ from those of transitional cell carcinoma, even when mixed tumors are deleted from the evaluation. Evidence of neurosecretory differentiation is found in most cases but systemic disease related to functioning tumors is unusual (222,223). Almost all patients have large, deeply invasive tumors at diagnosis. Cystoscopically, small cell carcinomas are polypoid or nodular, often ulcerated masses which cannot be distinguished from other high-grade cancers. They may occur at various locations and are not predominantly localized to the bladder base (219).

Pathologic Findings. Pure small cell carcinomas of the bladder are histologically indistinguishable from similar cancers arising at other sites (fig. 2-53). The tumors are composed of loosely cohesive sheets of small, often overlapping cells with scanty cytoplasm. Necrosis is common. Nuclei may be oat shaped or polygonal. In optimal preparations, chromatin is coarsely granular and evenly distributed, and nucleoli are usually small or absent. Mitoses are variable but may be numerous. Many tumor cells are seen in cytologic samples. They tend to aggregate in loose clusters and have eccentric nuclei with scant cytoplasm. Chromatin is coarse but evenly dispersed. Nucleoli are usually lacking. The cells of small cell carcinomas are significantly larger than those of lymphomas. Nonspecific dense core granules have been observed in almost all lesions examined by transmission electron microscopy. Immunohistochemical studies have revealed various polypeptides in many cases. These in-

clude neuron-specific enolase, adrenocorticotropic hormone, synaptophysin, chromogranin, and serotonin. Most small cell carcinomas contain cytokeratins and a few have S-100 protein.

Differential Diagnosis. Small cell carcinomas usually occur in association with other histologic types of urothelial cancer and are most properly classed among the mixed carcinomas. Pure small cell carcinomas can be differentiated from lymphomas and sarcomas by their cell size, aggregation, and lack of large nucleoli. Carcinomatous changes in the urothelium and immunohistochemical reactions for cytokeratins and polypeptides can be helpful. Small cell carcinomas metastatic to the bladder cannot be differentiated from primary bladder tumors without appropriate clinical information.

Mode of Dissemination. In contrast to other urothelial neoplasms, small cell carcinomas are often metastatic at the time of clinical detection (219). Like other small cell carcinomas, metastases preferentially involve lymph nodes, liver, and bone.

Staging. Almost all small cell carcinomas are large and deeply invasive at diagnosis. In one large series, only one tumor was less than stage T3a (220).

Prognosis. Despite poor differentiation and high stage, not all small cell carcinomas of the urinary bladder are fatal (219–221,224). Although most patients die of disease soon after diagnosis, survival without evidence of disease has been recorded at 5 years in a few and 10 to 20 percent of tumors had not progressed at the time of citation in the literature. Outcome depends primarily upon response to treatment rather than the size of the neoplasm or the type of therapy.

RARE NEOPLASMS

Carcinosarcoma

Carcinosarcoma is a neoplasm comprising histologically malignant epithelial and stromal components. Similar cancers are called *malignant mixed mesodermal tumors* in other publications. The etiology and pathogenesis are unknown but immunohistochemical studies strongly suggest that these cancers arise from a common group of cells which differentiate toward heterologous tissues (226,227). The epithelial component may be the primary source of neoplastic activity but

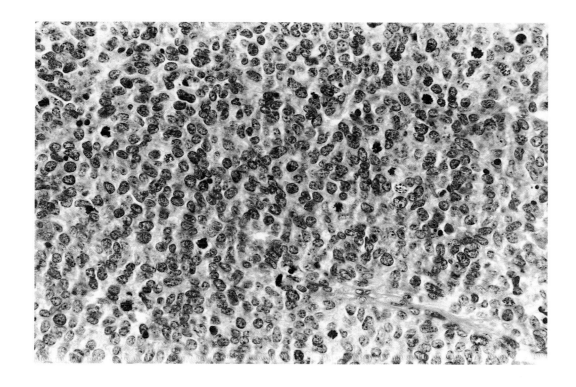

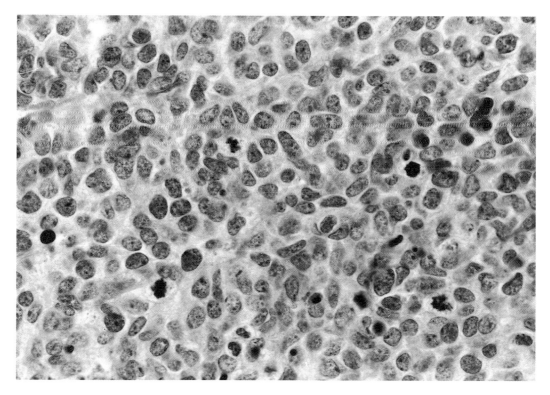

Figure 2-53
POORLY DIFFERENTIATED CARCINOMA, SMALL CELL TYPE
Top: At low magnification, these lesions are composed of uniform cells suggesting lymphoma or sarcoma.
Bottom: At higher magnification, numerous mitoses and lack of prominent nucleoli are conspicuous.

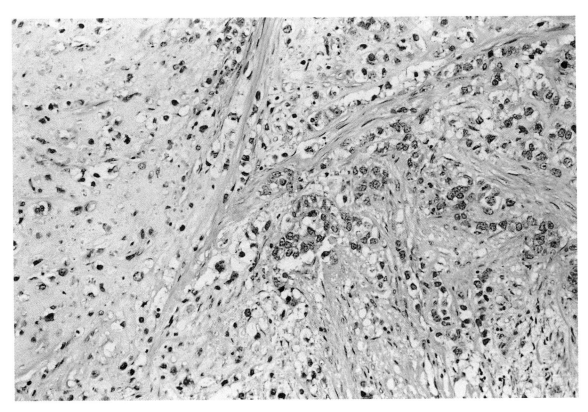

Figure 2-54
CARCINOSARCOMA
Glandular and chondrosarcomatous components are seen.

metastases composed of pure sarcomatous elements have been recorded (236). Rare cases have occurred following X-ray therapy (230).

Clinically, carcinosarcomas occur predominantly in men (male to female ratio of 3 to 1) aged 33 to 82 years (mean, 62 years) (240). Clinical signs and symptoms are nonspecific. Cystoscopically, the tumors are usually located at the bladder base where they appear polypoid and deceptively well circumscribed.

Pathologically, transitional cell carcinoma is the most common epithelial component. The most frequent stromal component is poorly differentiated and spindled but cartilaginous differentiation is very characteristic of bladder carcinosarcomas (fig. 2-54) (240). A variety of other histologic types of carcinomas and sarcomas have been recorded. If immunohistochemical studies performed on similar tumors arising at other sites are applied to the bladder, markers of epithelial differentiation can be expected in the sarcomatous compo-

nents of more than 50 percent of cases and markers of a mesenchymal phenotype will be common to the carcinomatous components (226,227).

The biphasic malignancy of carcinosarcomas distinguishes them from transitional cell carcinoma with spindle cell stroma, carcinomas with osseous or cartilaginous metaplasia, and sarcomas with pseudoepitheliomatous hyperplasia. Differentiation from sarcomatoid carcinoma is achieved if stromal elements other than poorly differentiated spindle cells are required for the diagnosis.

Carcinosarcomas are characteristically deeply infiltrative at initial presentation. An overall death rate of approximately 50 percent has been documented, but this figure is probably conservative since many reported cases had short follow-up and few patients have survived longer than 5 years (240). Most recorded deaths have resulted from complications of local growth rather than metastases. Metastases may contain both epithelial and mesenchymal components.

Carcinoid Tumor

Carcinoid tumors have been reported both as pure lesions and as small components of mixed carcinomas (238,239). Carcinoid tumors appearing in the bladder do not differ from those occurring at other sites. Diagnosis depends primarily upon recognition of the characteristic histologic patterns but can be corroborated with electron microscopy and studies to identify argentaffin and argyrophil cells. Carcinoid syndrome has not been reported among recorded cases. Despite its rather innocuous histologic appearance, carcinoid tumor of the urinary bladder is not always benign. At least one tumor-related death has been recorded.

Melanoma

Melanoma has been reported throughout the genitourinary tract, including the bladder (225, 229,232,237). These tumors do not differ histologically from similar lesions arising in the skin, and extravesical sources of a primary tumor must be excluded before the diagnosis can be confirmed. The pathogenesis is obscure. It is possible that rare individuals have bladders that contain melanocytes or that melanocytic differentiation infrequently occurs in otherwise normal bladders. Lesions are not localized to the bladder base and not all are pigmented. The disease has been uniformly fatal in recorded cases.

Lymphoepithelial Carcinoma

Cases of bladder carcinoma with a dense lymphoid infiltrate resembling lymphoepithelioma of the nasopharynx have been summarized in a single report (fig. 2-55) (244). Like other extremely rare tumors, the etiology and pathogenesis are probably more related to aberrations in individual host defense mechanisms than to specific carcinogenic influences. The diagnosis is confirmed using immunohistochemical reactions to identify the malignant epithelial component. Although the lymphoid infiltrate is benign, it may appear atypical by light microscopy. The reported tumors were large and invasive at diagnosis.

Plasmacytoid Carcinoma

Isolated reports have described bladder tumors composed of cells that resemble plasmacytes by light microscopy but are strongly positive for cytokeratin markers and negative for plasma-cyte markers by immunohistochemistry (235, 244). These tumors differ from lymphoepithelial carcinomas in that the tumor cells themselves, rather than a surrounding infiltrate, have lymphoma-like features. Unlike primary plasmacytomas of the bladder, these tumors do not produce or contain gamma globulins or light chains. Bone marrow, peripheral blood, and serum studies have been unremarkable. Recorded cases were inoperable at diagnosis.

Carcinoma with Spindle Cell Stroma

This tumor is distinguished by variable proportions of reactive stromal cells associated with transitional cell or squamous cell carcinoma (fig. 2-56) (229,233,242). The intimate admixture of elements and the occurrence of this histologic pattern in metastases and primary tumors militates against a chance association. In reported cases, the carcinoma was infiltrative or metastatic and of intermediate to high grade. The stromal reaction was comprised of loose aggregates of spindle cells reminiscent of proliferative fasciitis, inflammatory pseudotumor, or so-called giant cell cystitis. In fact, incompletely sampled cases have been misinterpreted as reactive processes. Immunohistochemical reactions for cytokeratins were negative in the spindle cell areas of all cases. Reactions for vimentin were uniformly positive. Muscle-specific actin was expressed in the spindle cells of most tumors. If tissue samples include both carcinomatous and spindle cell components, carcinoma with spindle cell stroma must be differentiated primarily from sarcomatoid carcinoma. The sharp demarcation between spindle and epithelial cells, lack of significant nuclear anaplasia among spindle cells, and negative reactions of the spindle cells to cytokeratin antibodies are distinguishing features.

Giant Cell Carcinoma

This rare malignant epithelial neoplasm resembles a giant cell carcinoma at other sites (fig. 2-57) (233,241). Both the large multinucleated cells and the smaller mononuclear cells contain epithelial markers. The giant cell component is prominent but is almost always associated with other poorly differentiated elements, such as spindle cells. These tumors should be differentiated

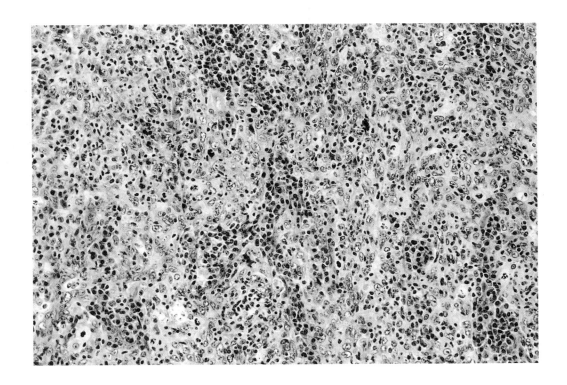

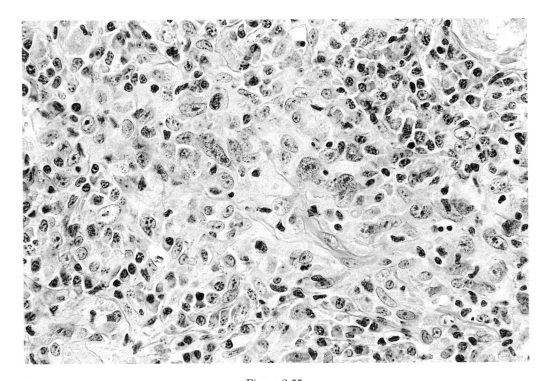

Figure 2-55
LYMPHOEPITHELIAL CARCINOMA

Top: At low magnification, the malignant epithelial elements are intimately intermixed with lymphoid tissue. (Courtesy of Dr. George Reichel, Lubbock, TX.)

Bottom: At higher magnification, the anaplastic epithelial cells are conspicuous. These cells reacted positively with antibodies to cytokeratins.

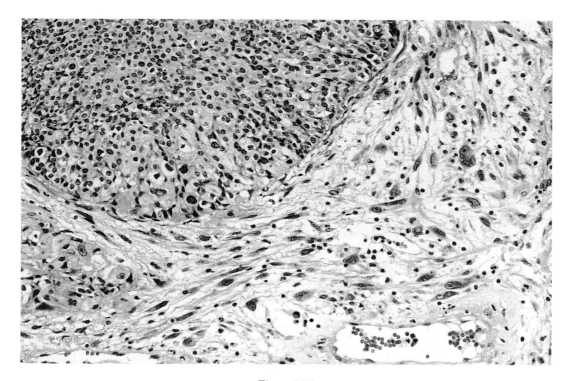

Figure 2-56
TRANSITIONAL CELL CARCINOMA WITH SPINDLE CELL STROMA
The marked atypia among the stromal cells is suggestive of neoplastic alteration. Immunohistochemical reactions for epithelial markers are negative, however. (Courtesy of Dr. Robert H. Young, Boston, MA.)

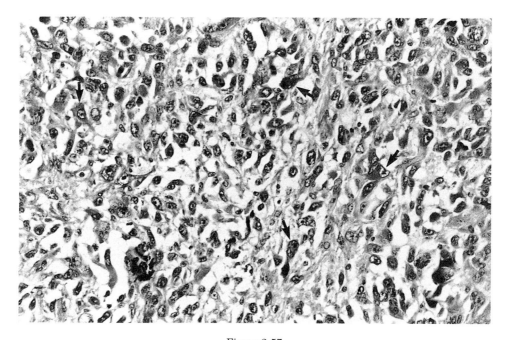

Figure 2-57
GIANT AND SPINDLE CELL CARCINOMA
Despite the name, the giant cells (arrows) are not particularly prominent. (Courtesy of Dr. Jonathan I. Epstein, Baltimore, MD.)

from transitional cell carcinomas with osteo-clast-type giant cells and the equally rare combination of transitional cell carcinoma and non-epithelial giant cell tumor of mesenchymal derivation (231,234,243).

METASTASES TO URINARY BLADDER

Extravesical tumors usually involve the urinary bladder by direct extension from adjacent pelvic organs such as the prostate gland, uterine cervix, and rectum. Metastases from distant sites are rare and almost always associated with widely disseminated disease (248). The most frequently recorded metastatic lesions have been melanomas and lymphomas, but a wide variety of malignancies have been observed (fig. 2-58). These include cancers of the stomach, breast, lung, kidney, pancreas, testis, appendix, ovary, uterus, gallbladder, and even tongue (245–253). Many cases are found at autopsy but patients may present with symptoms related to the metastatic bladder tumor. The urothelium is usually spared in metastatic bladder cancer, a situation that provides an important clue to the diagnosis. Bladder involvement by lesions that appear glandular or poorly differentiated but do not involve the urothelium should raise the suspicion of metastatic disease.

NONEPITHELIAL NEOPLASMS

Mesenchymal Neoplasms

Mesenchymal neoplasms are tumors differentiating toward muscle, nerve, bone, cartilage, fat, fibrous tissue, or blood vessels. They comprise less than 1 percent of all bladder neoplasms and may be histologically benign or malignant. The etiology and pathogenesis are unknown. With the exception of those with leiomyomas, most patients are men. Origin in the bladder usually produces hematuria and may result in dysuria or a palpable pelvic mass. Large tumors may produce urethral or ureteral obstruction and renal failure is a frequent serious complication. Mesenchymal tumors are ordinarily detected by pelvic examination and cystoscopy rather than cytology or radiography. Most present as polypoid growths with intact or focally ulcerated mucosal surfaces. Both benign and malignant tumors tend to grow

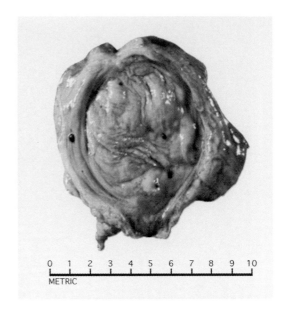

Figure 2-58
METASTATIC MELANOMA
Metastatic melanoma in the bladder with diffuse discoloration of the mucosa. The patient, a 31-year-old woman, had a melanoma removed from the skin approximately 1 year before her death from widespread metastases. (Plate IIIC from Fascicle 31a, 1st Series.)

locally. Dissemination in malignant lesions is usually a late event.

Mesenchymal neoplasms of the urinary bladder do not differ pathologically from similarly classified tumors arising at other sites and the pathologist confronted with such a case should consult a recent reference devoted to soft tissue tumors for details of histology, ultrastructure, and immunohistochemistry. Almost all histologic variants of mesenchymal tumors have been reported as primary bladder lesions, including leiomyoma, leiomyosarcoma, rhabdomyosarcoma, rhabdoid tumor, neurofibroma, ganglioneuroma, neurofibrosarcoma, granular cell tumor, osteosarcoma, chondrosarcoma, lipoma, liposarcoma, fibrosarcoma, benign and malignant fibrous histiocytomas, malignant mesenchymoma, adenofibroma, hemangioma, hemangiopericytoma, angiosarcoma, and lymphangioma (271, 278). Fibroma, rhabdomyoma, osteoma, and myxoma have been reported in the older literature but it is likely that the classification of these tumors would be disputed using current terminology (271). Mesenchymal tumors are rare in

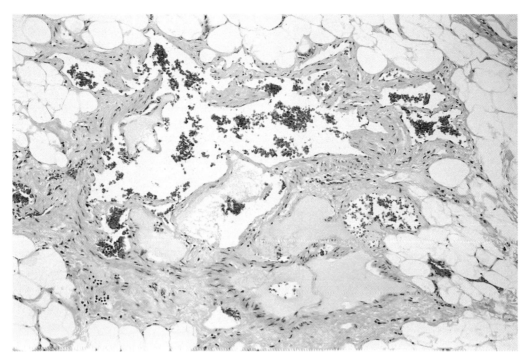

Figure 2-59
HEMANGIOMA OF THE URINARY BLADDER
This patient had clinical signs of the Klippel-Trenaunay syndrome.

the urinary bladder and only those that are most common, have peculiar features, or present especially difficult differential diagnostic problems are discussed.

Hemangioma. Hemangiomas of the bladder are generally considered congenital anomalies, although almost 50 percent of cases are detected in adults (256,265,278). Their importance is somewhat magnified in the bladder because transurethral resections have occasionally resulted in severe hemorrhage. Gross hematuria is the most frequent presenting sign, although bladder lesions may be discovered in patients with cutaneous, perineal, and genital hemangiomas. Vascular lesions of the bladder often occur in Klippel-Trenaunay syndrome (portwine hemangiomas, varicose veins, soft tissue and bone hemihypertrophy) (264). Patient age has varied from 5 weeks to 72 years. Lesions are usually single but may be multiple and occur anywhere in the bladder wall. They vary from a few millimeters to 10 cm in greatest dimension and are readily recognized cystoscopically. Histologically, most hemangiomas are of the cavernous type (fig. 2-59). Accurate interpretation is not difficult once the pathologist is mentally attuned to search for such rare lesions. Hemangiomas are differentiated from telangiectasias by their growth pattern, from arteriovenous malformations by lack of arterial structures, and from angiosarcomas by lack of significant endothelial atypia.

Myosarcoma. The most common mesenchymal tumors of the urinary bladder manifest features of muscle differentiation and can be considered myosarcomas (260,268,271,273,278). These neoplasms constitute less than 0.5 percent of all bladder tumors. In children, they are classified as *rhabdomyosarcomas* because some of the primitive cells comprising them have features of skeletal muscle differentiation (260). These bladder tumors have been observed in association with congenital anomalies of the brain and with nephroblastomas. A few have occurred in fetuses. Rhabdomyosarcomas in children most often affect boys (sex ratio, 3 to 1). They tend to grow as polypoid masses which may obstruct the urinary outflow. When this configuration resembles a bunch of grapes, the term *botryoid sarcoma* is used (fig. 2-60). Histologically, rhabdomyosarcomas characteristically have a "cambium" layer

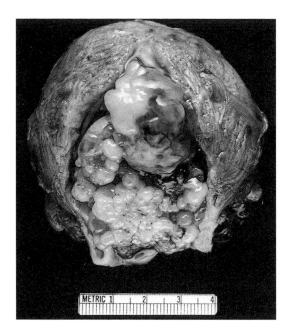

Figure 2-60
RHABDOMYOSARCOMA, BOTRYOID TYPE
The analogy to a bunch of grapes is apropos. (Courtesy of Dr. George M. Farrow, Rochester, MN.)

Table 2-8

IMMUNOHISTOCHEMISTRY IN THE DIFFERENTIAL DIAGNOSIS OF SPINDLE CELL TUMORS OF THE BLADDER

	CKs*	Actin	Desmin	Vim**
Leiomyosarcoma	–	+	±	+
Sarcomatoid carcinoma	+	–	–	±
Leiomyoma	–	+	+	+
IP/PSCN†	±	±	±	+

*CKs = cytokeratins.
**Vim = vimentin.
†IP = inflammatory pseudotumor; PSCN = postoperative spindle cell nodule.

of compressed rhabdomyoblasts immediately beneath an intact urothelium. Masses of stellate, round, and spindle cells occupy an edematous stroma rich in hyaluronic acid (fig. 2-61). The cytoplasm of the rhabdomyoblasts is scanty and cross striations are very difficult to identify in untreated cases. These tumors grow locally and recur if inadequately excised. Survival is increasingly favorable and several patients are alive more than 20 years after treatment.

Myosarcomas in adults generally have features of smooth muscle differentiation and are classified as *leiomyosarcomas* (268,271,273, 278). Patients of all ages may be affected but most are 40 to 60 years old. Men predominate in a ratio of 3 to 2. Tumors are often poorly circumscribed and invasive with ulcerated surfaces (figs. 2-62, 2-63). These cancers do not differ histologically from similar lesions at other sites except that the myxoid variant is reported with increasing frequency. Adult myosarcomas tend to grow locally but have a higher frequency of metastases than their childhood counterparts. The dismal prognosis reported in the older literature has not been observed in more recent series (255).

Differentiating leiomyosarcomas from other neoplasms and benign inflammatory conditions can be extremely difficult. Immunohistochemical and ultrastructural features are helpful but it should be emphasized that relatively few cases have been analyzed by these techniques (Table 2-8). Leiomyosarcomas are distinguished from sarcomatoid carcinomas by a lack of epithelial markers and islands of epithelial differentiation. They differ from leiomyomas primarily in their infiltrative growth pattern, although the increased mitotic rate and nuclear pleomorphism are often helpful clues. Distinction from inflammatory pseudotumors and postoperative spindle cell nodules may be difficult, especially since these benign inflammatory lesions can be large and infiltrative (see Non-neoplastic Tumorous Conditions). In the absence of a history of recent surgery, the most important clue is the destructive infiltrative margin characteristic of leiomyosarcomas. Other features indicating malignancy are areas of necrosis within the tumor rather than on its surface, high cellularity, nuclear pleomorphism, and abnormal mitoses. Some leiomyosarcomas, especially those of myxoid type, differ very little from some inflammatory pseudotumors and it is not yet completely clear whether a pathologic distinction can be made in every case. Doubtful cases are best considered low-grade neoplasms and treated accordingly.

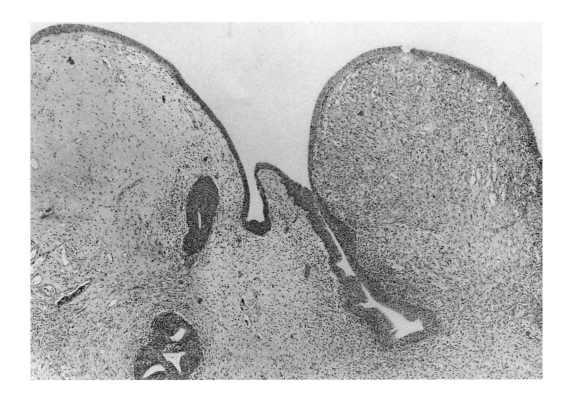

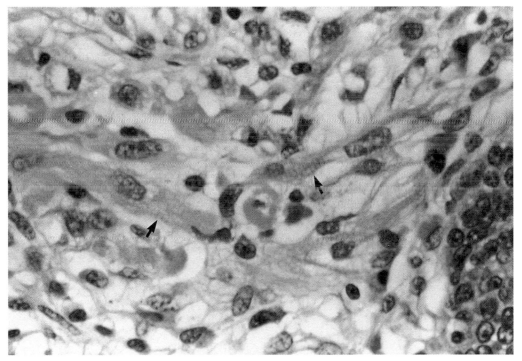

Figure 2-61
RHABDOMYOSARCOMA
Top: Polypoid surface of a rhabdomyosarcoma arising in the bladder of a child. (Courtesy of Dr. David Parham, Memphis, TN.)
Bottom: Higher magnification revealing a few cells with cross striations (arrows). (Fig. 2-62 from Murphy WM. Diseases of the urinary bladder, urethra, ureters, and renal pelves. In: Murphy WM, ed. Urological pathology. Philadelphia: WB Saunders, 1989:106.)

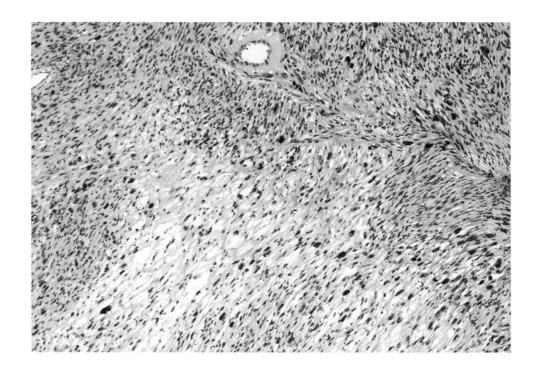

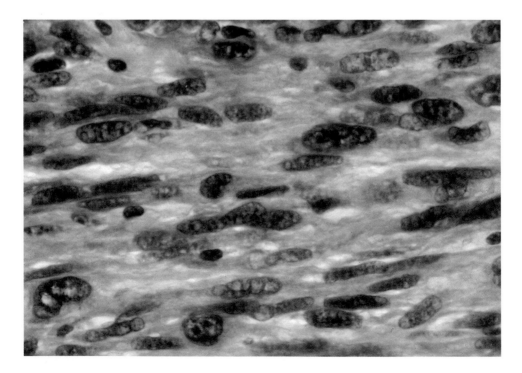

Figure 2-62
LEIOMYOSARCOMA OF THE BLADDER
Top: Even at low magnification, the nuclear pleomorphism of this high-grade tumor is evident.
Bottom: Higher magnification reveals typical smooth muscle cell nuclei.

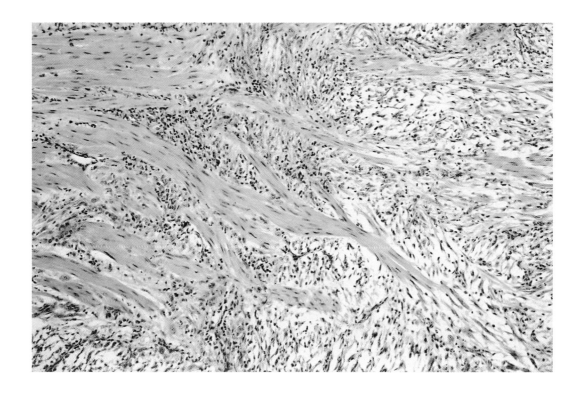

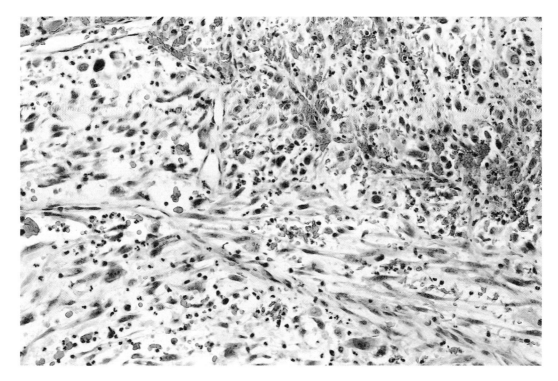

Figure 2-63
LEIOMYOSARCOMA, MYXOID TYPE

Top: This well-differentiated neoplasm looks like an inflammatory pseudotumor at low magnification.
Bottom: At higher magnification, there is significant nuclear atypia and necrosis.

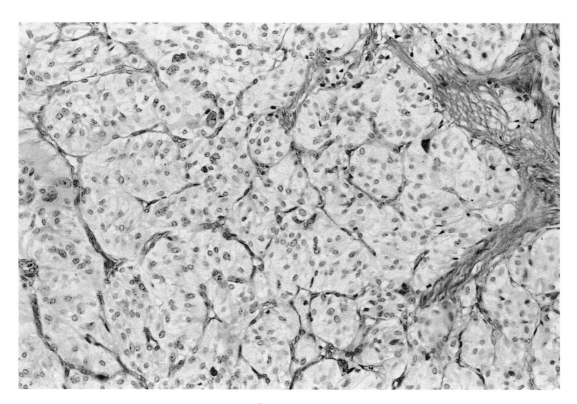

Figure 2-64
PHEOCHROMOCYTOMA
(Courtesy of Dr. Albert S. Hollingsworth, Anderson, SC.)

Pheochromocytoma (Paraganglioma)

Pheochromocytoma is the most common designation for a paraganglioma arising in the urinary bladder (271,278). These tumors comprise less than 0.1 percent of all bladder neoplasms. Rare cases have been associated with neurofibromatosis, transitional cell carcinoma, and renal cell carcinoma but bladder pheochromocytomas have not been observed as part of the multiple endocrine neoplasia syndrome. Patients have been aged 11 to 78 years (mean, 41 years). These tumors are slightly more common in females (sex ratio, 1.4 to 1). Hematuria is a common complaint but more than 50 percent of patients experience symptoms that can be directly related to the release of catecholamines from their tumors. Discomfort tends to be associated with a full bladder or voiding. The most characteristic symptom complex is the "micturition attack," consisting of bursting headache, anxiety, tremulousness, pounding sensation, blurred vision, sweating, and even syncope. Hypertension is observed in most individuals. Catecholamines or their metabolites are elevated in serum or urine in at least 50 percent of patients examined for these substances.

Pheochromocytomas, unlike most other bladder tumors, are not necessarily localized to the bladder base but occur anywhere in the organ. Most are single lesions measuring only a few millimeters in greatest dimension, but multiple and large tumors have been recorded. Small aggregates of paraganglionic cells occurring in the lamina propria may be mistaken for Brunn nests. Histologically, pheochromocytomas almost always assume the characteristic "zellballen" pattern but fibrous and ganglioneuromatous arrangements have been observed (fig. 2-64). Vascular invasion has been recorded. Cells tend to be round with amphophilic to acidophilic cytoplasm and ovoid nuclei. Occasional bizarre nuclei, such as seen in other neuroendocrine neoplasms, may be present. Mitoses are uncommon. Occasional foci of neuroblast-like cells occur. Ultrastructurally, dense core granules are common.

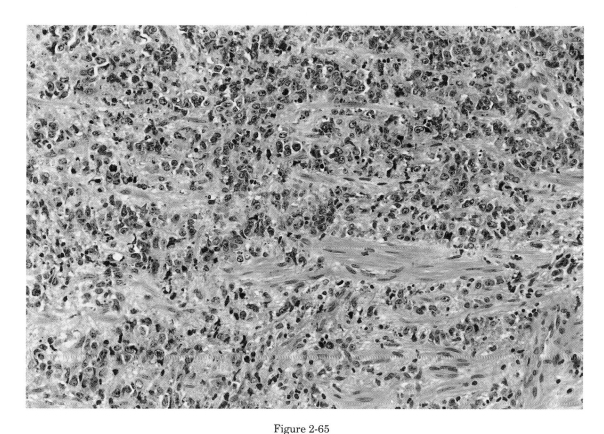

Figure 2-65
LYMPHOMA
The tumor cells separate and surround rather than destroy the smooth muscle fascicles of the bladder wall.

Characteristically, pheochromocytomas contain a combination of neuroendocrine and sustentacular cells which react with neuron-specific enolase and S-100 protein, respectively. Chromogranin is a commonly employed positive marker. Other substances identified in these tumors include adrenocorticotropin (ACTH), calcitonin, gastrin, glucagon, serotonin, somatostatin, vasoactive intestinal polypeptide, and glial fibrillary acidic protein (270). Flow cytometric studies performed on a few cases revealed aneuploid and tetraploid patterns (262).

The behavior of pheochromocytomas cannot be accurately predicted from pathologic examination alone. Multiple recurrences, nuclear anaplasia, vascular invasion, abnormal DNA ploidy, and an invasive growth pattern might identify patients at increased risk but none of these features are highly predictive of future progression. Nevertheless, between 5 to 15 percent of pheochromocytomas metastasize.

Lymphoma

Bladder involvement has been documented in 10 to 25 percent of lymphomas and leukemias but lymphoid neoplasms arising primarily in the urinary bladder are rare (263,271,278). The disease is usually detected in middle-aged women undergoing cystoscopy for nonspecific urinary symptoms but may present as a pelvic mass. Grossly, bladder lymphomas usually appear as discrete tumors rather than diffuse infiltrates. Most are large masses centered in the dome or lateral walls. Microscopically, infiltrating sheets of uniform cells surrounding and separating, rather than destroying, muscle fascicles are characteristic (fig. 2-65). Cytologic features do not differ from those of lymphomas at other sites. Well-differentiated lymphocytic lymphomas of B-cell type are the most common, although poorly differentiated lymphocytic, large cell, and even sarcomatous and signet ring varieties have been

273

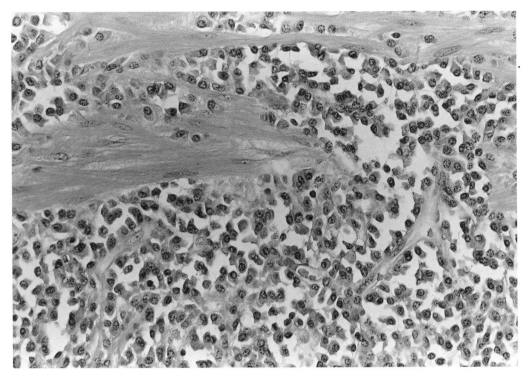

Figure 2-66
PLASMACYTOMA OF THE URINARY BLADDER

observed (258,261,274). A single case of primary Hodgkin disease of the bladder seems well documented (266). The prognosis of primary bladder lymphoma has been favorable, with many patients alive and well several years after treatment. Prolonged survival probably reflects the low grade and stage of most tumors. Well-differentiated lymphocytic lymphomas of the urinary bladder pose few differential diagnostic problems to knowledgeable observers once systemic disease is excluded. There appears to be no relationship to follicular cystitis and pseudolymphoma of the bladder has not been well documented. More poorly differentiated lymphomas can be differentiated from small cell cancers by reactions for intermediate filaments such as cytokeratins, leukocyte common antigen, and vimentin.

Plasmacytoma

Plasmacytomas arising in the urinary bladder are rare and all information concerning these neoplasms is derived from case reports (259,278, 279). The few recorded patients are both men and women ranging in age from 39 to 89 years.

Signs and symptoms are nonspecific. Like plasmacytomas at other extramedullary sites, these lesions look and act more like solid tumors than lymphoproliferative neoplasms. Depending on size and cellular activity, monoclonal immunoglobulins may occur in serum and urine; this finding should not necessarily indicate disseminated disease in the case of an unresected tumor. Plasmacytomas may present as single or multiple nodular masses in the bladder wall (fig. 2-66). Histologically, a wide range of mature and immature forms, including giant and multinucleated cells, may occur. Immunoglobulins A and G as well as both kappa and lambda light chains have been documented in individual cases. Although often difficult to identify immunohistochemically in paraffin-embedded tissue, the presence of immunoglobulins is an important distinguishing feature, especially since plasmacytomas can resemble various poorly differentiated cancers when examined using routine histologic preparations. Prognosis is favorable. Recurrences have been reported but no patient has died of a plasmacytoma arising in the bladder.

Germ Cell Tumors

Germ cell tumors arising in the urinary bladder include *choriocarcinoma, dermoid cyst, teratoma,* and *yolk sac tumor* (271,278). Most reports have described choriocarcinomas (254,267,269). These neoplasms occur as distinctive histologic components of poorly differentiated urothelial carcinomas, although metastases of pure choriocarcinoma have been observed. This suggests a histogenesis involving extreme heterogeneity of epithelial differentiation, perhaps in a host with peculiar deficiencies in tumor defenses. Bladder choriocarcinomas should be differentiated from high-grade transitional cell or poorly differentiated carcinomas with isolated syncytiotrophoblastic giant cells. Interestingly, the majority of patients are men and even the women are postmenopausal. Prognosis is dismal: all reported patients with more than a few months follow-up have died of their disease.

Dermoid cysts have been described in the bladders of women 30 to 49 years of age (257, 278). These tumors do not differ clinically or histologically from their ovarian counterparts. Isolated case reports of teratoma and yolk sac tumor have been recorded (273,276,277).

NON-NEOPLASTIC TUMOROUS CONDITIONS

Non-neoplastic tumorous conditions constitute a vast array of lesions described under various names by individuals with diverse views on the nature of disease. Some tumorous lesions are common and others rare. Most pose no diagnostic problems for experienced pathologists and are described primarily for the sake of completeness. A few are relatively new entities which require a discussion whose length may not be commensurate with their future importance. The following section briefly describes lesions that appear as discrete, space-occupying plaques or nodules arising in the urinary bladder. More complete discussions can be found in texts not limited to the pathology of tumors of the bladder (304,321).

Condyloma Acuminatum

Condyloma acuminatum is a characteristic proliferation of squamous cells that is highly associated with human papillomavirus (HPV) infection (287,305,322,323). Bladder involvement ordinarily occurs by direct extension from urethral lesions. Primary condyloma acuminatum of the urinary bladder is rare. The lesion does not differ histologically from similar tumors at other sites. Using sophisticated techniques that detect the presence of a few gene copies, viral DNA of HPV subtypes 6 and 11, but not 16 and 18, have been demonstrated in primary bladder condylomas. Structural viral antigens are rarely observed. Condyloma acuminatum may be distinguished from squamous cell papilloma in histologic preparations if the presence of typical koilocytes is required for the diagnosis. The lesions are very similar, however, and their relationship is unclear. Moderate nuclear atypia may occur in both lesions but areas of cellular anaplasia are not present. Condyloma acuminatum and squamous cell papilloma are distinguished from verrucous carcinoma primarily by the extent of bladder involvement since none of these lesions has unequivocally invasive margins and all lack significant cellular anaplasia.

Metaplasia

Metaplastic lesions of the urinary bladder exist in three basic types: squamous, intestinal, and nephrogenic. Osseous and cartilaginous metaplasias may also occur but are rare. Metaplastic changes can be considered reflections of a deranged urothelial response to injurious stimuli. They are often associated with structural defects and sources of chronic irritation. It is not uncommon for various types of metaplasia to coexist and for metaplasias to coexist with proliferative reactions of Brunn nests. The risk for subsequent cancer among patients with metaplasia varies with the type of metaplasia as well as its duration and extent.

Squamous Metaplasia. This is the replacement of normal urothelium with stratified squamous cells (fig. 2-67). Lesions resembling vaginal epithelium are so common in females that many authors consider this change to be normal (320). The vaginal type of squamous metaplasia apparently arises de novo. It is usually not associated with chronic irritation and the risk for subsequent carcinoma is very low (319). In contrast, the keratinizing type of squamous metaplasia (leukoplakia) is usually associated with sources of chronic irritation and occurs more commonly

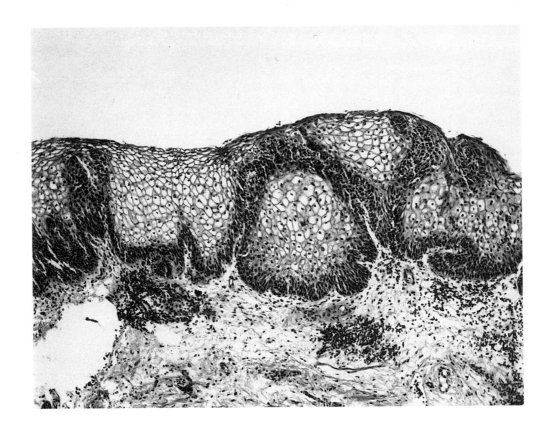

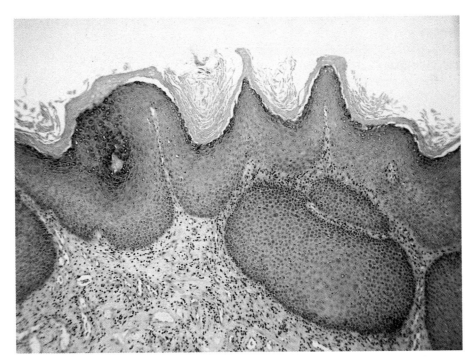

Figure 2-67
SQUAMOUS METAPLASIA OF THE URINARY BLADDER
Top: Vaginal type.
Bottom: Keratinizing type. (Both figures courtesy of Dr. George M. Farrow, Rochester, MN.)

in men (281). It is especially frequent in bladders with chronic indwelling catheters, stones, or calcareous material. Considerable cellular atypia, especially in the basilar layers, may occur and persist for long periods of time without the development of invasive carcinoma. The degree of intraepithelial atypia required for a pathologic diagnosis of squamous cell carcinoma in situ has not been determined. Areas of anaplastic nuclear change in the absence of invasion are distinctly unusual, however. Nodular and papillary squamous lesions suggestive of condyloma acuminatum or squamous cell papilloma may develop in the urinary bladder, especially among patients with sources of chronic irritation.

Intestinal Metaplasia. This describes the appearance of colonic-type glands or mucin-containing goblet cells in the urinary bladder (292, 304,305,317,323). This change exists in two major forms. Most commonly, a few colonic-type glands or isolated goblet cells appear in a proliferation of Brunn nests. This lesion is commonly called *cystitis glandularis* (fig. 2-68). Intestinal metaplasia of this type is easily recognized in histologic preparations and apparently has no significant association with bladder neoplasia. Rarely, relatively large areas of urothelium may be completely replaced by intestinal mucosa (284). The most extreme example occurs in exstrophy. The intestinal glands lack significant cytologic atypia but more closely resemble hyperplastic or early adenomatous changes than normal colonic mucosa (fig. 2-68). This type of intestinal metaplasia is highly associated with bladder carcinoma, usually of the glandular type. Whether focal or widespread, intestinal metaplasia seems to be an acquired change manifested in chronically irritated urothelium.

Nephrogenic Metaplasia (Nephrogenic Adenoma). This is a peculiar reactive process resulting in the formation of papillary and tubular growths reminiscent of immature urothelial or metanephric structures (288,293,302,305). Like squamous and intestinal metaplasia, these changes are almost always associated with sources of chronic irritation, such as recurrent infections. They are especially common in diverticula and at sites of previous surgery. The papillary component is usually mistaken for a transitional cell carcinoma cystoscopically but can be differentiated from a neoplasm histologically by the presence of a single layer of cytologically bland cuboidal cells lining the stalks (fig. 2-69). Significant nuclear atypia is unusual in nephrogenic metaplasia and focal even when present. When nephrogenic metaplasia occurs in diverticula and at previous surgical sites, the lesions ordinarily lack the papillary component and are composed solely of tubules. Such lesions may resemble prostatic carcinomas but can be distinguished by their histologic pattern and lack of prostatic antigens in immunohistochemical reactions. Nephrogenic metaplasia can be distinguished from clear cell carcinoma by its lack of widespread nuclear anaplasia (324). Despite a tendency to recur, nephrogenic metaplasia is not a significant risk factor for subsequent carcinoma.

Inflammation

The urinary bladder may manifest a complex array of reactions to a variety of injurious stimuli (305). Pathologic lesions are often poorly correlated with clinical disease even though their morphology may be distinctive. Inflammatory reactions seem to be host dependent, since the same stimulus can cause different lesions and different stimuli often result in the same lesions among individual patients. Many reactive processes have been termed "cystitis," even though most such lesions lack a significant component of leukocytic infiltration and some represent hyperplastic or metaplastic alterations of normal structures. The nodular lesions categorized as cystitis are different from other types of inflammation and are discussed separately. Lesions described in this section include postoperative spindle cell nodule, inflammatory pseudotumor, malakoplakia, and granulomas that arise primarily in the urinary bladder.

Postoperative Spindle Cell Nodule. This increasingly recognized myofibroblastic proliferation arises within a few months of a previous surgical procedure at the surgical site (296,308, 323). Most lesions involve the genital tract of women and the periurethral prostatic tissue of men. Postoperative spindle cell nodules (PSCN) of the urinary bladder are usually small (less than 1 cm), poorly defined nodules occurring in men followed for transitional cell carcinomas. These lesions histologically resemble nodular fasciitis and inflammatory pseudotumor (fig. 2-70). Characteristic changes include interlacing

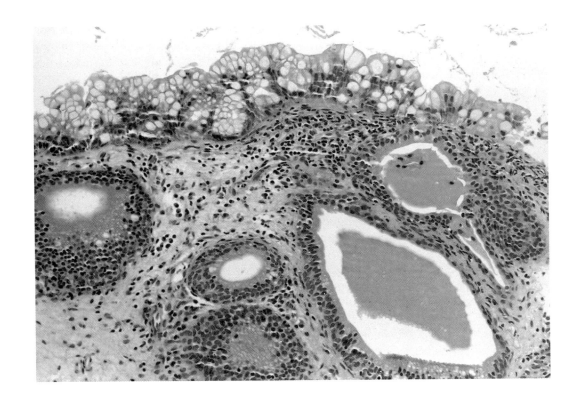

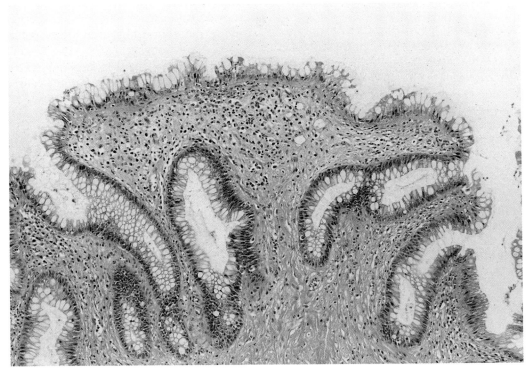

Figure 2-68
INTESTINAL METAPLASIA
Top: Surface goblet cells in association with glandular distention of Brunn nests.
Bottom: Intestinal metaplasia replacing urothelium.

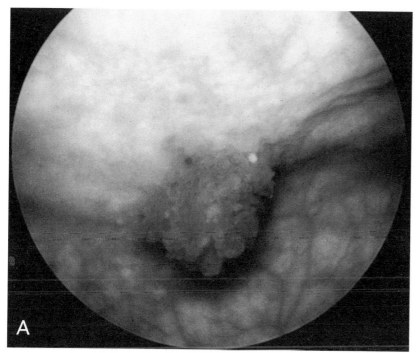

Figure 2-69
NEPHROGENIC METAPLASIA
A: Cystoscopic photograph emphasizing the papillary appearance. (Courtesy of Dr. Mark S. Soloway, Miami, FL.)
B: Papillary component of nephrogenic metaplasia. (Fig. 146 from Murphy WM. Atlas of bladder carcinoma. Chicago: American Society of Clinical Pathologists Press, 1986.)
C: Tubular component.

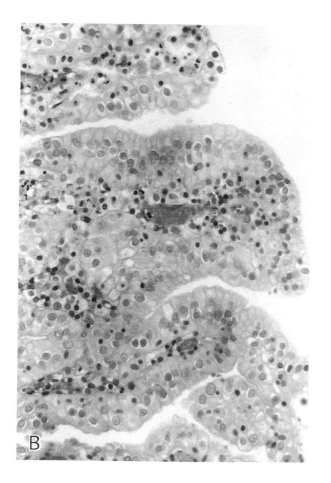

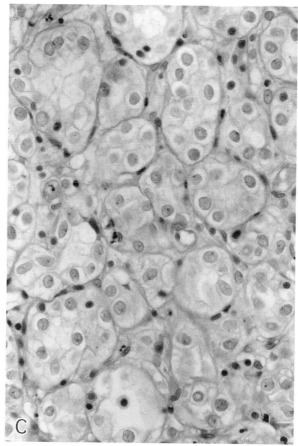

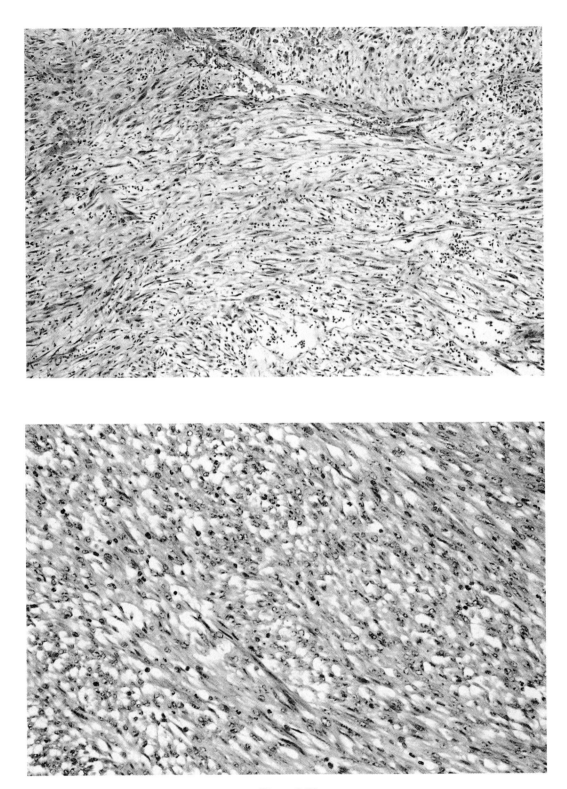

Figure 2-70
POSTOPERATIVE SPINDLE CELL NODULE

Top: A typical lesion with interlacing fascicles of myofibroblastic tissue.

Bottom: At higher magnification, the cells are uniform and intermixed with inflammatory elements. (Both figures courtesy of Dr. Charles Slonaker, Gulfport, MS.)

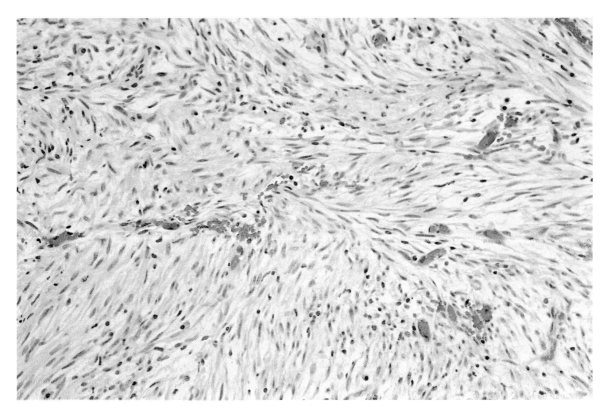

Figure 2-71
INFLAMMATORY PSEUDOTUMOR
These lesions are histologically similar to postoperative spindle cell nodules. Note the abundance of thin-walled blood vessels.

fascicles of spindle cells, areas rich in thin-walled blood vessels, and a sparse but uniformly distributed polymorphous leukocytic infiltrate. Mitoses may be numerous but are not atypical. Myxoid areas are often present. Infiltration of the detrusor muscle may occur but necrosis at the invading margin is not a feature of PSCN. Immunohistochemical and ultrastructural studies confirm a myofibroblastic differentiation but positive reactions to cytokeratins have also been recorded (Table 2-8) (318).

Inflammatory Pseudotumor. This is a nodular reaction of myofibroblasts which differs from PSCN primarily in the absence of a history of previous surgery (289,311,323). The name is misleading in that the lesions are tumors in the sense of space-occupying masses but an inflammatory etiology or pathogenesis has not been proven. The designation *pseudosarcomatous fibromyxoid tumor* is more accurate but is not widely accepted (310). Most lesions are observed in the

female genital tract and most patients with primary bladder lesions are women. Gross hematuria is the predominant presenting sign. In contrast to PSCN, these lesions range from 2 to 8 cm in greatest dimension and the myxoid component is so prominent as to suggest a "tissue culture" appearance (fig. 2-71). Tumor cells in the few cases examined have been diploid (298). Reported cases have not involved the trigone. The infiltrative growth pattern, histology, ultrastructure, immunohistochemistry, and clinical course of inflammatory pseudotumors are similar to PSCNs.

PSCNs and inflammatory pseudotumors probably represent similar processes despite differences in clinical presentation and variations in pathology among individual cases. Their histologic resemblance to benign myofibroblastic proliferations at other sites and their failure to progress even after inadequate treatment strongly support a reactive process, even though these lesions have an invasive growth pattern and occasional tumors recur. In most situations, differentiation from malignant spindle cell tumors should not be difficult, but it may not be possible to exclude a myxoid leiomyosarcoma in every case (Table 2-8). Underinterpretation of equivocal tumors should be avoided but may make little difference to the patient since it is likely that myxoid leiomyosarcomas that are so histologically innocuous that they might be confused with PSCN or inflammatory pseudotumor have a favorable outcome if adequately excised.

Malakoplakia. This is a peculiar host reaction to chronic infection stimulated by inability to completely metabolize certain bacteria and manifested by the accumulation of histiocytes and other inflammatory elements in plaques or nodules (286,305). The bladder is the most common site but lesions have been recognized throughout the genitourinary system as well as in many other organs. Patients range from 6 weeks to 96 years and are more often women than men. Malakoplakia occurs predominantly in the lamina propria. Sheets of histiocytes intermixed with variable numbers of lymphocytes, plasma cells, neutrophils, and eosinophils are characteristic (fig. 2-72). These lesions are often classified as granulomatous, although neither granulomas nor giant cells are usually present histologically. Diagnosis rests upon the identification of Michaelis-Gutmann bodies (301). These are mineralized intracellular or extracellular particles often consisting of a central core of partially digested bacteria coated with iron and calcium phosphate. Light microscopically, Michaelis-Gutmann bodies appear as target or ring-like structures (fig. 2-72).

Xanthogranulomatous Inflammation. This lesion is usually associated with the kidney but has been observed in the urinary bladder (316). Interestingly, most cases have been associated with urachal adenomas. Histologically, the lesions resemble malakoplakia but lack Michaelis-Gutmann bodies and tend to have Touton-type giant cells. Granuloma formation is not characteristic.

Isolated case reports of primary bladder *granulomas* have been recorded. These are inflammatory lesions of diverse histologic composition which may elicit signs and symptoms suggesting bladder disease or present clinically as discrete bladder tumors. They include paravesical suture granulomas, occurring after herniorrhaphy; granulomatous reactions resembling rheumatoid nodules, appearing after transurethral resections; and tubercular granulomas secondary to BCG treatment (305,323,325). Most reviews cite a single case of *plasma cell granuloma* (298). Nonspecific nodular infiltrates rich in eosinophils have been labeled *eosinophilic granuloma* and *eosinophilic cystitis* (283,305,314).

"Cystitis"

A variety of hyperplasias, metaplasias, and reactive processes have been labeled "cystitis." Some, like interstitial cystitis, giant cell cystitis, and eosinophilic cystitis, are poorly defined in histopathologic terms and are not further discussed (305). Mass lesions labeled cystitis include cystitis glandularis et cystica, cystitis follicularis, bullous and polypoid cystitis, fibroepithelial polyp, and emphysematous cystitis.

Cystitis Glandularis et Cystica. This proliferation of Brunn nests most likely represents a reaction to bladder injury (295,305,320,323). The "glands" consist of layers of basal and intermediate transitional cells lined by superficial urothelial cells compressed into columnar shapes (fig. 2-73). Superficial transitional cells secrete and store small amounts of mucin and this material commonly accumulates in the lumina of gland-like structures formed by transitional cells. Some authors prefer the term *proliferative cystitis* to describe lesions composed entirely of transitional cells, reserving the term cystitis glandularis for lesions with focal intestinal metaplasia. Some degree of cystic dilatation is usually present. Prostatic antigens have been demonstrated in a few cells (306). Rarely, the cells may be markedly atypical in the absence of previous or coincident bladder cancer (305). Florid examples of cystitis glandularis et cystica may form nodular masses in the lamina propria. Such lesions have been considered either variants of inverted papilloma or hamartoma by some authors (fig. 2-74) (300,305). Cystitis glandularis et cystica is distinguished from the nested type of transitional cell carcinoma by its nodular, noninfiltrative growth pattern and lack of cellular anaplasia. Well-documented cases of adenocarcinoma associated with cystitis glandularis et cystica have rarely been observed and this lesion is not considered a risk factor for subsequent bladder cancer.

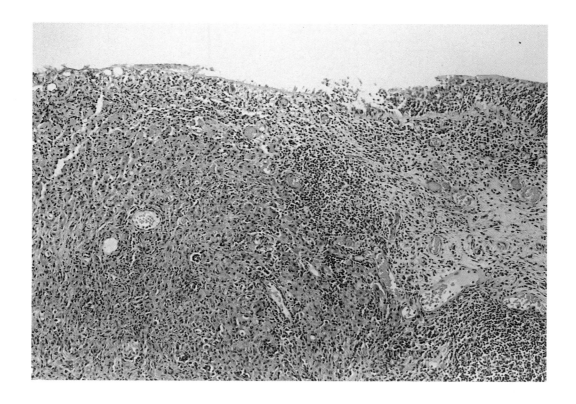

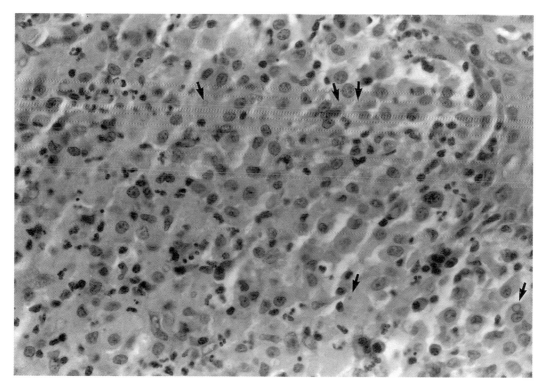

Figure 2-72
MALAKOPLAKIA

Top: Plaque-like lesion eroding the bladder mucosa.
Bottom: At higher magnification, the target-shaped Michaelis-Gutmann bodies (arrows) are prominent.

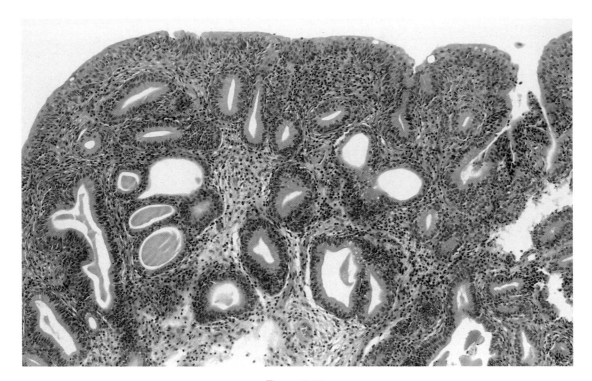

Figure 2-73
CYSTITIS GLANDULARIS ET CYSTICA

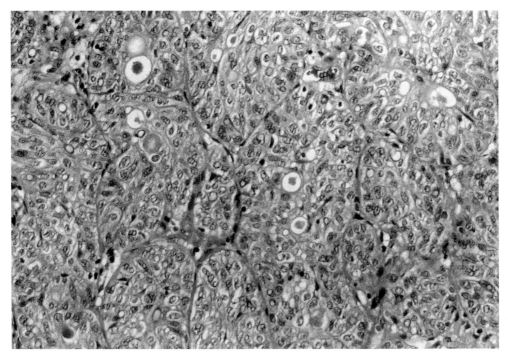

Figure 2-74
FLORID CYSTITIS GLANDULARIS
(Courtesy of Dr. Brian Montgomery, Fairhope, AL.)

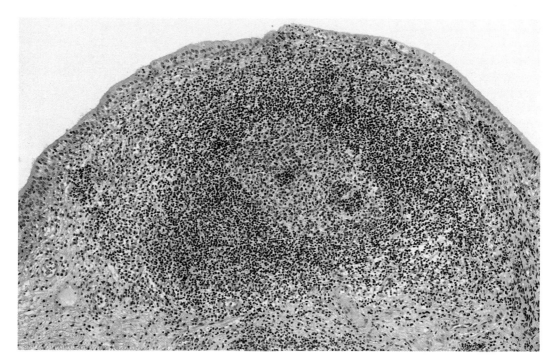

Figure 2-75
CYSTITIS FOLLICULARIS

Cystitis Follicularis. Cystitis follicularis describes the appearance of lymphoid follicles within the lamina propria. The lymphoid tissue is histologically unremarkable but the attenuated overlying urothelium often develops slight to moderate cellular atypia (fig. 2-75) (305,323). These lesions are often associated with urinary tract infection, especially with *Salmonella* sp.

Bullous and Polypoid Cystitis. The lamina propria of the bladder may be edematous or focally fibrotic. Edema is especially common after physical trauma produced by chronic indwelling catheters and radiation therapy. It has also been described in association with neoplasia. Diffuse edema is labeled *bullous cystitis*, and the more localized form, *polypoid cystitis* (fig. 2-76)(305,323). When the lamina propria of polypoid areas is filled with fibrous connective tissue, the lesion is termed *fibroepithelial polyp*. The association of this rare lesion with Beckwith-Wiedemann syndrome suggests that it may be a separate entity rather than a variant of bullous or polypoid cystitis (320,323). Like similar lesions elsewhere, the cores of fibroepithelial polyps may

have numerous, occasionally bizarre, stellate giant cells and focal muscle fibers, suggesting a hamartomatous tumor.

Emphysematous Cystitis. This describes the presence of gas-filled spaces in the bladder wall (305,309,323). Lesions usually result from collections of gas produced by microorganisms, most commonly *Escherichia coli* and *Enterobacter aerogenes*. Many patients are diabetics with neurogenic bladders.

Amyloidosis

Amyloidosis describes the presence of amyloid fibrils and associated ground substance in the urinary bladder. The disease is more often primary than systemic and most often type A lambda (291,294,305,323). Patients present with gross hematuria, often associated with nodular mucosal lesions misinterpreted clinically as carcinoma. Amyloid involving the urinary bladder characteristically occurs as large masses of acidophilic proteinaceous material associated with hemorrhage in the lamina propria (figs. 2-77, 2-78). Vascular involvement occurs but is not

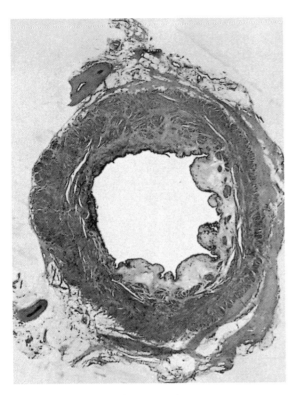

Figure 2-76
BULLOUS CYSTITIS
Cross section of bladder showing bullous edema. This patient had a carcinoma of the bladder, but the tumor does not appear in this section. (Fig. 76 from Fascicle 31a, 1st Series.)

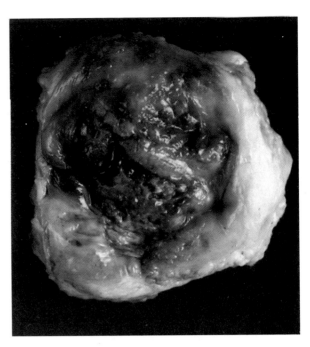

Figure 2-77
AMYLOIDOSIS OF URINARY BLADDER
(Courtesy of Dr. George M. Farrow, Rochester, MN.)

usually prominent. The diagnosis is easily confirmed once the condition is suspected and it is prudent to perform reactions for amyloid in any case where amorphous acidophilic material occurs in the lamina propria. As in many conditions involving attenuation of the urothelium, atypical epithelial changes may occur. These may assume unwarranted significance if too much emphasis is placed upon a clinical diagnosis of carcinoma and the amyloid deposition is overlooked.

Cysts, Rests, Choristomas, Hamartomas

Cysts. Most bladder cysts are urachal. Persistent urachal remnants are most likely a normal phenomenon and clinically important only when complicated by infection, neoplasia, or cystic dilatation (290,305,312).

Urachal cysts are ordinarily small, multilocular, asymptomatic structures which may occur anywhere along the urachal tract as well as within the bladder (fig. 2-79). Depending on size,

urachal cysts may be lined by urothelium or cuboidal, flat, or atrophic cells. Cysts and sinuses of apparent müllerian and urothelial derivation have also been recorded (313,323).

Endometriosis. Endometriosis presenting as a primary bladder tumor is an uncommon lesion virtually confined to women in the menstrual years; estrogen stimulation seems to be required (305,323). Men with vesical endometriosis develop the lesion after treatment with estrogen following pelvic surgery for adenocarcinoma of the prostate gland. The pathologic features are characteristic of endometrium (fig. 2-80). Rarely, cancers may arise in association with vesical endometriosis (280,315). In several cases with areas resembling ectopic endocervix, *endocervicosis* of the urinary bladder has been reported (285).

Ectopic Prostate. This ordinarily presents as a polypoid mass at the bladder base (305,323). Histologic recognition is not difficult and can be confirmed using immunohistochemical reactions for prostatic antigens. Similar lesions occur after transurethral resections and probably represent regrowths of adenomatous prostatic tissue into defects caused by the surgery. Diagnostic problems

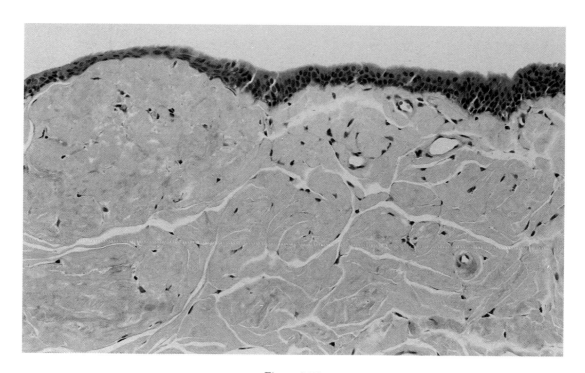

Figure 2-78
AMYLOIDOSIS
In contrast to other body sites, amyloid in the urinary bladder usually occurs as globular masses of amorphous acidophilic material.

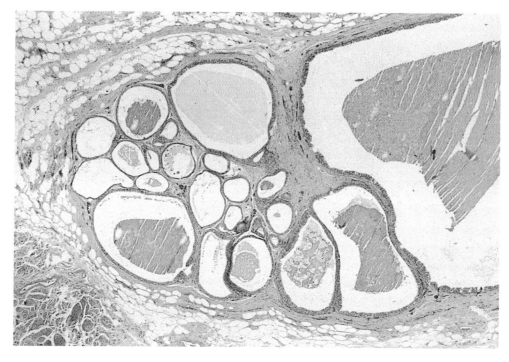

Figure 2-79
URACHAL CYST
(Courtesy of Dr. Lawrence Parrott, Camden, SC.)

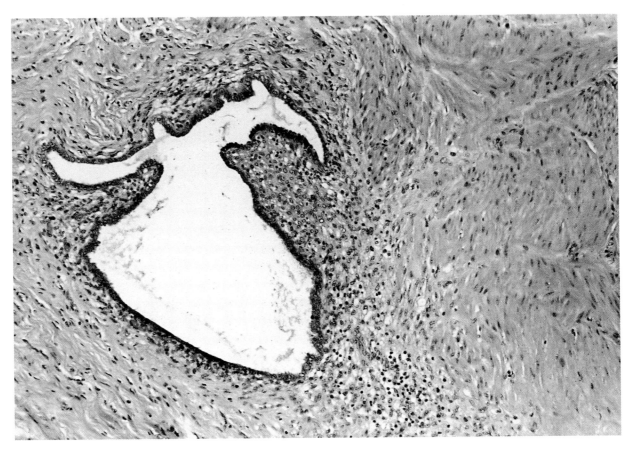

Figure 2-80
ENDOMETRIOSIS OF THE URINARY BLADDER

occasionally arise when the prostatic tissue contains few glands or arises at bladder sites distant from the prostate (303).

Paraganglionic Tissue. Rarely, prominent paraganglionic tissue occurs in the bladder (323). These areas may cause diagnostic concern to the unwary, especially if the hyperplastic cells occur in a small biopsy. Accurate interpretation can be facilitated using immunohistochemical reactions.

Extramedullary Hematopoiesis. Tumors composed of hematopoietic cells may occur in various organs, including the urinary bladder

(297). A history of a myeloproliferative disorder should be sought but is not essential to accurate pathologic interpretation.

Hamartomas. Hamartomas have been described in the urinary bladder (282,307,323). Almost all have occurred in children. Nodular accumulations of Brunnian glands with or without metaplasia, are so predominant that the correct classification of these lesions becomes controversial. As previously mentioned, certain cases of fibroepithelial polyp may represent hamartomatous malformation (321).

REFERENCES

Normal Anatomy

1. Coon JS, Weinstein RS, Summers JL. Blood group precursor T-antigen expression in human urinary bladder carcinoma. Am J Clin Pathol 1982;77:692–9.
2. Edwards BF, Rossitto PV, Baker WC, et al. Transitional cell cytokeratins as a second parameter in flow cytometry of bladder cancer. World J Urol 1987;5:123–6.
3. Fradet Y, Cordon-Cardo C, Whitmore WF Jr, Melamed MR, Old LJ. Cell surface antigens of human bladder tumors: definition of tumor subsets by monoclonal antibodies and correlation with growth characteristics. Cancer Res 1986;46:5183–8.
4. Guirguis R, Schiffmann E, Liu B, Birkbeck D, Engel J, Liotta L. Detection of autocrine motility factor in urine as a marker of bladder cancer. JNCI 1988;80:1203–11.
5. Keep JC, Piehl M, Miller A, Oyasu R. Invasive carcinomas of the urinary bladder. Am J Clin Pathol 1989; 91:575–9.
6. Kissane JM. Development and structure of the urogenital system. In: Murphy WM, ed. Urological pathology. Philadelphia: WB Saunders, 1989:14–16.
7. Koss LG. Tumors of the urinary bladder. Atlas of Tumor Pathology, 2nd Series, Fascicle 11 (Suppl). Washington, D.C.: Armed Forces Institute of Pathology, 1985:S-1–3.
8. Limas C, Lange P. A, B, H antigen detectability in normal and neoplastic urothelium: influence of methodologic factors. Cancer 1982;49:2476–84.
9. Messing EM. Clinical implications of the expression of epidermal growth factor receptors in human transitional cell carcinoma. Cancer Res 1990;50:2530–7.
10. Reuter VE. Urinary bladder and ureter. In: Sternberg SS, ed. Histology for pathologists. New York: Raven Press 1992:709–19.
11. Russell PJ, Brown JL, Grimmond SM, Raghavan D. Molecular biology of urological tumours. Br J Urol 1990;65:121–30.

Classification

12. Ash JE. Epithelial tumors of the bladder. J Urol 1940,44:135–45.
13. Bergkvist A, Ljungqvist A, Moberger G. Classification of bladder tumours based on the cellular pattern. Acta Chir Scand 1965;130:371–8.
14. Broders AC. Epithelium of the genito-urinary organs. Ann Surg 1922;75:574–604.
15. Dukes CE, Masina F. Classification of epithelial tumours of the bladder. Br J Urol 1949;21:273–95.
16. Koss LG. Tumors of the urinary bladder. Atlas of Tumor Pathology, 2nd Series, Fascicle 11. Washington, D.C.: Armed Forces Institute of Pathology, 1975.
17. Miller A, Mitchell JP, Brown NJ. The Bristol Bladder Tumour Registry. Br J Urol 1969;41(Suppl):1–64.
18. Mostofi FK, Sobin LH, Torloni H. Histological typing of urinary bladder tumours. International histological classification of tumours, No. 10. Geneva: World Health Organization, 1973.
19. Murphy WM. Diseases of the urinary bladder, urethra, ureters, and renal pelves. In: Murphy WM, ed. Urological pathology. Philadelphia: WB Saunders, 1989:64–96.

Bladder Neoplasia

20. Anwar K, Naiki H, Nakakuki K, Inuzuka M. High frequency of human papillomavirus infection in carcinoma of the urinary bladder. Cancer 1992;70:1967–73.
21. Boring CC, Squires TS, Tong T, Montgomery S. Cancer statistics, 1994. CA Cancer J Clin 1994;44:7–26.
22. Boyd PJ, Burnand KG. Site of bladder-tumour recurrence. Lancet 1974;2:1290–2.
23. Chetsanga C, Malmström PU, Gyllensten U, Moreno-Lopez J, Dinter Z, Pettersson U. Low incidence of human papillomavirus type 16 DNA in bladder tumor detected by the polymerase chain reaction. Cancer 1992;69:1208–11.
24. Chowaniec J. Aetiology: epidemiological and experimental considerations. In: Skrabanek P, Walsh A, eds. Bladder cancer, Vol 60. Geneva: UICC Technical Report Series 1981:118–43.
25. Cutler SJ, Heney NM, Friedell GH. Longitudinal study of patients with bladder cancer: factors associated with disease recurrence and progression. In: Bonney WW, ed. Bladder cancer. Baltimore: Williams & Wilkins, 1982:35–46. (AUA monographs, Vol 1).
26. Droller MJ. Transitional cell cancer: upper tracts and bladder. In: Walsh PC, Gittes RF, Perlmutter AD, Stamey TA, eds. Campbell's urology. 5th ed. Philadelphia: WB Saunders, 1986:1343–440.
27. El-Bolkainy MN, Tawfik HN, Kamel IA. Histopathologic classification of carcinomas in the schistosomal bladder. In: El-Bolkainy MN, Chu EW, eds. Detection of bladder cancer associated with schistosomiasis. Cairo: Al-Ahram Press, 1981:106–23.
28. Farrow GM, Utz DC, Rife CC. Morphological and clinical observations of patients with early bladder cancer treated with total cystectomy. Cancer Res 1976;36(7 Pt 2):2495–501.
29. Fitzpatrick JM, Reda M. Bladder carcinoma in patients 40 years old or less. J Urol 1986;135:53–4.
30. Ibrahim AS, El-Bolkainy MN. Epidemiologic survey of rural population. In: El-Bolkainy MN, Chu EW, eds. Detection of bladder cancer associated with schistosomiasis. Cairo: Al-Ahram Press, 1981:29–46.
31. Jordan AM, Weingarten J, Murphy WM. Transitional cell neoplasms of the urinary bladder: can biologic potential be predicted from histologic grading? Cancer 1987;60:2766–74.
32. Kaubisch S, Lum BL, Reese J, Freiha F, Torti FM. Stage T1 bladder cancer: grade is the primary determinant for risk of muscle invasion. J Urol 1991;146:28–31.
33. Kaye KW, Lange PH. Mode of presentation of invasive bladder cancer: reassessment of the problem. J Urol 1982;128:31–3.

34. Koss LG. Diagnostic cytology and its histopathologic bases. Vol 2. 4th ed. Philadelphia: JB Lippincott, 1992:46.

35. _____, Melamed MR, Kelly RE. Further cytologic and histologic studies of bladder lesions in workers exposed to para-aminodiphenyl: progress report. JNCI 1969;43:233–43.

36. Lower GM Jr. Concepts in causality: chemically induced human urinary bladder cancer. Cancer 1982;49:1056–66.

37. Mostofi FK, Sobin LH, Torloni H. Histological typing of urinary bladder tumours. International Classification of Tumours, No. 10. Geneva: World Health Organization, 1973.

38. Murphy WM. Diseases of the urinary bladder, urethra, ureters, and renal pelves. In: Murphy WM, ed. Urological pathology. Philadelphia: WB Saunders, 1989:64–96.

39. _____, Soloway MS. Developing carcinoma (dysplasia) of the urinary bladder. Pathol Annu 1982;17(Pt 1):197–217.

40. Schulte PA, Ringen K, Hemstreet GP, et al. Risk factors for bladder cancer in a cohort exposed to aromatic amines. Cancer 1986;58:2156–62.

41. Shinka T, Sawada Y, Morimoto S, Fujinaga T, Nakamura J, Ohkawa T. Clinical study on urothelial tumors of dye workers in Wakayama City. J Urol 1991;146:1504–07.

42. Sidransky D, Frost P, Von Eschenbach A, Oyasu R, Preisinger AC, Vogelstein B. Clonal origin of bladder cancer. N Engl J Med 1992;326:737–40.

43. Weldon TE, Soloway MS. Susceptibility of urothelium to neoplastic cellular implantation. Urology 1975;5:824–7.

44. Wynder EL, Augustine A, Kabat GC, Hebert JR. Effect of the type of cigarette smoked on bladder cancer risk. Cancer 1988;61:622–7.

45. _____, Goldsmith R. The epidemiology of bladder cancer: a second look. Cancer 1977;40:1246–68.

Transitional Cell Neoplasms

46. Alroy J, Miller AW III, Coon JS IV, James KK, Gould VE. Inverted papilloma of the urinary bladder. Cancer 1980;46:64–70.

47. Althausen AF, Prout GR Jr, Dal JJ. Non-invasive papillary carcinoma of the bladder associated with carcinoma in situ. J Urol 1976;116:575–80.

48. American Joint Committee on Cancer (AJCC). Manual for staging of cancer. 3rd ed. Philadelphia: JB Lippincott, 1988:197.

49. Antonakopoulos GN, Hicks RM, Berry RJ. The subcellular basis of damage to the human urinary bladder induced by irradiation. J Pathol 1984;143:103–16.

50. Arends MJ, Wyllie AH. Apoptosis: mechanisms and roles in pathology. Int Rev Exp Pathol 1991;32:223–54.

51. Ash JE. Epithelial tumors of the bladder. J Urol 1940;44:135–45.

52. Babu VR, Lutz MD, Miles BJ, Farah RN, Weiss L, Van Dyke DL. Tumor behavior in transitional cell carcinoma of the bladder in relation to chromosomal markers and histopathology. Cancer Res 1987;47:6800–5.

53. Badalament RA, Hermansen DK, Kimmel M, et al. The sensitivity of bladder wash flow cytometry, bladder wash cytology, and voided cytology in the detection of bladder carcinoma. Cancer 1987;60:1423–7.

54. Bander NH. Monoclonal antibodies in urologic oncology. Cancer 1987;60:658–67.

55. Bergkvist A, Ljungqvist A, Moberger G. Classification of bladder tumours based on the cellular pattern. Acta Chir Scand 1965;130:371–8.

56. Blomjous CE, Schipper NW, Vos W, Baak JP, de Voogt HJ, Meijer CJ. Comparison of quantitative and classic prognosticators in urinary bladder carcinoma. A multivariate analysis of DNA flow cytometric, nuclear morphometric and clinicopathological features. Virchows Arch [A] 1989;415:421–8.

57. _____, Vos W, Schipper NW, et al. The prognostic significance of selective nuclear morphometry in urinary bladder carcinoma. Hum Pathol 1990;21:409–13.

58. Broders AC. Epithelium of the genito-urinary organs. Ann Surg 1922;75:574–604.

59. Buckley I. Oncogenes and the nature of malignancy. Adv Cancer Res 1988;50:71–94.

60. Campo E, Algaba F, Palacin A, Germa R, Sole-Balcells FJ, Cardesa A. Placental proteins in high-grade urothelial neoplasms: an immunohistochemical study of human chorionic gonadotropin, human placental lactogen, and pregnancy-specific beta-1-glycoprotein. Cancer 1989;63:2497–504.

61. Carbin BE, Ekman P, Gustafson H, Christensen NJ, Silfverswärd C, Sandstedt B. Grading of human urothelial carcinoma based on nuclear atypia and mitotic frequency. II. Prognostic importance. J Urol 1991;145:972–6.

62. Caro DJ, Tessler A. Inverted papilloma of the bladder: a distinct urological lesion. Cancer 1978;42:708–13.

63. Chopin DK, Whitmore KE, Abbou CC, DeKernion JB. Immunopathology of urothelial lesions: immunological markers as predictive for clinical aggressiveness. World J Urol 1987;5:133–7.

64. Coon JS, McCall A, Miller AW III, Farrow GM, Weinstein RS. Expression of blood-group-related antigens in carcinoma in situ of the urinary bladder. Cancer 1985;56:797–804.

65. Coon JS, Weinstein RS, Summers JL. Blood group precursor T-antigen expression in human urinary bladder carcinoma. Am J Clin Pathol 1982;77:692–9.

66. Cutler SJ, Heney NM, Friedell GH. Longitudinal study of patients with bladder cancer: factors associated with disease recurrence and progression. In: Bonney WM, ed. Bladder cancer. Baltimore: Williams & Wilkins, 1982:35–46. (AUA monographs, Vol 1.).

67. Czerniak B, Cohen GL, Etkind P, et al. Concurrent mutations of coding and regulatory sequences of the Ha-ras gene in urinary bladder carcinomas. Hum Pathol 1992;23:1199–204.

68. Delladetsima J, Antonakopoulos GN, Dapolla V, Kittas C. Intraepithelial lumina in urothelial bladder neoplasms: a histochemical, immunohistochemical and electron microscopy study. APMIS 1989;97:406–12.

69. DeMeester LJ, Farrow GM, Utz DC. Inverted papillomas of the urinary bladder. Cancer 1975;36:505–13.

70. de Prez C, de Launoit Y, Kiss R, et al. Computerized morphonuclear cell image analyses of malignant disease in bladder tissues. J Urol 1990;143:694–9.

71. Donhuijsen K, Schmidt U, Richter HJ, Leder LD. Mucoid cytoplasmic inclusions in urothelial carcinomas. Hum Pathol 1992;23:860–4.

72. Droller MJ. Transitional cell cancer: upper tracts and bladder. In: Walsh PC, Gittes RF, Perlmutter AD, Stamey TA, eds. Campbell's urology. 5th ed. Philadelphia: WB Saunders, 1986:1343–440.

73. _____, Walsh PC. Intensive intravesical chemotherapy in the treatment of flat carcinoma in situ: is it safe? J Urol 1985;134:1115–7.

74. Eble JN, Young RH. Stromal osseous metaplasia in carcinoma of the bladder. J Urol 1991;145:823–5.

75. Farrow GM, Utz DC. Observations on microinvasive transitional cell carcinoma of the urinary bladder. Clinics in Oncol 1982;1:609–15.

76. _____, Utz DC, Rife CC. Morphological and clinical observations of patients with early bladder cancer treated with total cystectomy. Cancer Res 1976; 36:2495–501.

77. Farsund T, Hoestmerk JG, Laerum OD. Relation between flow cytometric DNA distribution and pathology in human bladder cancer: a report on 69 cases. Cancer 1984;54:1771–7.

78. Feitz WF, Beck HL, Smeets AW, et al. Tissue-specific markers in flow cytometry of urological cancers: cytokeratins in bladder carcinoma. Int J Cancer 1985;36:349–56.

79. Fradet Y, Tardif M, Bourget L, Robert J. Laval University Urology Group. Clinical cancer progression in urinary bladder tumors evaluated by multiparameter flow cytometry with monoclonal antibodies. Cancer Res 1990;50:432–7.

80. Friedell GH, MCauley RL. Untreated bladder cancer: 31 autopsy cases. J Urol 1968;100:293–6.

81. Garden RJ, Liu BC, Redwood SM, Weiss RE, Droller MJ. Bacillus Calmette-Guerin abrogates in vitro invasion and motility of human bladder tumor cells via fibronectin interaction. J Urol 1992;148:900–5.

82. Gibas Z, Prout GR, Pontes JE, Connolly JG, Sandberg AA. A possible specific chromosome change in transitional cell carcinoma of the bladder. Cancer Genet Cytogenet 1986;19:229–38

83. Harewood LM. The significance of urothelial dysplasia as diagnosed by cup biopsies. Aust NZ J Surg 1986; 56:199–203.

84. Harris M, Eyden BP, Joglekar VM. Rhabdoid tumour of the bladder: a histological, ultrastructural, and immunohistochemical study. Histopathology 1987;11:1083–92.

85. Heney NM, Koontz WW, Barton B, et al. Intravesical thiotepa versus mitomycin C in patients with Ta, T1 and TIS transitional cell carcinoma of the bladder: a phase III prospective randomized study. J Urol 1988;140:1390–3.

86. Hormanck P, Sobin LH, eds. TNM classification of malignant tumours. 4th ed. 2nd revision. Berlin: Springer-Verlag, 1992.

87. Herr HW, Wartinger DD, Fair WR, Oettgen HF. Bacillus Calmette-Guerin therapy for superficial bladder cancer: a 10-year followup. J Urol 1992;147:1020–3.

88. Hicks RM, Wakefield JJ. Membrane changes during urothelial hyperplasia and neoplasia. Cancer Res 1976;36(7 Pt 2):2502–7.

89. Hug EB, Donnelly SM, Shipley WU, et al. Deoxyribonucleic acid flow cytometry in invasive bladder carcinoma: a possible predictor for successful bladder preservation following transurethral surgery and chemotherapy-radiotherapy. J Urol 1992;148:47–51.

90. Iles RK, Chard T. Human chorionic gonadotropin expression by bladder cancers: biology and clinical potential. J Urol 1991;145:453–8.

91. Jakse G, Loidl W, Seeber G, Hofstädter F. Stage T1, grade 3 transitional cell carcinoma of the bladder: an unfavorable tumor? J Urol 1987;137:39–43.

92. Jordan AM, Weingarten J, Murphy WM. Transitional cell neoplasms of the urinary bladder: can biological potential be predicted from histologic grading? Cancer 1987;60:2766–74.

93. Juhl BR, Hartzen SH, Hainau B. A, B, H antigen expression in transitional cell carcinomas of the urinary bladder. Cancer 1986;57:1768–75.

94. Kaubisch S, Lum BL, Reese J, Freiha F, Torti FM. Stage T1 bladder cancer: grade is the primary determinant for risk of muscle invasion. J Urol 1991;146:28–31.

95. Kaye KW, Lange PH. Mode of presentation of invasive bladder cancer: reassessment of a problem. J Urol 1982;128:31–3.

96. Klän R, Huland E, Baisch H, Huland H. Sensitivity of urinary quantitative immunocytology with monoclonal antibody 486 P3/12 in 241 unselected patients with bladder carcinoma. J Urol 1991;145:495–7.

97. Klein G. The approaching era of the tumor suppressor genes. Science 1987;238:1539–45.

98. Koss LG. Diagnostic cytology and its histopathologic bases, Vol 2. 4th ed. Philadelphia: JB Lippincott, 1992:890–1017.

99. _____. Mapping of the urinary bladder: its impact on the concepts of bladder cancer. Hum Pathol 1979;10:533–48.

100. _____. Tumors of the urinary bladder. Atlas of Tumor Pathology, 2nd Series, Fascicle 11. Washington, D.C.: Armed Forces Institute of Pathology 1975:46–52.

101. _____, Wersto RP, Simmons DA, Deitch D, Herz F, Freed SZ. Predictive value of DNA measurements in bladder washings: comparison of flow cytometry, image cytophotometry, and cytology in patients with a past history of urothelial tumors. Cancer 1989;64:1916–24.

102. Kunze E, Schauer A, Schmitt M. Histology and histogenesis of two different types of inverted urothelial papillomas. Cancer 1983;51:348–58.

103. Lamb D. Correlation of chromosome counts with histological appearances and prognosis in transitional-cell carcinoma of bladder. Br Med J 1967;1:273–7.

104. Lamm DL, van der Meijden PM, Morales A, et al. Incidence and treatment of complications of bacillus Calmette-Guerin intravesical therapy in superficial bladder cancer. J Urol 1992;147:596–600.

105. Larsen MP, Steinberg GD, Brendler CB, Epstein JI. Use of Ulex europaeus agglutinin I (UEA1) to distinguish vascular and "pseudovascular" invasion in transitional cell carcinoma of bladder with lamina propria invasion. Mod Pathol 1990;3:83–8.

106. Lerman RI, Hutter RV, Whitmore WF Jr. Papilloma of the urinary bladder. Cancer 1970;25:333–42.

107. Levi PE, Cooper EH, Anderson CK, Williams RE. Analyses of DNA content, nuclear size and cell proliferation of transitional cell carcinoma in man. Cancer 1969;23:1074–85.

108. Lipponen PK, Eskelinen MJ, Nordling S. Nucleolar organizer regions (AgNORs) as predictors in transitional cell bladder cancer. Br J Urol 1991;64:1139–44.

109. _____, Kosma VM, Collan Y, Kulju T, Kosunen O, Eskelinen M. Potential of nuclear morphometry and volume-corrected mitotic index in grading transitional cell carcinoma of the urinary bladder. Eur Urol 1990;17:333–7.

110. Longin A, Fontaniere B, Berger-Dutrieux N, Devonec M, Laurent JC. A useful monoclonal antibody (BL2-10D1) to identify tumor cells in urine cytology. Cancer 1990;65:1412–7.

111. Melamed MR, Voutsa NG, Grabstald H. Natural history and clinical behavior of in situ carcinoma of the human urinary bladder. Cancer 1964;17:1533–45.

112. Morales A. Long-term results and complications of intracavitary bacillus Calmette-Guerin therapy for bladder cancer. J Urol 1984;132:457–9.

113. Morris GF, Mathews MB. Regulation of proliferating cell nuclear antigen during the cell cycle. J Biol Chem 1989;264:13856–64.

114. Mostofi FK, Sobin LH, Torloni H. Histological typing of urinary bladder tumours. International Classification of Tumours, No. 10. Geneva: World Health Organization, 1973.

115. Murphy WM. Current status of urinary cytology in the evaluation of bladder neoplasms. Hum Pathol 1990;21:886–96.

116. _____. Diseases of the urinary bladder, urethra, ureters, and renal pelves. In: Murphy WM ed. Urological pathology. Philadelphia: WB Saunders, 1989:64–96.

117. _____. Urothelial neoplasia. In: Weinstein RS, Gardner WA, eds. Pathology and pathobiology of the urinary bladder and prostate. Baltimore: Williams and Wilkins 1992:77–111. (Weinstein RS, Gardner WA, eds. Monographs in pathology, No. 34).

118. _____, Chandler RW, Trafford RM. Flow cytometry of deparaffinized nuclei compared to histological grading for the pathological evaluation of transitional cell carcinomas. J Urol 1986;135:694–7.

119. _____, Deana DG. The nested variant of transitional cell carcinoma: a neoplasm resembling proliferation of Brunn's nests. Mod Pathol 1992;5:240–3.

120. _____, Emerson LD, Chandler RW, Moinuddin SM, Soloway MS. Flow cytometry versus urinary cytology in the evaluation of patients with bladder cancer. J Urol 1986;136:815–9.

121. _____, Nagy GK, Rao MK, et al. "Normal" urothelium in patients with bladder cancer. A preliminary report from the National Bladder Cancer Collaborative Group A. Cancer 1979;44:1050–8.

122. _____, Soloway MS. Developing carcinoma (dysplasia) of the urinary bladder. Pathol Annu 1982;17(Pt 1):197–217.

123. _____, Soloway MS, Finebaum PJ. Pathological changes associated with topical chemotherapy for superficial bladder cancer. J Urol 1981;126:461–4.

124. _____, Vandevoorde JP. Determination of baseline values for urinary carcinoembryonic antigen-like substances. Am J Clin Pathol 1977;67:455–8.

125. Nemoto R, Uchida K, Hattori K, et al. S phase fraction of human bladder tumor measured in situ with bromodeoxyuridine labeling. J Urol 1988;139:286–9.

126. Norming U, Nyman CR, Tribukait B. Comparative histopathology and deoxyribonucleic acid flow cytometry of random mucosal biopsies in untreated bladder carcinoma. J Urol 1991;145:1164–8.

127. Okamura K, Miyake K, Koshikawa T, Asai J. Growth fractions of transitional cell carcinomas of the bladder defined by the monoclonal antibody Ki-67. J Urol 1990;144:875–8.

128. Olumi AF, Tsai YC, Nichols PW, et al. Allelic loss of chromosome 17p distinguishes high grade from low grade transitional cell carcinomas of the bladder. Cancer Res 1990;50:7081–3.

129. Ørntoft TF, Hvid H, Clausen H, Hakomori S, Dabelsteen E. Loss of blood group ABO-related antigen expression in urothelium from patients with chronic cystitis. Lab Invest 1989;60:305–10.

130. _____, Nielsen MJ, Wolf H, et al. Blood group ABO and Lewis antigen expression during neoplastic progression of human urothelium: immunohistochemical study of type 1 change structures. Cancer 1987;60:2641–8.

131. Orozco RE, Martin AA, Murphy WM. Carcinoma in-situ of the urinary bladder: clues to host involvement in human carcinogenesis. Cancer 1994;74:115–22.

132. _____, Vander Zwaag R, Murphy WM. The pagetoid variant of urothelial carcinoma in situ. Hum Pathol 1993;24:1199–202.

133. Paschkis R. Über adenome der harnblase. Z Urol Nephrol 1927;21:315–25.

134. Pauwels RP, Smeets AW, Schapers RF, Geraedts JP, Debruyne FMJ. Grading in superficial bladder cancer. II. Cytogenetic classification. Br J Urol 1988;61:135–9.

135. Presti JC Jr, Reuter VE, Galan T, Fair WR, Cordon-Cardo C. Molecular genetic alterations in superficial and locally advanced human bladder cancer. Cancer Res 1991;51:5405–9.

136. Prout GR Jr, Griffin PP, Daly JJ, Heney NM. Carcinoma in situ of the urinary bladder with and without associated vesical neoplasms. Cancer 1983;52:524–32.

137. Rife CC, Farrow GM, Utz DC. Urine cytology of transitional cell neoplasms. Urol Clin North Am 1979;6:599–612.

138. Ro JY, Ayala AG, Wishnow KI, Ordóñez NG. Sarcomatoid bladder carcinoma: clinicopathologic and immunohistochemical study on 44 cases. Surg Pathol 1988;1:359–74.

139. Russell PJ, Brown JL, Grimmond SM, Raghavan D. Molecular biology of urological tumours. Br J Urol 1990;65:121–30.

140. Schade RO, Swinney J. The association of urothelial abnormalities with neoplasia: a 10-year followup. J Urol 1983;129:1125–6.

141. Sella A, Dexeus FH, Chong C, Ro JY, Logothetis CJ. Radiation therapy-associated invasive bladder tumors. Urology 1989;33:185–8.

142. Seo IS, Clark SA, McGovern FD, Clark DL, Johnson EH. Leiomyosarcoma of the urinary bladder: 13 years after cyclophosphamide therapy for Hodgkin's disease. Cancer 1985;55:1597–603.

143. Sheinfeld J, Reuter VE, Melamed MR, et al. Enhanced bladder cancer detection with the Lewis X antigen as a marker of neoplastic transformation. J Urol 1990;143:285–8.

144. Sherman AB, Koss LG, Wyschogrod D, Melder KH, Eppich EM, Bales CE. Bladder cancer diagnosis by computer image analysis of cells in the sediment of voided urine using a video scanning system. Anal Quant Cytol Histol 1986;8:177–86.

145. Shevchuk MM, Fenoglio CM, Richart RM. Carcinoembryonic antigen localization in benign and malignant transitional epithelium. Cancer 1981;47:899–905.

146. Shields PG, Harris CC. Molecular epidemiology and the genetics of environmental cancer. JAMA 1991;266:681–7.

147. Shipley WU, Kaufman SD, Prout GR Jr. Intraoperative radiation therapy in patients with bladder cancer: a review of techniques allowing improved tumor doses and providing high cure rates without loss of bladder function. Cancer 1987;60:1485-8.

148. Sidransky D, Frost P, Von Eschenbach A, Oyasu R, Preisinger AC, Vogelstein B. Clonal origin of bladder cancer. N Engl J Med 1992;326:737–40.

149. _____, Von Eschenback A, Tsai YC, et al. Identification of p53 gene mutations in bladder cancers and urine samples. Science 1991;251:706–9.

150. Smeets AW, Pauwels RP, Beck JL, et al. Tissue-specific markers in flow cytometry of urological cancers. III. Comparing chromosomal and flow cytometric DNA analysis of bladder tumors. Int J Cancer 1987;39:304–10.

151. Sowter C, Slavin G, Sowter G, Rosen D, Hendry W. Morphometry of bladder carcinoma: morphometry and grading complement each other. Anal Cell Pathol 1991;3:1–9.

152. Stillwell TJ, Benson RC Jr. Cyclophosphamide-induced hemorrhagic cystitis: a review of 100 patients. Cancer 1988;61:451–7.

153. Stöckle M, Tanke HJ, Mesker WE, Ploem JS, Jonas U, Hohenfellner R. Automated DNA-image cytometry: a prognostic tool in infiltrating bladder carcinoma? World J Urol 1987;5:127–32.

154. Summers DE, Rushin JM, Frazier HA, Cotelingam JD. Inverted papilloma of the urinary bladder with granular eosinophilic cells. An unusual neuroendocrine variant. Arch Pathol Lab Med 1991;115:802–6.

155. Summers JL, Falor WH, Ward R. A 10-year analysis of chromosomes in non-invasive papillary carcinoma of the bladder. J Urol 1981;125:177–8.

156. Talbert ML, Young RH. Carcinomas of the urinary bladder with deceptively benign-appearing foci: a report of three cases. Am J Surg Pathol 1989;13:374–81.

157. Tribukait B. Flow cytometry in assessing the clinical aggressiveness of genito-urinary neoplasms. World J Urol 1987;5:108–22.

158. _____. Flow cytometry in surgical pathology and cytology of tumors of the genitourinary tract. In: Koss LG, Coleman DV, eds. Advances in clinical cytology, Vol II. New York: Masson, 1984:163–89.

159. Tsai YC, Nichols PW, Hiti AL, Williams Z, Skinner DG, Jones PA. Allelic losses of chromosomes 9, 11, and 17 in human bladder cancer. Cancer Res 1990;50:44–7.

160. Tsujihashi H, Nakanishi A, Matsuda H, Uejima S, Kurita T. Cell proliferation of human bladder tumors determined by BrdUrd and Ki-67 immunostaining. J Urol 1991;145:846–9.

161. van der Poel HG, Boon ME, Kok LP, et al. Morphometry, densitometry and pattern analysis of plastic-embedded histologic material from urothelial cell carcinoma of the bladder. Anal Quant Cytol Histol 1991;13:307–15.

162. _____, Schaafsma HE, Vooijs GP, Debruyne FMJ, Shalken JA. Quantitative light microscopy in urological oncology. J Urol 1992;148:1–13.

163. Wahren B, Nilsson B, Zimmerman R. Urinary CEA for prediction of survival time and recurrence in bladder cancer. Cancer 1982;50:139–45.

164. Waldman FM, Carroll PR, Cohen MB, Kerschmann R, Chew K, Mayall BH. 5 - bromodeoxyuridine incorporation and PCNA expression as measures of cell proliferation in transitional cell carcinoma of the urinary bladder. Mod Pathol 1993;6:20–4.

165. Wick MR, Brown BA, Young RH, Mills SE. Spindle-cell proliferations of the urinary tract: an immunohistochemical study. Am J Surg Pathol 1988;12:379–89.

166. Wishnow KI, Johnson DE, Ro JY, Swanson DA, Babaian RJ, von Eschenbach AC. Incidence, extent and localization of unsuspected pelvic lymph node metastasis in patients undergoing radical cystectomy for bladder cancer. J Urol 1987;137:408–10.

167. Wolinska WH, Melamed MR, Klein FA. Cytology of bladder papilloma. Acta Cytol 1985;29:817–22.

168. Wood DP Jr, Montie JE, Pontes JE, Levin HS. Identification of transitional cell carcinoma of the prostate in bladder cancer patients: a prospective study. J Urol 1989;141:83–5.

169. Woosley JT. Measuring cell proliferation. Arch Pathol Lab Med 1991;115:555–7.

170. Yamada T, Fukui I, Yokokawa M, Oshima H. Changing expression of ABH blood group and cryptic T-antigens of noninvasive and superficially invasive papillary transitional cell carcinoma of the bladder from initial occurrence to malignant progression. Cancer 1988,61.721–6.

171. Young RH, Eble JN. Unusual forms of carcinoma of the urinary bladder. Hum Pathol 1991;22:948–65.

172. _____, Wick MR, Mills SE. Sarcomatoid carcinoma of the urinary bladder: a clinicopathologic analysis of 12 cases and review of the literature. Am J Clin Pathol 1988;90:653–61.

173. _____, Zukerberg LR. Microcystic transitional cell carcinoma of the urinary bladder: a report of four cases. Am J Clin Pathol 1991;96:635–9.

174. Zukerberg LR, Armin AR, Pisharodi L, Young RH. Transitional cell carcinoma of the urinary bladder with osteoclast-type giant cells: a report of two cases and review of the literature. Histopathology 1990;17:407–11.

Squamous Cell Carcinoma

175. Bejany DE, Lockhart JL, Rhamy RK. Malignant vesical tumors following spinal cord injury. J Urol 1987;138:1390–2.

176. Benson RC Jr, Swanson SK, Farrow GM. Relationship of leukoplakia to urothelial malignancy. J Urol 1984;131:507–11.

177. Costello AJ, Tiptaft RC, England HR, Blandy JP. Squamous cell carcinoma of bladder. Urology 1984;22:234–6.

178. El-Bolkainy MN, Mokhtar NM, Ghoneim MA, Hussein MH. The impact of schistosomiasis on the pathology of bladder carcinoma. Cancer 1981;48:2643–8.

179. el-Sebai I, Sherif M, el-Bolkainy MN, Mansour MA, Ghoneim MA. Verrucous squamous carcinoma of bladder. Urology 1974;4:407–10.

180. Faysal MH. Squamous cell carcinoma of the bladder. J Urol 1981;126:598–9.

181. Friedell GH, Bell JR, Burney SW, Soto EA, Tiltman AJ. Histopathology and classification of urinary bladder carcinoma. Urol Clin North Am 1976;3:53–70.

182. Hermanek P, Sobin LH, eds. TNM classification of malignant tumours. 4th ed. 2nd revision. Berlin: Springer-Verlag, 1992.

183. Horner SA, Fisher HA, Barada JH, Eastman AY, Migliozzi J, Ross JS. Verrucous carcinoma of the bladder. J Urol 1991;145:1261–3.

184. Kerley SW, Persons DL, Fishback JL. Human papillomavirus and carcinoma of the urinary bladder. Mod Pathol 1991;4:316–9.

185. Koss LG. Tumors of the urinary bladder. Atlas of Tumor Pathology, 2nd Series, Fascicle 11. Washington, D.C.: Armed Forces Institute of Pathology, 1975:46–52.

186. _____. Tumors of the urinary tract and prostate in urinary sediment. In: Diagnostic cytology and its histopathologic bases. 4th ed. Philadelphia: JB Lippincott, 1992:964.

187. Locke JR, Hill DE, Walzer Y. Incidence of squamous cell carcinoma in patients with long-term catheter drainage. J Urol 1985;133:1034–5.

188. Lundgren R, Elfving P, Heim S, Kristoffersson U, Mandahl N, Mitelman F. A squamous cell bladder carcinoma with karyotypic abnormalities reminiscent of transitional cell carcinoma. J Urol 1989;142:374–6.

189. Morgan RJ, Cameron KM. Vesical leukoplakia. Br J Urol 1980;52:96–100.

190. Murphy WM. Atlas of bladder carcinoma. Chicago: ASCP Press, 1986:51–8, 85.
191. Rundle JS, Hart AJ, McGeorge A, Smith JS, Malcolm AJ, Smith PM. Squamous cell carcinoma of bladder. A review of 114 patients. Br J Urol 1982;54:522–6.
192. Schroder LE, Weiss MA, Hughes C. Squamous cell carcinoma of bladder: an increased incidence in blacks. Urology 1986;28:288–91.
193. Shaaban AA, Tribukait B, El-Bedeiwy AF, Ghoneim MA. Characterization of squamous cell bladder tumors

194. Tannenbaum SI, Carson CC III, Tatum A, Paulson DF. Squamous carcinoma of urinary bladder. Urology 1983;22:597–9.
195. Walther M, O'Brien DP III, Birch HW. Condylomata acuminata and verrucous carcinoma of the bladder: case report and literature review. J Urol 1986;135:362–5.
196. Winkler HZ, Nativ O, Hosaka Y, Farrow GM, Lieber MM. Nuclear deoxyribonucleic acid ploidy in squamous cell bladder cancer. J Urol 1989;141:297–302.

by flow cytometric deoxyribonucleic acid analysis: a report of 100 cases. J Urol 1990;144:879–83.

Mixed Carcinoma

197. Koss LG. Tumors of the urinary bladder. Atlas of Tumor Pathology, 2nd Series, Fascicle 11. Washington, D.C.: Armed Forces Institute of Pathology, 1975:46–52.
198. Murphy WM. Diseases of the urinary bladder, urethra, ureters, and renal pelves. In: Murphy WM, ed. Urological pathology. Philadelphia: WB Saunders, 1989:64–96.

Adenocarcinoma

199. Abenoza P, Manivel C, Fraley EE. Primary adenocarcinoma of urinary bladder: clinicopathologic study of 16 cases. Urology 1987;29:9–14.
200. Bullock PS, Thoni DE, Murphy WM. The significance of colonic mucosa (intestinal metaplasia) involving the urinary tract. Cancer 1987;59:2086–90.
201. Daroca PJ Jr, Mackenzie F, Reed RJ, Keane JM. Primary adenovillous carcinoma of the bladder. J Urol 1976;115:41–5.
202. Eble JN, Hull MT, Rowland RG, Hostetter M. Villous adenoma of the urachus with mucusuria: a light and electron microscopic study. J Urol 1986;135:1240–4.
203. Epstein JI, Kuhajda FP, Lieberman PH. Prostate-specific acid phosphatase immunoreactivity in adenocarcinomas of the urinary bladder. Hum Pathol 1986;17:939–42.
204. Goyanna R, Emmett JL, McDonald JR. Exstrophy of the bladder complicated by adenocarcinoma. J Urol 1951;65:391–400.
205. Grignon DJ, Ro JY, Ayala AG, Johnson DE, Primary signet-ring cell carcinoma of the urinary bladder. Am J Clin Pathol 1991;95:13–20.
206. _____, Ro JY, Ayala AG, Johnson DE. Ordóñez NG. Primary adenocarcinoma of the urinary bladder: a clinicopathologic analysis of 72 cases. Cancer 1991; 67:2165–72.
207. Hermanek P, Sobin LH, eds. TNM Classification of malignant tumours. 4th ed. 2nd revision. Berlin: Springer-Verlag, 1992.
208. Koss LG. Tumors of the urinary tract and prostate in urinary sediment. In: Diagnostic cytology and its histopathologic bases. 4th ed. Philadelphia: JB Lippincott, 1992:964.

209. Miller DC, Gang DL, Gavris V, Alroy J, Ucci AA, Parkhurst EC. Villous adenoma of the urinary bladder: a morphologic or biologic entity? Am J Clin Pathol 1983;79:728–31.
210. Murphy WM. Atlas of bladder carcinoma. Chicago: ASCP Press, 1986:59–65.
211. _____. Diseases of the urinary bladder, urethra, ureters, and renal pelves. In: Murphy WM, ed. Urological pathology. Philadelphia: WB Saunders, 1989:35–37,39–41, 85.
212. Newbould M, McWilliam LJ. A study of vesical adenocarcinoma, intestinal metaplasia and related lesions using mucin histochemistry. Histopathol 1990;17:225–30.
213. O'Brien AM, Urbanski SJ. Papillary adenocarcinoma in situ of bladder. J Urol 1985;134:544–6.
214. Pallesen G. Neoplastic Paneth cells in adenocarcinoma of the urinary bladder: a first case report. Cancer 1981;47:1834–7.
215. Sinard J, Macleary L, Melamed J. Hepatoid adenocarcinoma in the urinary bladder. Unusual localization of a newly recognized tumor type. Cancer 1994;73:1919–25.
216. Song J, Farrow GM, Lieber MM. Primary adenocarcinoma of the bladder: favorable prognostic significance of deoxyribonucleic acid diploidy measured by flow cytometry. J Urol 1990;144:1115–8.
217. Thomas DG, Ward AM, Williams JL. A study of 52 cases of adenocarcinoma of the bladder. Br J Urol 1971;43:4–15.
218. Ward AM. Glandular neoplasia within the urinary tract. The aetiology of adenocarcinoma of the urothelium with a review of the literature. I. Introduction: the origin of glandular epithelium in the renal pelvis, ureter and bladder. Virchows Arch Pathol Anat Physiol Klin Med 1971;352:296–311.

Poorly Differentiated Carcinoma, Small Cell Carcinoma

219. Blomjous CE, Vos W, De Voogt HJ, Van der Valk P, Meijer CJ. Small cell carcinoma of the urinary bladder: a clinicopathologic, morphometric, immunohistochemical, and ultrastructural study of 18 cases. Cancer 1989;64:1347–57.
220. Grignon DJ, Ro JY, Ayala AG, et al. Small cell carcinoma of the urinary bladder: a clinicopathologic analysis of 22 cases. Cancer 1992;69:527–36.
221. Mills SE, Wolfe JT, Weiss MA, et al. Small cell undifferentiated carcinoma of the urinary bladder. A light-

microscopic immunocytochemical, and ultrastructural study of 12 cases. Am J Surg Pathol 1987;11:606–17.
222. Partanen S, Asikainen U. Oat-cell carcinoma of the urinary bladder with ectopic adrenocorticotropic hormone production. Hum Pathol 1985;16:313–5.
223. Reyes CV, Soneru I. Small cell carcinoma of the urinary bladder with hypercalcemia. Cancer 1985;56:2530–3.
224. Young RH, Eble JN. Unusual forms of carcinoma of the bladder. Hum Pathol 1991;22:948–65.

Rare Neoplasms

225. Ainsworth AM, Clarke WH, Mastrangelo M, Conger KB. Primary malignant melanoma of the urinary bladder. Cancer 1976;37:1928–36.

226. Bitterman P, Chun B, Kurman RJ. The significance of epithelial differentiation in mixed mesodermal tumors of the uterus. A clinicopathologic and immunohistochemical study. Am J Surg Pathol 1990;14:317–28.

227. George E, Manivel JC, Dehner LP, Wick MR. Malignant mixed müllerian tumors: an immunohistochemical study of 47 cases, with histogenetic considerations and clinical correlation. Hum Pathol 1991;22:215–23.

228. Ironside JW, Timperley WR, Madden JW, Royds JA, Taylor CB. Primary melanoma of the urinary bladder presenting with intracerebral metastases. Br J Urol 1985;57:593–4.

229. Jacobsen AB, Nesland JM, Fosså SD, Pettersen EO. Human chorionic gonadotropin, neuron specific enolase and deoxyribonucleic acid flow cytometry in patients with high grade bladder carcinoma. J Urol 1990;143:706–9.

230. Kanno J, Sakamoto A, Washizuka M, Kawai T, Kasuga T. Malignant mixed mesodermal tumor of bladder occurring after radiotherapy for cervical cancer: report of a case. J Urol 1985;133:854–6.

231. Kitazawa M, Kobayashi H, Ohnishi Y, Kimura K, Sakurai S, Sekine S. Giant cell tumor of the bladder associated with transitional cell carcinoma. J Urol 1985;133:472–5.

232. Kojima T, Tanaka T, Yoshimi N, Mori H. Primary malignant melanoma of the urinary bladder. Arch Pathol Lab Med 1992;116:1213–6.

233. Koss LG. Tumors of the urinary bladder. Atlas of Tumor Pathology, 2nd Series, Fascicle 11. Washington, D.C.: Armed Forces Institute of Pathology, 1975:46–52.

234. Lidgi S, Embon OM, Turani H, Sazbon AI. Giant cell reparative granuloma of the bladder associated with transitional cell carcinoma. J Urol 1989;142:120–2.

235. Sahin AA, Myhre M, Ro JY, Sneige N, Dekmezian RH, Ayala AG. Plasmacytoid transitional cell carcinoma: report of a case with initial presentation mimicking multiple myeloma. Acta Cytol 1991;35:277–80.

236. Smith JA Jr, Herr HW, Middleton RG. Bladder carcinosarcoma: histologic variation in metastatic lesions. J Urol 1983;129:829–31.

237. Stein BS, Kendall AR. Malignant melanoma of the genitourinary tract. J Urol 1984;132:859–68.

238. Walker BF, Someren A, Kennedy JC, Nicholas EM. Primary carcinoid tumor of the urinary bladder. Arch Pathol Lab Med 1992;116:1217–20.

239. Yang CH, Krzyzaniak K, Brown WJ, Kurtz SM. Primary carcinoid tumor of urinary bladder. Urology 1985;26:594–7.

240. Young RH. Carcinosarcoma of the urinary bladder. Cancer 1987;59:1333–9.

241. _____, Eble JN. Unusual forms of carcinoma of the urinary bladder. Hum Pathol 1991;22:948–65.

242. _____, Wick MR. Transitional cell carcinoma of the urinary bladder with pseudosarcomatous stroma. Am J Clin Pathol 1988;89:216–9.

243. Zukerberg LR, Armin AR, Pisharodi L, Young RH, et al. Transitional cell carcinoma of the urinary bladder with osteoclast-type giant cells: a report of two cases and review of the literature. Histopathology 1990;17:407–11.

244. _____, Harris NL, Young RH. Carcinomas of the urinary bladder simulating malignant lymphoma: a report of five cases. Am J Surg Pathol 1991;15:569–76.

Metastases to Urinary Bladder

245. Berger Y, Nissenblatt M, Salwitz J, Lega B. Bladder involvement in metastatic breast carcinoma. J Urol 1992;147:137–9.

246. Chen KT, Spaulding RW. Appendiceal carcinoma masquerading as primary bladder carcinoma. J Urol 1991;145:821–2.

247. Ferris DO, Beare JB. Wilms' tumor: report of a case with unusual postoperative metastasis. Staff Meet Mayo Clin Proc 1947;22:94–8.

248. Goldstein AG. Metastatic carcinoma to the bladder. J Urol 1967;98:209–15.

249. Remis RE, Halverstadt DB. Metastatic renal cell carcinoma to the bladder: case report and review of the literature. J Urol 1986;136:1294–6.

250. Sufrin G, Keogh B, Moore RH, Murphy GP. Secondary involvement of the bladder in malignant lymphoma. J Urol 1977;118:251–3.

251. Viddeleer AC, Lycklama À Nijeholt GA, Beekhuis-Brussee JA. A late manifestation of testicular seminoma in the bladder of a renal transplant recipient: a case report. J Urol 1992;148(2 Pt 1):401–2.

252. Young RH. Unusual variants of primary bladder carcinoma and secondary tumors of the bladder. In: Young RH, ed. Pathology of the urinary bladder. New York: Churchill Livingstone, 1989:128–30.

253. _____, Johnston WH. Serous adenocarcinoma of the uterus metastatic to the urinary bladder mimicking primary bladder neoplasia: a report of a case. Am J Surg Pathol 1990;14:877–80.

Nonepithelial Neoplasms

254. Abratt RP, Temple-Camp CR, Pontin AR. Choriocarcinoma and transitional cell carcinoma of the bladder—a case report and review of the clinical evolution of the disease in reported cases. Eur J Surg Oncol 1989;15:149–53.

255. Ahlering TE, Weintraub P, Skinner DG. Management of adult sarcomas of the bladder and prostate. J Urol 1988;140:1397–9.

256. Caro DJ, Brown JS. Hemangioma of bladder. Urology 1976;7:479–81.

257. Cauffield EW. Dermoid cysts of the bladder. J Urol 1956;75:801–4.

258. Chaitin BA, Manning JT, Ordóñez NG. Hematologic neoplasms with initial manifestations in lower urinary tract. Urology 1984;23:35–42.

259. De Bruyne R, Peters O, Goossens A, Braeckman J, Denis LJ. Primary IgG-lambda immunocytoma of the urinary bladder. Eur J Surg Oncol 1987;13:361–4.

260. Dehner LP. Pathology of the urinary bladder in children. In: Young RH, ed. Pathology of the urinary bladder. New York: Churchill Livingstone, 1989:179–211.

261. Forrest JB, Saypol DC, Mills SE, Gillenwater JY. Immunoblastic sarcoma of the bladder. J Urol 1983;130:350–1.

262. Grignon DJ, Ro JY, Mackay B, et al. Paraganglioma of the urinary bladder: immunohistochemical, ultrastructural, and DNA flow cytometric studies. Hum Pathol 1991;22:1162–9.

263. Guthman DA, Malek RS, Chapman WR, Farrow GM. Primary malignant lymphoma of the bladder. J Urol 1990;144:1367–9.

264. Hockley NM, Bihrle R, Bennett RM III, Curry JM. Congenital genitourinary hemangiomas in a patient with the Klippel-Trenaunay syndrome: management with the neodymium:YAG laser. J Urol 1989;141:940–1.

265. Kahle PJ, Maltry E, Vickery G. Hemangioma of the bladder: report of an additional case. J Urol 1942;47:267–9.

266. Marconis JT. Primary Hodgkin's (paragranulomatous type) disease of the bladder. J Urol 1959;81:275–81.

267. Masui T, Asamoto M, Imaida K, Fukushima S, Okamura T, Ohtaguro K. Primary choriocarcinoma of the urinary bladder. Jpn J Clin Oncol 1988;18:59–64.

268. Mills SE, Bova GS, Wick MR, Young RH. Leiomyosarcoma of the urinary bladder: a clinicopathologic and immunohistochemical study of 15 cases. Am J Surg Pathol 1989;13:480–9.

269. Morton KD, Burnett RA. Choriocarcinoma arising in transitional cell carcinoma of bladder: a case report. Histopathology 1988;12:325–8.

270. Moyana TN, Kontozoglou T. Urinary bladder paragangliomas: an immunohistochemical study. Arch Pathol Lab Med 1988;112:70–2.

271. Murphy WM. Diseases of the urinary bladder, urethra, ureters, and renal pelves. In: Murphy WM, ed. Urological pathology. Philadelphia: WB Saunders, 1989:104–9.

272. Ohsawa M, Aozasa K, Horiuchi K, Kanamaru A. Malignant lymphoma of bladder. Report of three cases and review of the literature. Cancer 1993;72:1969–74.

273. Pollack AD. Malignant teratoma of the urinary bladder: report of a case. Am J Pathol 1936;12:561–8.

274. Siegel RJ, Napoli VM. Malignant lymphoma of the urinary bladder. A case with signet-ring cells simulating urachal adenocarcinoma. Arch Pathol Lab Med 1991;115:635–7.

275. Swartz DA, Johnson DE, Ayala AG, Watkins DL. Bladder leiomyosarcoma: a review of 10 cases with 5-year follow-up. J Urol 1985;133:200–2.

276. Taylor G, Jordan M, Churchill B, Mancer K. Yolk sac tumor of the bladder. J Urol 1983;129:591–4.

277. Vance RP, Geisinger KR, Randall MB, Marshall RB. Immature neural elements in immature teratomas: an immunohistochemical and ultrastructural study. Am J Clin Pathol 1988;90:397–11.

278. Walker AN, Mills SE, Young RH. Mesenchymal and miscellaneous other primary tumors of the urinary bladder. In: Young RH, ed. Pathology of the urinary bladder. New York: Churchill Livingstone, 1989:139–78.

279. Yang C, Motteram R, Sandeman TF. Extramedullary plasmacytoma of the bladder: a case report and review of literature. Cancer 1982;50:146–9.

Non-neoplastic Tumorous Conditions

280. al-Izzi MS, Horton LW, Kelleher J, Fawcett D. Malignant transformation in endometriosis of the urinary bladder. Histopathology 1989;14:191–8.

281. Benson RC Jr, Swanson SK, Farrow GM. Relationship of leukoplakia to urothelial malignancy. J Urol 1984;131:507–11.

282. Billis A, Lima AC, Queiroz LS, Cia EM, Oliveira ER, Pinto W Jr. Adenoma of bladder in siblings with renal dysplasia. Urology 1980;16:299–302.

283. Brown EW. Eosinophilic granuloma of the bladder. J Urol 1960;83:665–8.

284. Bullock PS, Thoni DE, Murphy WM. The significance of colonic mucosa (intestinal metaplasia) involving the urinary tract. Cancer 1987;59:2086–90.

285. Clement PB, Young RH. Endocervicosis of the urinary bladder: a report of six cases of a benign müllerian lesion that may mimic adenocarcinoma. Am J Surg Pathol 1992;16:533–42.

286. Damjanov I, Katz SM. Malakoplakia. Pathol Annu 1981;16(Pt 2):103–26.

287. Del Mistro A, Koss LG, Braunstein J, Bennett B, Saccomano G, Simons KM. Condylomata acuminata of the urinary bladder: natural history, viral typing, and DNA content. Am J Surg Pathol 1988;12:205–15.

288. Devine P, Ucci AA, Krain H, et al. Nephrogenic adenoma and embryonic kidney tubules share PNA receptor sites. Am J Clin Pathol 1984;81:728–32.

289. Dietrick DD, Kabalin JN, Daniels GF Jr, Epstein AB, Fielding IM. Inflammatory pseudotumor of the bladder. J Urol 1992;148:141–4.

290. Eble JN. Abnormalities of the urachus. In: Young RH, ed. Pathology of the urinary bladder. New York: Churchill Livingstone 1989;213–44.

291. Ehara H, Deguchi T, Yanagihara M, Yokota T, Uchino F, Kawada Y. Primary localized amyloidosis of the bladder: an immunohistochemical study of a case. J Urol 1992;147:458–60.

292. Erturk E, Erturk E, Sheinfeld J, Davis RS. Metaplastic cystitis complicated with von Brunn nests, cystitis cystica, and intestinal type of glandular metaplasia. Urology 1988;32:165–7.

293. Friedman NB, Kuhlenbeck H. Adenomatoid tumors of the bladder reproducing renal structures (nephrogenic adenomas). J Urol 1950;64:657–70.

294. Fujihara S, Glenner GG. Primary localized amyloidosis of the genitourinary tract: immunohistochemical study on eleven cases. Lab Invest 1981;44:55–60.

295. Goldstein AM, Fauer RB, Chinn M, Kaempf MJ. New concepts on formation of Brunn's nests and cysts in urinary tract mucosa. Urology 1978;11:513–7.

296. Huang WL, Ro JY, Grignon DJ, Swanson D, Ordonez NG, Ayala AG. Postoperative spindle cell nodule of the prostate and bladder. J Urol 1990;143:824–6.

297. Iyengar V, Smith DK, Jablonski DV, Gallivan MV. Extramedullary hematopoiesis in the urinary bladder in a case of agnogenic myeloid metaplasia. J Urol Pathol 1993;1:419–23.

298. Jones EC, Clement PB, Young RH. Inflammatory pseudotumor of the urinary bladder. A clinicopathological, immunohistochemical, ultrastructural and flow cytometric study of 13 cases. Am J Surg Pathol 1993;17:264–74.

299. Jufe R, Molinolo AA, Fefer SA, Meiss RP. Plasma cell granuloma of the bladder: a case report. J Urol 1984;131:1175–6.

300. Kunze E, Schauer A, Schmitt M. Histology and histogenesis of two different types of inverted urothelial papillomas. Cancer 1983;51:348–58.

301. McClurg FV, D'Agostino AN, Martin JH, Race GJ. Ultrastructural demonstration of intracellular bacteria in three cases of malakoplakia of the bladder. Am J Clin Pathol 1973;60:780–8.

302. McIntire TL, Soloway MS, Murphy WM. Nephrogenic adenoma. Urology 1987;29:237–41.

303. Morey AF, Kreder KJ, Wikert GA, Cooper G, Dresner ML. Ectopic prostate tissue at the bladder dome. J Urol 1989;141:942–3.

304. Mostofi FK. Potentialities of bladder epithelium. J Urol 1954;71:705–14.

305. Murphy WM. Diseases of the urinary bladder, urethra, ureters, and renal pelves. In: Murphy WM, ed. Urological pathology. Philadelphia: WB Saunders, 1989:42–64.

306. Nowels K, Kent E, Rinsho K, Oyasu R. Prostate specific antigen and acid phosphatase-reactive cells in cystitis cystica and glandularis. Arch Pathol Lab Med 1988;112:734–7.

307. Park C, Kim H, Lee YB, Song JM, Ro JY. Hamartoma of the urachal remnant. Arch Pathol Lab Med 1989;113;1393–5.

308. Proppe KH, Scully RE, Rosai J. Postoperative spindle cell nodules of genitourinary tract resembling sarcomas: a report of eight cases. Am J Surg Pathol 1984;8:101–8.

309. Quint HJ, Drach GW, Rappaport WD, Hoffman CJ. Emphysematous cystitis: a review of the spectrum of disease. J Urol 1992;147:134–7.

310. Ro JY, Ayala AG, Ordonez NG, Swanson DA, Babaian RJ. Pseudosarcomatous fibromyxoid tumor of the urinary bladder. Am J Clin Pathol 1986;86:583–90.

311. Roth JA. Reactive pseudosarcomatous response in urinary bladder. Urology 1980;16:635–7.

312. Schubert GE, Pavkovic MB, Bethke-Bedürftig BA. Tubular urachal remnants in adult bladders. J Urol 1982;127:40–2.

313. Steele AA, Byrne AJ. Paramesonephric (müllerian) sinus of urinary bladder. Am J Surg Pathol 1982;6:173–6.

314. Thijssen A, Gerridzen RG. Eosinophilic cystitis presenting as invasive bladder cancer: comments on pathogenesis and management. J Urol 1990;144:977–9.

315. Vara AR, Ruzics EP, Moussaback O, Martin DC. Endometrioid adenosarcoma of the bladder arising from endometriosis. J Urol 1990;143:813–5.

316. Walther M, Glenn JF, Vellios F. Xanthogranulomatous cystitis. J Urol 1985;134:745–6.

317. Wells M, Anderson K. Mucin histochemistry of cystitis glandularis and primary adenocarcinoma of the urinary bladder. Arch Pathol Lab Med 1985;109:59–61.

318. Wick MR, Brown BA, Young RH, Mills SE. Spindle-cell proliferations of the urinary tract. An immunohistochemical study. Am J Surg Pathol 1988;12:379–89.

319. Widran J, Sanchez R, Gruhn J. Squamous metaplasia of the bladder: a study of 450 patients. J Urol 1974;112:479–82.

320. Wiener DP, Koss LG, Sablay B, Freed SZ. The prevalence and significance of Brunn's nests, cystitis cystica and squamous metaplasia in normal bladders. J Urol 1979;122:317–21.

321. Williams MP, Ibrahim SK, Rickwood AM. Hamartoma of the urinary bladder in an infant with Beckwith-Wiedemann syndrome. Br J Urol 1990;65:106–7.

322. Wilson RW, Chenggis ML, Unger ER. Longitudinal study of human papilloma virus infection of the female urogenital tract by in situ hybridization. Arch Pathol Lab Med 1990;114:155–9.

323. Young RH. Non-neoplastic epithelial abnormalities and tumorlike lesions. In: Young RH, ed. Pathology of the urinary bladder. New York: Churchill Livingstone, 1989:1–64.

324. _____, Scully RE. Nephrogenic adenoma: a report of 15 cases, review of the literature, and comparison with clear cell adenocarcinoma of the urinary tract. Am J Surg Pathol 1986;10:268–75.

325. Zilberman M, Laor E, Moriel E, Reid RE, Farkas A. Paravesical granulomas masquerading as bladder neoplasms: late complications of inguinal hernia repair. J Urol 1990;143:489–91

❖❖❖

3
TUMORS OF THE URETHRA

NORMAL ANATOMY

The urethra develops from the caudal portion of the urogenital sinus (18,37). In females, failure of fusion of the genital swelling and growth of the genital tubercle results in a short organ emptying into a vestibule shared with the vagina. The mature female urethra is lined predominantly with squamous epithelium and receives ducts from multiple paraurethral glands (Skene glands), homologues of the prostatic glands in the male (38). The mucosa is surrounded by a thick muscular wall containing scanty erectile tissue. In males, growth of the genital tubercle and fusion of the genital swellings produce an elongated urethra which becomes surrounded by the prostate gland and fuses with the phallic ectoderm to form prostatic, membranous, and penile portions. The prostatic and membranous parts of the mature male urethra are lined predominantly by transitional mucosa but areas of epithelium are frequent in the prostatic portion. Pseudo-stratified columnar and squamous epithelium appear in the penile portion.

The transitional cells of the normal urethra are more compact and have less cytoplasmic clearing than those of the urinary bladder. In usual histologic preparations, their nuclei seem larger, with slightly more granular chromatin. Whether these changes reflect normal development or acquired alterations is unclear but they are important when the urethral mucosa is evaluated for dysplastic (atypical hyperplastic) changes. Paired bulbourethral glands (Cowper glands), the male homologue of Bartholin glands, form inferior to the prostate and empty into the proximal penile urethra through discrete ducts. Tubular periurethral glands (glands of Littré) lubricate the penile urethra at multiple sites along its course. Regardless of location, these accessory urethral glands are rich in mucus-secreting cells. The posterior prostatic portion of the male urethra is elevated by the utricle (uterus masculinus) and terminal portions of the ejaculatory ducts, which together form the verumontanum (colliculus seminalis). Depending on its location, the male urethra is surrounded by the musculature of the bladder neck, the prostate gland, the urogenital diaphragm (external sphincter), or the corpus spongiosum.

EPITHELIAL NEOPLASMS

Epithelial neoplasms of the urethra are almost exclusively carcinomas (28). If squamous cell papilloma is considered an inflammatory reaction similar to condyloma acuminatum, benign epithelial neoplasms are rare. The etiology, pathogenesis, methods of detection and monitoring, histologic classification, and staging of urethral cancers are essentially the same as for their bladder counterparts and are not reiterated (see chapter 2). Reactions to therapy and epithelial atypias have been less thoroughly studied but are probably similar to those in the bladder. The literature suggests that carcinomas arising in the urethra differ from those originating in the urinary bladder in the following respects: lower incidence; higher frequency in women; greater percentage of high-grade invasive tumors; greater percentage of squamous cell carcinomas; greater likelihood of high stage at diagnosis; and poorer prognosis (9,12,22,24).

Primary carcinomas of the urethra comprise less than 1 percent of all urothelial neoplasms. Patients are usually women (male to female ratio, 1 to 4) with a mean age of 60 years (9,12). Chronic irritation, urethral stricture, urethral diverticula, and chronic infections with sexually transmitted diseases have been considered predisposing factors. Human papillomavirus activity has been demonstrated in the neoplastic cells of rare cases (25). Bladder cancer is a commonly associated condition and more than a few cases reported as urethral carcinoma represent secondary involvement by multifocal carcinoma in situ of the bladder (2,10,17). A bleeding urethral mass is the most common presenting complaint in women; obstruction is most often observed in men. Patients of both sexes may have dysuria, pain, and discharge.

Histologically, epithelial neoplasms of the urethra are almost all transitional cell, squamous cell, or adenocarcinomas, although other types have been reported (fig. 3-1) (15). The histologic subtype varies with the location of the lesion. Distal urethral tumors are usually squamous cell carcinoma, especially in women. More proximal carcinomas tend to be transitional cell or adenocarcinomas. In women, lesions often occupy the entire urethra; in men, over 75 percent of primary urethral carcinomas occur in the membranous and penile regions.

The differential diagnosis of primary urethral tumors follows the guidelines established for bladder neoplasms. Most carcinomas present no diagnostic problems. Primary ductal prostatic carcinomas commonly present as papillary lesions in the urethra. Careful examination reveals the uniform nuclei; the finely granular, evenly distributed chromatin; and the prominent nucleoli characteristic of high-grade prostatic carcinomas. Immunohistochemical reactions for prostatic antigens can be used if necessary.

Regardless of sex, urethral carcinomas tend to grow locally (9,12,19). Metastases to distant organs are unusual but preferentially involve lymph nodes when present. The prognosis for proximal urethral tumors is poor. The median survival time is less than 2 years and the death rate is greater than 50 percent in most reports. Carcinomas arising in the penile urethra are associated with a more favorable prognosis, perhaps because their location allows complete surgical resection prior to dissemination.

Carcinoma in Situ

Carcinoma in situ (CIS) rarely occurs as a primary urethral neoplasm but has been documented in over 30 percent of urethras following cystoprostatectomy for bladder cancer (10,11, 44). If the entire urethra is not removed at the time of radical surgery, pathologic evaluation is essential to subsequent patient care, beginning with an examination of the prostate gland, since patients whose prostates contain bladder carcinoma are at especially high risk for subsequent involvement of the residual urethra (10). The best current method for monitoring the urethra after cystoprostatectomy is urinary cytology (fig. 3-2) (11,28). Tumor cells in urethral washings are

usually more poorly preserved than similar elements in bladder washings but can be distinguished by their eccentricity, high nuclear-cytoplasmic ratios, pleomorphism, and granular chromatin. Neoplastic cells in specimens obtained at periodic intervals from asymptomatic patients signal the presence of focal carcinoma in situ. These lesions are rarely detectable at subsequent urethroscopy and biopsy confirmation prior to complete urethrectomy is usually not possible. In such cases, the pathologist should submit the entire urethra for histologic examination. Using cytology, lesions in residual urethras have been detected while still in situ (11). Lesions presenting with gross hematuria or a palpable mass have often been invasive, with a correspondingly poorer prognosis (44).

Clear Cell Carcinoma

This is a relatively rare tumor with distinctive histogenetic and histologic features (22,28,45). Cases have been reported in the bladder but are most frequent in the female urethra, where they may arise from periurethral ducts or diverticula. Reactions for prostatic antigens, a characteristic of periurethral ducts, have been positive in the few cases examined (36). Unlike other urethral carcinomas, association with sources of chronic irritation have not been strong. The histologic features are most reminiscent of clear cell carcinoma of the uterus or vagina and many authors favor a müllerian differentiation, if not derivation. Histologic changes suggestive of mesonephric or nephrogenic differentiation also occur but derivation from these sources has been rejected by most authorities (36,45).

Patients with clear cell carcinoma range in age from 35 to 73 years (mean, 51 years). Almost all are women. Most cancers arise at periurethral sites. Gross hematuria, dysuria, pain, and discharge are the usual presenting complaints. A visible mass was present in nearly every case.

The pathology of clear cell carcinoma is distinctive (fig. 3-3). Tumors are composed predominantly of sheets of uniform, ovoid cells with moderately well-defined borders and amphophilic to acidophilic cytoplasm. Papillary, tubular, and even cystic areas are common and all may be partially lined by "hobnailed" cells. A single layer of neoplastic cells usually lines the papillae

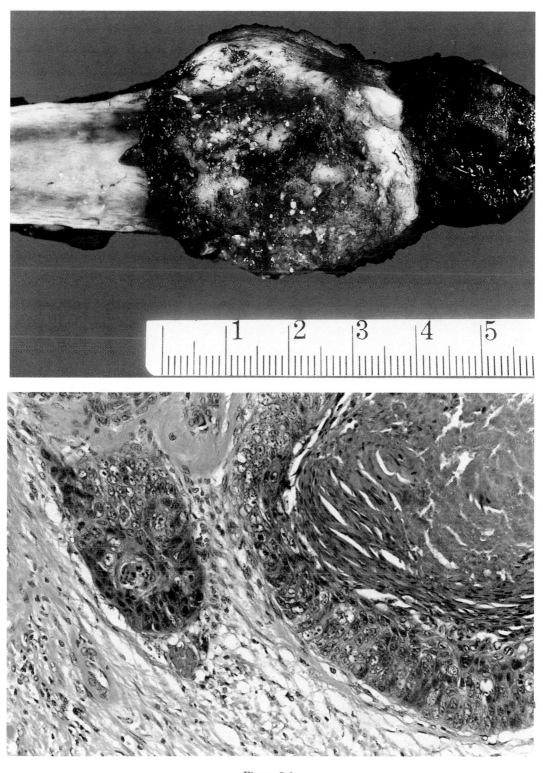

Figure 3-1
SQUAMOUS CELL CARCINOMA OF THE URETHRA

Top: Gross specimen.
Bottom: Histologically, the tumor produced large amounts of keratin. (Fig. 2-76 from Murphy WM. Urological pathology. Philadelphia: WB Saunders, 1989:119.)

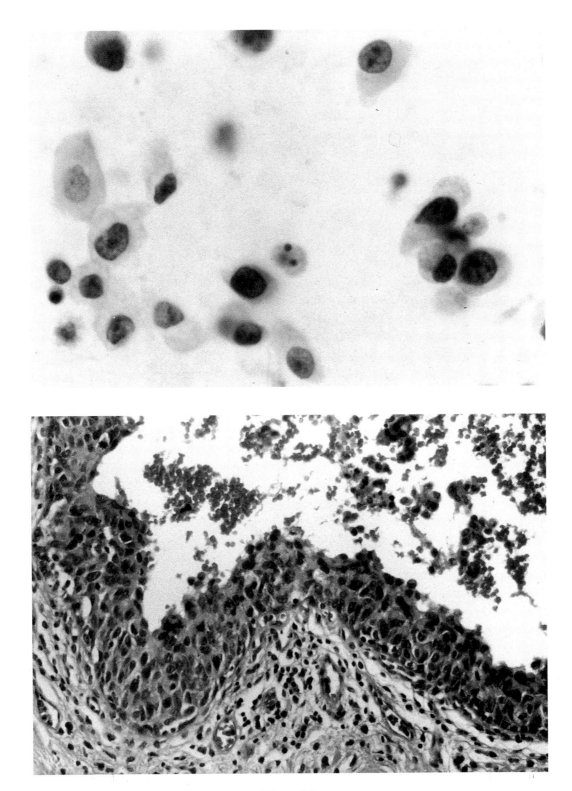

Figure 3-2
CARCINOMA IN SITU IN THE URETHRAL STUMP

Top: These lesions are usually detected in cytologic specimens such as this, where the tumor cells have hyperchromatic, eccentric nuclei and relatively high nuclear-cytoplasmic ratios.

Bottom: Multiple sections of the urethrectomy specimen are usually required to detect the focal carcinoma in situ.

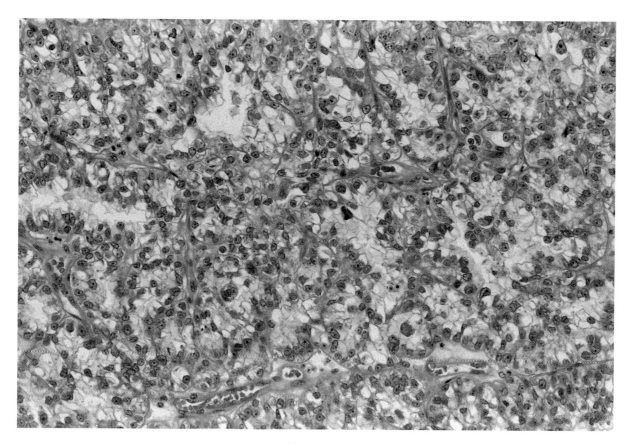

Figure 3-3
CLEAR CELL CARCINOMA OF THE URETHRA

or tubules. Clear cells rich in glycogen are characteristic but are rarely the predominant element in our experience. Prostate-specific antigen, prostatic acid phosphatase, small amounts of luminal mucin, and psammoma bodies have been observed. The nuclei of the clear cells tend to be round and uniform, with slightly irregular borders; finely granular, evenly distributed chromatin; and prominent nucleoli. Mitoses are readily found. Cytologic and ultrastructural studies have confirmed the histologic findings.

Clear cell carcinoma must be differentiated from other types of adenocarcinoma, mesonephric carcinoma, nephrogenic metaplasia, and metastatic carcinomas. The histologic pattern of sheets, papillae, and tubules without significant mucin distinguishes these tumors from other urothelial adenocarcinomas. Mesonephric carcinoma is a controversial tumor which may not exist as a separate entity and is almost always

difficult to confirm. The hobnailed pattern suggestive of this lesion is common to other neoplasms, has never predominated in reported cases of clear cell carcinoma, and cannot be considered strong evidence of mesonephric differentiation. Further, clear cell carcinomas tend to arise at anterior and posterior sites rather than the lateral locations expected of a tumor arising in mesonephric remnants. Nephrogenic metaplasia is histologically similar to clear cell carcinoma and it is possible that nephrogenic and clear cell patterns differentiate simultaneously. Nephrogenic metaplasia is not known to manifest prostatic antigens nor has clear cell carcinoma been observed among patients followed for nephrogenic metaplasia. Cellular anaplasia is rare in nephrogenic metaplasia and never occurs in large portions of the lesion. Metastatic carcinomas, especially from kidney or prostate gland, may be difficult to distinguish from clear cell carcinoma on histologic grounds alone. Radiographic studies may be required in selected cases.

The prognosis of clear cell carcinoma is unclear. Most reported patients were treated with radical surgery but followed for less than 5 years. Metastases occurred in at least 15 percent of cases. The survival rate was less than 60 percent. Tumor-related deaths have occurred after apparently adequate surgical excision and after many years of follow-up.

MELANOMA

The urethra is the most common site of primary melanoma in the genitourinary tract (14,32). The etiology and pathogenesis are unknown. Melanomas are more common in women (male to female ratio, 1 to 2.6) and occur in blacks as well as whites. Most patients are 50 to 70 years of age (mean, 64 years). Lesions usually occur in the distal urethra where they may produce symptoms of dysuria or hematuria. Lesions in the urethra may be secondary to melanomas of the glans penis or labia. The pathology does not differ from that at other body sites. Most urethral melanomas are localized at diagnosis. Even so, prognosis is poor with few patients surviving more than 5 years.

OTHER URETHRAL NEOPLASMS

A variety of neoplasms of the urethra have been reported as individual cases. They include carcinoid, cloacogenic carcinoma, villous adenoma, rhabdomyosarcoma, lymphoma, plasmacytoma, granular cell tumor, hemangioma, leiomyoma, and intravascular angiomatosis (Masson angiomatosis) (15,28,30,39,43). The pathology of these lesions is characteristic of each type of tumor and does not differ from that of similar neoplasms at other body sites.

NON-NEOPLASTIC TUMOROUS CONDITIONS

Condyloma Acuminatum

Condyloma acuminatum is an inflammatory reaction manifested by a proliferation of squamous epithelium. The urethra is ordinarily involved by direct extension from lesions arising at adjacent sites but primary urethral condylomas occur. Evidence of infection with human papillomavirus (HPV) can be demonstrated in almost every case and it is generally accepted that condylomata acuminata are caused by infection with HPV. Using sophisticated techniques to detect gene copies, HPV types 6 or 11 have been most commonly identified; a few lesions have contained other types (4,23). In contrast to the almost universal evidence of viral exposure, many lesions fail to manifest viral structural antigens and even when present, these antigens occur in only a tiny percentage of the cells examined (29). Condyloma acuminatum rarely coexists with, and does not appear to be a direct precursor of, cancer.

Condyloma acuminatum is common, especially in men, where it accounts for up to 30 percent of tumorous lesions of the urethra (9,24). Most patients are 20 to 40 years of age. Lesions grow slowly and are often asymptomatic. Multiplicity and recurrence are common.

The pathologic features of condyloma acuminatum do not differ from those of similar lesions arising elsewhere (fig. 3-4). Condylomas may be either papillary or flat and characteristically manifest koilocytotic areas. Significant cytologic atypia is unusual. The relationship to squamous cell papilloma is unclear. While many authors differentiate these histologically similar lesions on the basis of koilocytotic areas and evidence of HPV, viral studies have been performed on very few cases and papillary squamous lesions lacking koilocytosis occasionally contain the virus.

Polyps

Polyps of the urethra exist in two major types: fibrous and prostatic (27,41). *Fibrous polyps* are almost certainly congenital anomalies arising in the posterior urethra at the verumontanum. The condition most commonly occurs in male infants and boys 3 to 10 years of age but has been observed in late-term fetuses and older men (5,16). Most patients complain of obstructive symptoms; a few have hematuria or urinary tract infections.

Pathologically, the name is descriptive. The lesions are polypoid growths protruding into the urethra from a relatively narrow stalk (fig. 3-5). The stalk is rich in fibrous connective tissue and blood vessels. It often contains glands, smooth

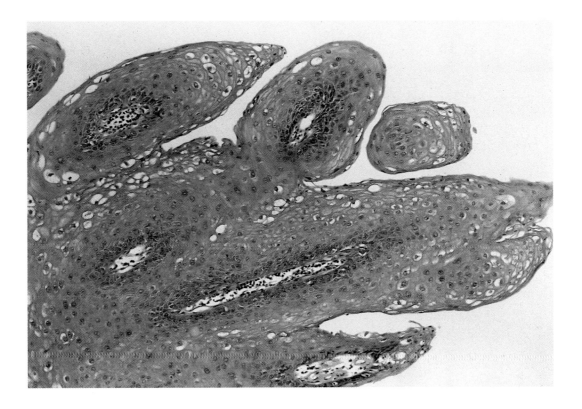

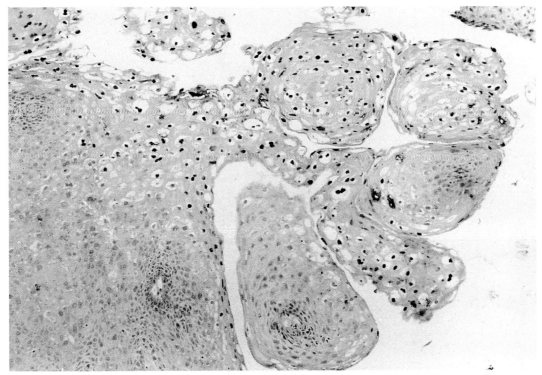

Figure 3-4
CONDYLOMA ACUMINATUM OF THE PENILE URETHRA
Top: Typical koilocytotic change occurs in the upper layers of epithelium.
Bottom: Human papillomavirus structural antigens are numerous in this tissue.

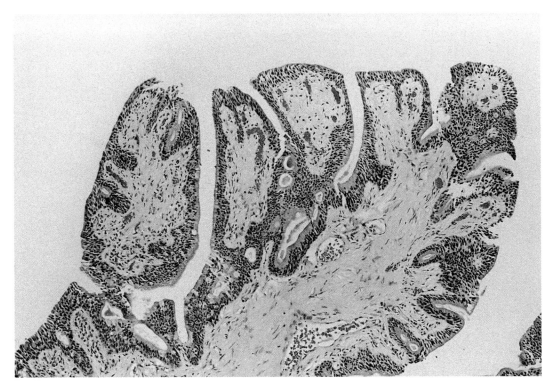

Figure 3-5
FIBROUS POLYP OF THE URETHRA

muscles, and nerves. The overlying epithelium is almost always transitional but may contain areas of ulceration or squamous metaplasia.

Prostatic polyps (ectopic prostate, adenomatous polyp, papillary adenoma) are usually reactive lesions associated with urethral injury, although hamartomatous and even neoplastic etiologies cannot be completely excluded (1,41). These tumors may arise at various sites, most commonly in the area of the verumontanum in men 13 to 31 years of age. Patients may have obstructive symptoms or hematuria. Hemospermia has been observed in a surprisingly large number, suggesting an element of ejaculatory duct in the "prostatic" epithelium.

The lesions are composed predominantly of histologically unremarkable prostate glands arranged in either polypoid or papillary configurations (fig. 3-6). Polypoid growths consist of nodular accumulations of prostate tissue usually covered with a double layered, prostatic type epithelium; papillary lesions comprise similar epithelium without the submucosal nodules. Corpora amylacea may be present.

Sporadic cases of polypoid urethral lesions not conforming to the two major types have been reported (27,33,41). Growths histologically identical to polypoid cystitis are observed in the urethra. Significant cellular atypia may rarely occur in papillary prostatic lesions. Both recurrences and a resemblance to the so-called endometrioid variant of prostatic duct carcinoma have been noted but the biologic potential of these rare lesions is unknown.

Diverticula

Diverticula of the urethra are saccular invaginations of mucosa, most commonly detected in women aged 20 to 60 years (3,6,28). The lesions are either congenital or acquired but are rarely observed in infants. Most remain asymptomatic for prolonged periods with clinical symptoms arising from complications such as obstruction, infection, stones, metaplasia, neoplasia, and even endometriosis. Most diverticula are small but lesions larger than 10 cm in greatest dimension have been recorded. Pathologic findings depend

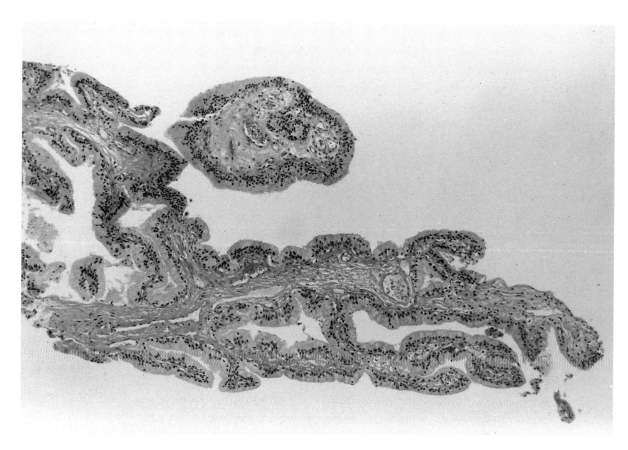

Figure 3-6
PROSTATIC POLYP OF THE URETHRA

upon the type of complication, usually comprising inflammatory reactions of varying severity. Urethral diverticula seem particularly prone to develop nephrogenic metaplasia and most carcinomas arising in diverticula have been adenocarcinomas (8,21).

Caruncle

A caruncle is an inflammation of the urethral lamina propria which may assume a nodular form (28). Most lesions occur in the posterior or lateral portions of the female urethra. The etiology is obscure but a likely possibility is obstruction with subsequent destruction of paraurethral glands. Bacterial infection is not an important etiologic factor. Patients are women, often in the postmenopausal years, who usually complain of pain and spotting (42). Pathologically, urethral caruncles are nodular or pedunculated lesions comprising a dense polymorphous infiltrate rich in lymphocytes and small blood vessels (fig. 3-7). Epithelial hyperplasia and metaplasia may occur but caruncles have not been considered a risk factor for subsequent carcinoma (7). Subtyping on the basis of the predominant type of inflammatory pattern has not significantly improved our understanding of the process. The differential diagnosis becomes a problem only when epithelial hyperplasia is exuberant and occurs in finger-like projections. In such cases, islands of epithelium may seem to be deep in the lamina propria. These nests maintain their cytologic organization and lack significant cellular atypia.

Almost any lesion occurring in the urothelium or its supporting tissues may arise in the urethra. Neoplasms have been discussed in chapter 2. The most common non-neoplastic tumorous conditions include *nephrogenic metaplasia* and *amyloidosis* (20,40).

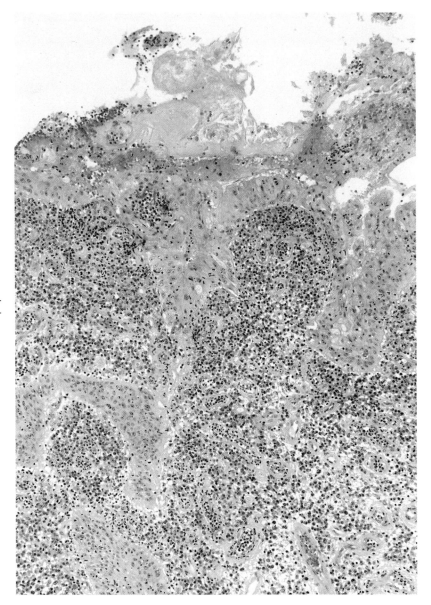

Figure 3-7
URETHRAL CARUNCLE
The inflammatory debris and epithelial hyperplasia might suggest carcinoma to the unwary.

TUMORS OF
ACCESSORY URETHRAL GLANDS

Accessory urethral glands are of two basic types: paraurethral and bulbourethral. Paraurethral glands are relatively simple tubuloalveolar mucosal invaginations lined by transitional, pseudostratified columnar, and mucus-secreting cells (13). They are variable in number and size and secrete a seromucinous fluid into the urethra at multiple sites along its course. Paraurethral glands in females (Skene glands) are homologues of prostatic tissue, as judged by their expression of prostatic antigens (38). In males, paraurethral glands describe those structures arising in the penile urethra (glands of Littré). Bulbourethral glands (Cowper glands) are paired seromucinous organs arising from the urogenital sinus that become embedded in the urogenital diaphragm of males. In contrast to paraurethral glands, these structures are larger, more discrete, and empty into the bulbous urethra via well-formed ducts.

Tumors of accessory urethral glands are predominantly *cysts* and *adenocarcinomas* (28). With the exception of clear cell carcinomas and

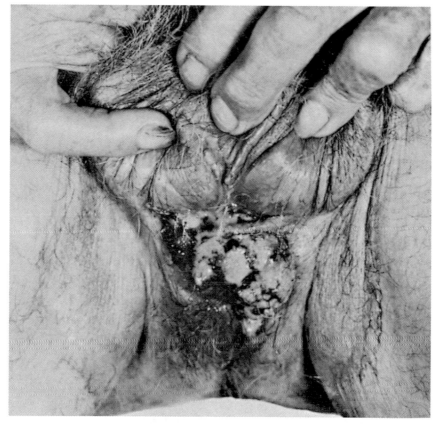

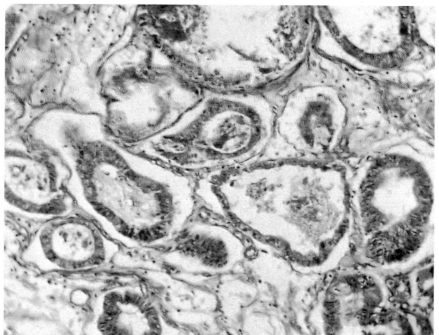

Figure 3-8
CARCINOMA OF COWPER GLANDS
Top: Gross specimen. (Fig. 266 from Fascicle 8, 2nd Series.)
Bottom: Adenocarcinoma. (Fig. 267 from Fascicle 8, 2nd Series.)

caruncles, most accessary gland lesions arise in the bulbourethral glands and are rare. Given their size and variable distribution, it is not surprising that tumors attributed to the paraurethral glands have been difficult to confirm (26,34). Cysts have been lined with transitional, pseudostratified columnar, and squamous epithelium. The most common neoplasm is clear cell carcinoma in women (36). Mucus-secreting adenocarcinomas and adenoid cystic carcinomas have also been reported (28).

The site of origin of bulbourethral gland tumors has been somewhat easier to establish (27, 28). Cysts may be either congenital or acquired (31). Congenital cysts are attributed to developmental fusion and acquired cysts to inflammatory obstruction of the bulbourethral ducts. Carcinomas are even less common than cysts. These neoplasms may remain localized for prolonged periods, eventually causing symptoms related to urethral obstruction or painful defecation. Histologically, bulbourethral gland neoplasms are mucus-secreting adenocarcinomas or adenoid cystic carcinomas (fig. 3-8) (27,35). Prognosis is unclear, especially since large tumors in this region are difficult to confirm as bulbourethral and many cases were reported before the advent of modern treatment and life support techniques.

REFERENCES

1. Baroudy AC, O'Connell JP. Papillary adenoma of the prostatic urethra. J Urol 1984;132:120–2.
2. Bégin LR, Dêschenes J, Mitmaker B. Pagetoid carcinomatous involvement of the penile urethra in association with high-grade transitional cell carcinoma of the urinary bladder. Arch Pathol Lab Med 1991;115:632–5.
3. Davis BL, Robinson DG. Diverticula of the female urethra: assay of 120 cases. J Urol 1970;104:850–3.
4. Del Mistro A, Braunstein JD, Halwer M, Koss LG. Identification of human papillomavirus types in male urethral condylomata acuminata by in situ hybridization. Hum Pathol 1987;18:936–40.
5. Downs RA. Congenital polyps of the prostatic urethra. A review of the literature and report of two cases. Br J Urol 1970;42:76–85.
6. Duckett JW, Snow BW. Disorders of the urethra and penis. In: Walsh PC, Gittes RF, Perlmutter AD, Stamey TA, eds. Campbell's urology. 5th ed. Philadelphia: WB Saunders, 1986;2000–30.
7. Elbadawi A, Malhoski WE, Frank IN. Mucinous urethral caruncle. Urology 1978;12:587–90.
8. Gonzalez MO, Harrison ML, Boileau MA. Carcinoma in diverticulum of female urethra. Urology 1985;26:328–32.
9. Grabstald H. Tumors of the urethra in men and women. Cancer 1973;32:1236–55.
10. Hardeman SW, Soloway MS. Urethral recurrence following radical cystectomy. J Urol 1990;144:666–9.
11. Hickey DP, Soloway MS, Murphy WM. Selective urethrectomy following cystoprostatectomy for bladder cancer. J Urol 1986;136:828–30.
12. Hopkins SC, Nag SK, Soloway MS. Primary carcinoma of male urethra. Urology 1984;23:128-133.
13. Huffman JW. The detailed anatomy of the periurethral ducts in the adult human female. Am J Obstet Gynecol 1948;55:86–101.
14. Katz JI, Grabstald H. Primary malignant melanoma of the female urethra. J Urol 1976;116:454–7.
15. Lucman L, Vadas G. Transitional cloacogenic carcinoma of the urethra. Cancer 1973;31:1508–10.
16. Madden NP, Turnock RR, Rickwood AM. Congenital polyps of the posterior urethra in neonates. J Pediatr Surg 1986;21:193–4.
17. Mahadevia PS, Koss LG, Tar IJ. Prostatic involvement in bladder cancer: prostate mapping in 20 cystoprostatectomy specimens. Cancer 1986;58:2096–102.
18. Maizels M. Normal development of the urinary tract. In: Walsh PC, Gittes RF, Perlmutter AD, Stamey TA, eds. Campbell's urology. 5th ed. Philadelphia: WB Saunders, 1986:1638–64.
19. Mayer R, Fowler JE Jr, Clayton M. Localized urethral cancer in women. Cancer 1987;60:1548–51.
20. McIntire TL, Soloway MS, Murphy WM. Nephrogenic adenoma: a review. Urology 1987;29:237–41.
21. Medeiros LJ, Young RH. Nephrogenic adenoma arising in urethral diverticula: a report of five cases. Arch Pathol Lab Med 1989;113:125–8.
22. Meis JM, Ayala AG, Johnson DE. Adenocarcinoma of the urethra in women: a clinicopathologic study. Cancer 1987;60:1038–52.
23. Melchers WJ, Schift R, Stolz E, Lindeman J, Quint WG. Human papillomavirus detection in urine samples from male patients by the polymerase chain reaction. J Clin Microbiol 1989;27:1711–4.
24. Melicow MM, Roberts TW. Pathology and natural history of urethral tumors in males: a review of 142 cases. Urology 1978;11:83–9.
25. Mevorach RA, Cos LR, di Sant'Agnese PA, Stoler M. Human papilloma-virus type 6 in grade I transitional cell carcinoma of the urethra. J Urol 1990;143:126–8.
26. Miller EV. Skene's duct cyst. J Urol 1984;131:966–7.

27. Mostofi FK, Price EB Jr. Tumors of the male genital system. Atlas of Tumor Pathology, 2nd Series, Fascicle 8. Washington, D.C.:Armed Forces Institute of Pathology, 1973:263–6.

28. Murphy WM. Diseases of the urinary bladder, urethra, ureters, and renal pelves. In: Murphy WM, ed. Urological pathology. Philadelphia: WB Saunders, 1989:112–24.

29. _____, Fu YS, Lancaster WD, Jenson AB. Papillomavirus structural antigens in condyloma acuminatum of the male urethra. J Urol 1983;130:84–5.

30. Raju GC, Roopnarinesingh A, Woo J. Villous adenoma of female urethra. Urology 1987;29:446–7.

31. Redman JF, Rountree GA. Pronounced dilatation of Cowper's gland duct manifest as a perineal mass: a recommendation for management. J Urol 1988;139:87–8.

32. Sanders TJ, Venable DD, Sanusi ID. Primary malignant melanoma of the urethra in a black man: a case report. J Urol 1986;135:1012–4.

33. Schinella R, Thurm J, Feiner H. Papillary pseudotumor of the prostatic urethra: proliferative papillary urethritis. J Urol 1974;111:38–40.

34. Silverman ML, Eyre RC, Zinman LA, Corsson AW. Mixed mucinous and papillary adenocarcinoma involving male urethra, probably originating in periurethral glands. Cancer 1981;47:1398–402.

35. Small JD, Albertsen PC, Graydon RJ, Ricci A Jr, Sardella WV. Adenoid cystic carcinoma of Cowper's glands. J Urol 1992;147:699–701.

36. Spencer JR, Brodin AG, Ignatoff JM. Clear cell adenocarcinoma of the urethra: evidence for origin within periurethral ducts. J Urol 1990;143:122–5.

37. Tanagho EA. Anatomy of the lower urinary tract. In: Walsh PC, Gittes RF, Perlmutter AD, Stamey TA, eds. Campbell's urology. 5th ed. Philadelphia: WB Saunders, 1986:46–94.

38. Tepper SL, Jagirdar J, Heath D, Geller SA. Homology between the female paraurethral (Skene's) glands and the prostate. Arch Pathol Lab Med 1984;108:423–5.

39. Vapnek JM, Turzan CW. Primary malignant lymphoma of the female urethra: report of a case and review of the literature. J Urol 1992;147:701–3.

40. Vasudevan P, Stein AM, Pinn VW, Rao CN. Primary amyloidosis of urethra. Urology 1981;17:181–3.

41. Walker AN, Mills SE. Papillary and polypoid tumors of the prostatic urethra. In: Damjanov I, Cohen AH, Mills SE, Young RH, eds. Progress in reproductive and urinary tract pathology. New York: Field and Wood Medical Publishers, Inc., 1989:113–37.

42. Walther HWE. Caruncle of the urethra in the female with special reference to the importance of histological examination in the differential diagnosis. J Urol 1943;50:380–8.

43. Witjes JA, De Vries JD, Schaafsma HE, Bogman MJ, Barentsz JO, Corten RL. Extramedullary plasmacytoma of the urethra: a case report. J Urol 1991;145:826–8.

44. Wolinska WH, Melamed MR, Schellhammer PF, Whitmore WF Jr. Urethral cytology following cystectomy for bladder carcinoma. Am J Surg Pathol 1977;1:225–34.

45. Young RH, Scully RE. Clear cell adenocarcinoma of the bladder and urethra: a report of three cases and review of the literature. Am J Surg Pathol 1985;9:816–26.

✧✧✧

4
TUMORS OF THE URETERS AND RENAL PELVES

NORMAL ANATOMY

The ureters and renal pelves form by elongation and branching of diverticular outgrowths from the mesonephric ducts (43,53). Initial branches are absorbed by dilatation of the advancing ureters to form the renal pelves but later branches are retained as renal calyces and terminal portions of collecting ducts. The mature structures function as conduits for the passage of urine. Each is lined by a folded epithelium supported by a lamina propria and surrounded by a muscular wall with a fibrous adventitia.

The structural components of the ureter and renal pelvis are similar to those of the urinary bladder but certain features deserve further elaboration. Except for its distal portion, the wall of the ureter consists of interlacing bundles of smooth muscles that are not arranged into distinct longitudinal and circular layers (26). When portions of the ureteral wall appear in surgical resections of adjacent organs, this lack of organization might be a source of diagnostic difficulty, especially when the ureteral mucosa is not present. In contrast to the bladder, the mucosa of the upper collecting system is normally arranged in folds, creating crypts from which rounded aggregates of cells may be avulsed into urinary specimens during catheterization or ureteroscopy. These "papillary" clusters may cause diagnostic confusion in the cytologic evaluation of low-grade transitional cell tumors if too much emphasis is placed on papillary aggregation as a sign of neoplastic growth. The nuclei of urothelial cells from the upper collecting system are larger and more irregular than their bladder counterparts. These features also occur in dysplasia and both normal and slightly reactive ureteral mucosa can be easily confused with dysplastic epithelium, especially in frozen sections performed at the time of cystectomy for bladder cancer. Considering the embryologic development of the renal collecting ducts, it is not surprising that urothelium extending into them may be a possible confounding factor to determining the origin of small glandular neoplasms arising in this area.

Almost all tumors previously described in the urinary bladder and urethra have been observed in the ureters or renal pelves (6,46). Neoplasms arising in these structures differ very little from their bladder counterparts and will be only briefly summarized. A few non-neoplastic tumorous conditions are especially important in the pathologic evaluation of ureteral lesions and require a more detailed discussion.

EPITHELIAL NEOPLASMS

Epithelial neoplasms arising in the ureters and renal pelves are uncommon lesions whose clinical behavior and pathologic features have remained essentially unchanged over the past half century (6,14,23,24,33,46). Age, sex ratio, frequency of histologic types, and prognosis do not differ significantly from those of similar tumors arising in the bladder (39). Important variations from bladder neoplasms include: a lower frequency of all types; a stronger association with certain types of chemical agents, such as phenacetin; a stronger association with obstruction to urinary outflow; a decreased value of cytology and endoscopy for detection and monitoring; and an increased frequency of synchronous or metachronous urothelial neoplasms at other sites.

Etiologic and pathogenetic factors influencing the development of upper collecting system neoplasms are similar to those described for the bladder. Associations with phenacetin abuse and Balkan nephropathy seem particularly strong (32,54). A history of infection or urinary stones has been obtained in 15 to 20 percent of cases (24). Transitional cell neoplasms of the upper collecting system are frequently associated with similar lesions at other sites. Renal pelvic and ureteral tumors occur simultaneously in 6 to 38 percent of cases and 10 to 50 percent of patients with upper collecting system lesions have had previous, coincident, or subsequent bladder tumors.

Epithelial neoplasms of the upper collecting system constitute less than 5 percent of all urothelial tumors (6,14,23,24,33,46). They have

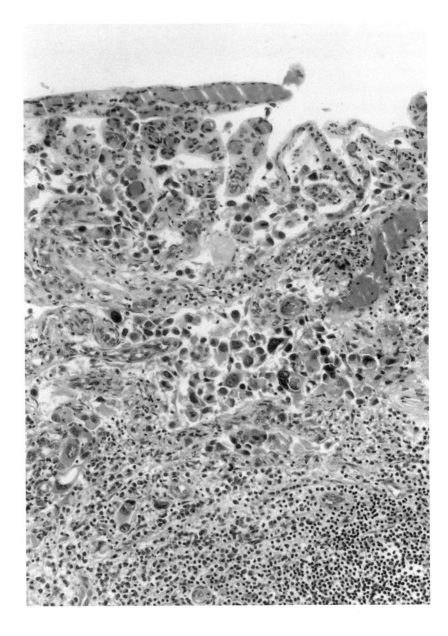

Figure 4-1
TRANSITIONAL CELL
CARCINOMA OF THE
RENAL PELVIS

been recorded in patients of all ages, most commonly in men aged 50 to 70 years. Any part of the system may be involved but the distal third of the ureter and the extrarenal portion of the renal pelvis are most commonly affected. Single lesions are the rule, although multiple tumors are not rare. Signs and symptoms are nonspecific: most patients have hematuria (90 percent) or flank pain (20 percent). Upper tract neoplasms can be recognized by urinary cytology and endoscopy but most tumors are localized by radiography (5,29,46).

Epithelial neoplasms arising in the ureters and renal pelves do not differ pathologically from those of the bladder (figs. 4-1–4-3). All histologic types, including inverted papilloma and rare variants of carcinoma, have been recorded with similar frequencies (6,7,11,17,37,38,46,47,57, 60). Expression of blood group antigens, DNA ploidy, and cell kinetics have been similar (1,25, 48,50, 52). Grading and staging systems developed for bladder lesions have been slightly modified to apply to similar tumors arising in the upper collecting system (28). Reactions to therapy and the

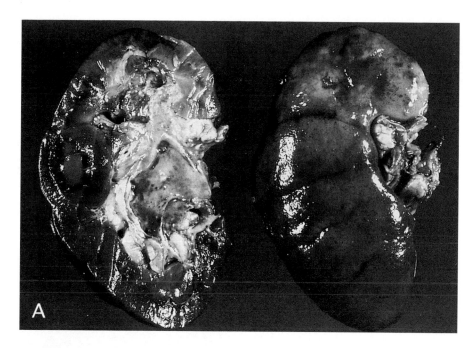

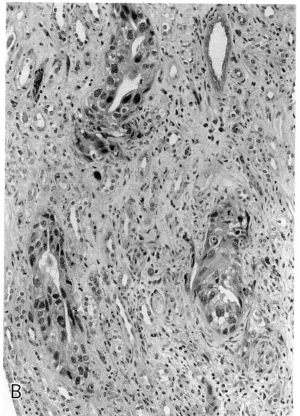

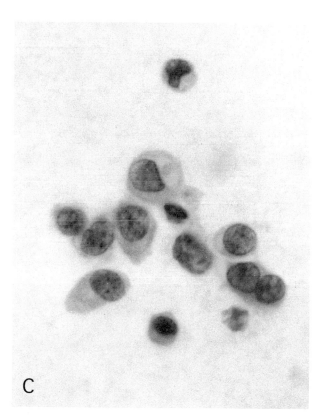

Figure 4-2
TRANSITIONAL CELL CARCINOMA WITH EXTENSIVE INVOLVEMENT OF COLLECTING DUCTS
A: The upper pole of this gross specimen is abnormal but a distinct pelvic mass is difficult to discern.
B: Transitional cell carcinoma in collecting ducts.
C: Malignant cells in the renal pelvic washing.

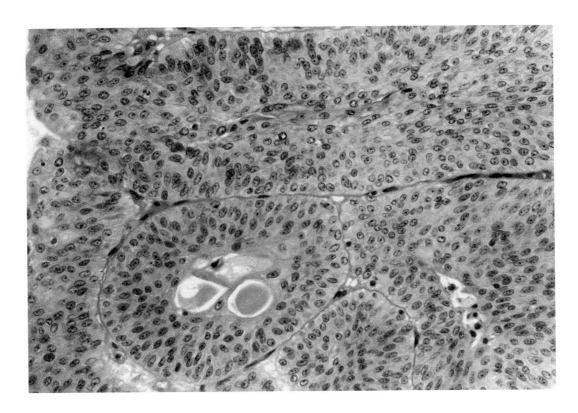

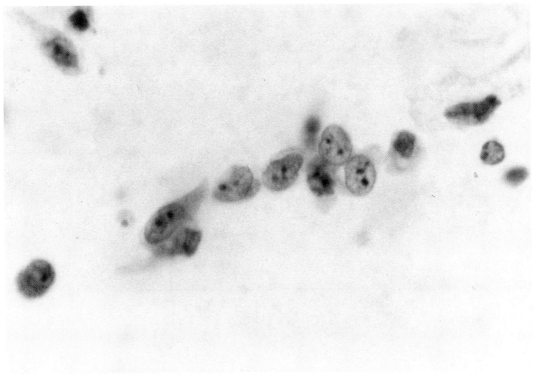

Figure 4-3
TRANSITIONAL CELL CARCINOMA OF URETER

Top: Histology.
Bottom: Tumor cells in bladder washing.

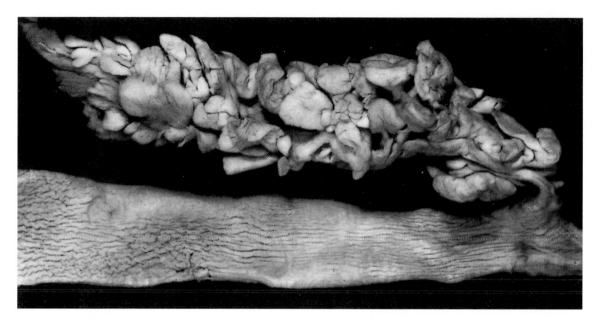

Figure 4-4
FIBROEPITHELIAL POLYP OF URETER
This fibroepithelial polyp of the ureter was removed from a 38-year-old woman. The solitary, elongated, and lobulated polyp is attached to the ureteral wall by a slender stalk. (Fig. 257 from Fascicle 12, 2nd Series.)

features of epithelial atypias are difficult to study in the ureters and renal pelves and current knowledge in this regard is fragmentary. Like bladder tumors, upper collecting system neoplasms grow initially by extension into adjacent structures. Involvement of the distal renal collecting ducts, especially by high-grade carcinomas, is common (42). Metastases usually involve regional structures, including lymph nodes, peritoneum, and liver (5). Metastases to the upper collecting system generally involve the ureters and arise from cancers of the kidney, breast, and lymph nodes (12). Prognosis varies with grade and stage. A nonfunctioning ipsilateral kidney or multiple areas of carcinoma in situ are grave prognostic signs.

Guidelines for the differential diagnosis of epithelial neoplasms arising in the ureters and renal pelves are similar to those for lesions arising in the bladder. Certain tumors of the renal pelvis must be distinguished from carcinomas of the renal collecting ducts (36). In addition to location, renal pelvic neoplasms are more solid and the transitional cell variety is often accompanied by an in situ component. Mucin may be

less prominent. Immunohistochemical reactions also vary, with urothelial carcinomas less reactive for peanut agglutinin and *Ulex europaeus*.

OTHER NEOPLASMS

In addition to carcinosarcoma, a variety of non-epithelial neoplasms have been observed in the ureters and renal pelves (9,11). These tumors do not differ histologically from similar lesions at other body sites. They include hemangioma, hemangiomyoma, leiomyoma, neurofibroma, leiomyosarcoma, angiosarcoma, choriocarcinoma, and Wilms tumor (3,13,34,41,51,56,58,62-65).

NON-NEOPLASTIC TUMOROUS CONDITIONS

Polyps

Polyps of the ureters and renal pelves are usually acquired rather than congenital (6,10, 15,46,66). Few cases have been associated with predisposing conditions although many etiologic factors have been proposed. Most polyps are hamartomatous growths which tend to arise in the proximal portions of the left ureter of men.

Single tumors are the rule but multiple or branched lesions have been observed (fig. 4-4). Signs and symptoms occur if the ureter is obstructed. Pathologically, these polyps grow as intraluminal lesions and consist of a broad core of loose connective tissue covered by normal or denuded urothelium. The connective tissue core may be rich in smooth muscle, collagen, or blood vessels and may even contain small numbers of lipid-laden macrophages. The composition of the stalks is variable but there is no evidence that the nature of polyps is altered by the relative proportions of blood vessels, smooth muscles, or connective tissue comprising their cores.

Retroperitoneal Fibrosis

Retroperitoneal fibrosis is an inflammatory process that must often be considered in the differential diagnosis of ureteral tumors (4,6,46). Most cases are of unknown etiology although a close association with ergot compounds such as methysergide has been documented. The disease develops insidiously, eventuating in a dense fibrosis that causes medial deviation of the ureters and ureteral obstruction. Depending upon the stage of disease, fibrosis may not be the predominant component in a biopsy specimen. A nonspecific pattern of chronic inflammation often occurs. Perhaps more importantly, any condition that attenuates urothelium may cause dysplastic epithelial changes, rarely mimicking those of carcinoma in situ (46).

A wide range of non-neoplastic tumorous conditions are observed in the ureters and renal pelves. Most lesions are described in single case reports, with or without a review of the literature. These lesions do not differ pathologically from similar conditions occurring at other body sites. They include amyloidosis, endometriosis, nephrogenic metaplasia, schistosomal infection produc-

ing ureteritis cystica, ectopic ureter presenting as an abdominal mass, mycetoma, plasma cell granuloma, hamartoma, hematoma (Antopol-Goldman lesion), cholesteatoma, and paraffinoma (8,16, 20–22,30,31,35,40,44,45,59).

INTESTINAL CONDUITS

Intestinal conduits have been fashioned in both children and adults for diversion and short-term storage of urine in cases of congenital anomalies and neoplasia (2,19,27,46,49,55). Surgical procedures for repair are well established and long-term results are favorable. Complications depend upon the nature of the primary disease, patient age, and the type of conduit. Colonic conduits are associated with an increased frequency of intestinal adenocarcinomas but a low frequency of reflux and stenosis. Ileal conduits rarely develop primary intestinal neoplasms but commonly reflux. Even so, renal failure has been recorded in less than 10 percent of cases and decreased renal function in less than 30 percent.

Pathologically, the epithelium of intestinal conduits is usually chronically inflamed, atrophic, and partially denuded (46). Ileal conduits are especially prone to colonization by *Candida* sp. but lack well-formed Peyer patches (61). Intestinal conduits are best monitored using urinary cytology, especially since almost all malignancies occurring in these structures are of high cytologic grade (fig. 4-5) (46,67). Malignant cells in urinary specimens are best detected using procedures that include direct smears. In contrast to bladder specimens, neoplastic elements appearing in conduits tend to be more degenerated. They must be further differentiated from the abundant aggregates of intestinal cells ordinarily present in these samples.

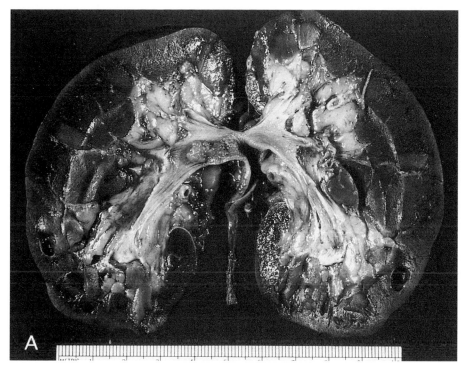

Figure 4-5
TRANSITIONAL
CELL CARCINOMA,
LOW GRADE,
OF RENAL PELVIS
A: Gross specimen containing a discrete renal pelvic tumor.
B: The neoplastic cells of an ileal conduit are surrounded by degenerated inflammatory and ileal mucosal cells.
C: Histology.

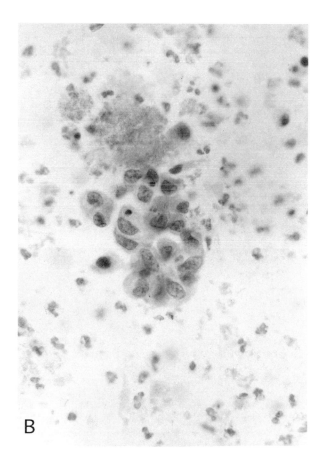

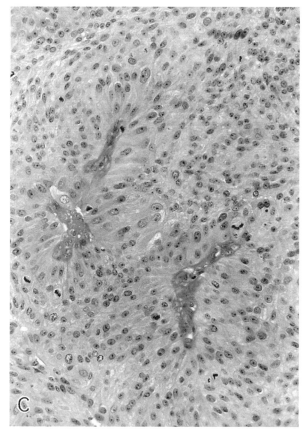

REFERENCES

1. al-Abadi H, Nagel R. Transitional cell carcinoma of the renal pelvis and ureter: prognostic relevance of nuclear deoxyribonucleic acid ploidy studied by slide cytometry: an 8-year survival time study. J Urol 1992;148:31–7.

2. Altwein JE, Jonas U, Hohenfellner R. Long-term follow-up of children with colon conduit urinary diversion and ureterosigmoidostomy. J Urol 1977;118:832–6.

3. Anderson JB, Lee JJ, Hancock RA, Black SR. Hemangioma of the kidney pelvis. J Urol 1953;70:869–73.

4. Baker LR, Mallinson WJ, Gregory MC, et al. Idiopathic retroperitoneal fibrosis. A retrospective analysis of 60 cases. Br J Urol 1987;60:497–503.

5. Batata MA, Whitmore WF, Hilaris BS, Tokita N, Grabstald H. Primary carcinoma of the ureter: a prognostic study. Cancer 1975;35:1626–32.

6. Bennington JL, Beckwith JB. Tumors of the kidney, renal pelvis, and ureter. Atlas of Tumor Pathology, 2nd Series, Fascicle 12. Washington, D.C.: Armed Forces Institute of Pathology, 1975;243–336.

7. Blacher EJ, Johnson DE, Abdul-Karim FW, Ayala AG. Squamous cell carcinoma of renal pelvis. Urology 1985;25:124–6.

8. Bradford JA, Ireland EW, Giles WB. Ureteric endometriosis: 3 case reports and a review of the literature. Aust NZ J Obstet Gynaecol 1989;29:421–4.

9. Byard RW, Bell ME, Alkan MK. Primary carcinosarcoma: a rare cause of unilateral ureteral obstruction. J Urol 1987;137:732–3.

10. Chang HH, Ray P, Ockuly E, Guinan P. Benign fibrous ureteral polyps. Urology 1987;30:114–8.

11. Chen KT, Workman RD, Flam MS, DeKlotz RJ. Carcinosarcoma of renal pelvis. Urology 1983;22:429–31.

12. Cohen WM, Freed SZ, Hasson J. Metastatic cancer to the ureter: a review of the literature and case presentations. J Urol 1974;112:188–9.

13. Coup AJ. Angiosarcoma of the ureter. Br J Urol 1988;62:275–6.

14. Das AK, Carson CC, Bolick D, Paulson DF. Primary carcinoma of the upper urinary tract: effect of primary and secondary therapy on survival. Cancer 1990;66:1919–23.

15. de Jonge JP, von Kortzfleisch D, Blessing MH, Stöker W. Fibroepithelioma of the renal pelvis. Urol Int 1988;43:56–9.

16. Eisenberg RL, Hedgcock MW, Shanser JD. Aspergillus mycetoma of the renal pelvis associated with ureteropelvic junction obstruction. J Urol 1977;118:466–7.

17. Essenfeld H, Manivel JC, Benedetto P, Albores-Saavedra J. Small cell carcinoma of the renal pelvis: a clinicopathological, morphological and immunohistochemical study of 2 cases. J Urol 1990;144(2 Pt 1):344–7.

18. Everett HS, Wayburn, GJ. A unique case of submucosal epithelial nests in the ureter and renal pelvis. J Urol 1946;56:310–18.

19. Filmer RB, Spencer JR. Malignancies in bladder augmentations and intestinal conduits. J Urol 1990;143:671–8.

20. Finan BF, Mollitt DL, Golladay ES, Redman JF. Giant ectopic ureter presenting as abdominal mass in infant. Urology 1987;30:246–7.

21. Fitko R, Gallagher L, Gonzalez-Crussi F, Oyasu R. Urothelial leiomyomatous hamartoma of the kidney. Am J Clin Pathol 1991;95:481–3.

22. Freedberg LE, Stables DP, Bloustein PA, Donohue R. Cholesteatoma of renal pelvis. Urology 1977;10:263–5.

23. Gilbert JB. Studies of the natural history of genitourinary tumors. I: Primary cancer of ureter: autopsy study with review of the literature. Am J Surg 1937;36:711–6.

24. Grabstald H, Whitmore WF, Melamed MR. Renal pelvic tumors. JAMA 1971;218:845–54.

25. Hall L, Faddoul A, Saberi A, Edson M. The use of red cell surface antigen to predict the malignant potential of transitional cell carcinoma of the ureter and renal pelvis. J Urol 1982;127:23–5.

26. Hanna MK, Jeffs RD, Sturgess JM, Barkin M. Ureteral structure and ultrastructure. Part I. The normal human ureter. J Urol 1976;116:718–24.

27. Helander KG, Ahren C, Philipson BM, Samuelsson BM, Ojerskog B. Structure of mucosa in continent ileal reservoirs 15 to 19 years after construction. Hum Pathol 1990;21:1235–8.

28. Hermanek P, Sobin LH eds. TNM classification of malignant tumours. 4th ed. 2nd revision. Berlin: Springer-Verlag, 1992.

29. Huffman JL, Bagley DH, Lyon ES, Morse MJ, Herr HW, Whitmore WF Jr. Endoscopic diagnosis and treatment of upper-tract urothelial tumors: a preliminary report. Cancer 1985;55:1422–8.

30. Itoh H, Namiki M, Yoshioka T, Itatani H. Plasma cell granuloma of the renal pelvis. J Urol 1982;127:1177–8.

31. Jakse G, Mikuz G. Nephrogenic adenoma of the ureter. Eur Urol 1983;9:60–2.

32. Johansson S, Angervall L, Bengtsson U, Wahlqvist L. Uroepithelial tumors of the renal pelvis associated with abuse of phenacetin-containing analgesics. Cancer 1974;33:743–53.

33. Kakizoe T, Fujita J, Murase T, Matsumoto K, Kishi K. Transitional cell carcinoma of the bladder in patients with renal pelvic and ureteral cancer. J Urol 1980;124:17–9.

34. Kao VC, Graff PW, Rappaport H. Leiomyoma of the ureter: a histologically problematic rare tumor confirmed by immunohistochemical studies. Cancer 1969;24:535–42.

35. Kelleher J, Wilson S, Witherow RO. Paraffinoma of the ureter. Br J Urol 1987;59:92–3.

36. Kennedy SM, Merino MJ, Linehan WM, Roberts JR, Robertson CN, Neumann RD. Collecting duct carcinoma of the kidney. Hum Pathol 1990;21:449–56.

37. Kobayashi S, Ohmori M, Akaeda T, Ohmori H, Miyaji Y. Primary adenocarcinoma of the renal pelvis: report of two cases and brief review of literature. Acta Pathol Jpn 1983;33:589–97.

38. Kvist E, Lauritzen AF, Bredesen J, Luke M, Sjølin KE. A comparative study of transitional cell tumors of the bladder and upper urinary tract. Cancer 1988;61:2109–12.

39. Kyriakos M, Royce RK. Multiple simultaneous inverted papillomas of the upper urinary tract: a case report with a review of ureteral and renal pelvic inverted papillomas. Cancer 1989;63:368–80.

40. Levitt S, Waisman J, deKernion J. Subepithelial hematoma of the renal pelvis (Antopol-Goldman lesion): a case report and review of the literature. J Urol 1984;131:939–41.

41. Loomis RC. Primary leiomyosarcoma of the kidney: report of a case and review of the literature. J Urol 1972;107:557–60.

42. Mahadevia PS, Karwa GL, Koss LG. Mapping of urothelium in carcinomas of the renal pelvis and ureter: a report of nine cases. Cancer 1983;51:890–7.

43. Maizels M. Normal development of the urinary tract. In: Walsh PC, Gittes RF, Pearlmutter AD, Stamey TA, eds. Campbell's urology. 5th ed. Philadelphia: WB Saunders, 1986:1638–64.

44. Miller R, Bowley NB. Localized amyloidosis of the ureter. J Urol 1984;131:112–3.

45. Murphy MN, Alguacil-Garcia A, MacDonald RG. Primary amyloidosis of renal pelvis with duplicate collecting system. Urology 1986;27:470–3.

46. Murphy WM. Diseases of the urinary bladder, urethra, ureters, and renal pelves. In: Murphy WM, ed. Urological pathology. Philadelphia: WB Saunders, 1989:124–34.

47. _____, von Buedingen RP, Poley RW. Primary carcinoma in situ of renal pelvis and ureter. Cancer 1974;34:1126–30.

48. Nativ O, Winkler HZ, Reiman HM Jr, Lieber MM. Squamous cell carcinoma of the renal pelvis: nuclear deoxyribonucleic acid ploidy studied by flow cytometry. J Urol 1990,144.23–6.

49. Neal DE. Complications of ileal conduit diversion in adults with cancer followed up for at least five years. Br Med J (Clin Res Ed) 1985;290:1695–7.

50. Nemoto R, Hattori K, Sasaki A, Miyanaga N, Koiso K, Harada M. Estimations of the S phase fraction in situ in transitional cell carcinoma of the renal pelvis and ureter with bromodeoxyuridine labelling. Br J Urol 1989;64:339–44.

51. Ogata S, Mizoguchi H, Arita M, Sakamoto S, Ogata J. A case of hemangiomyoma of the ureter in a child. Eur Urol 1985;11:355–6.

52. Oldbring J, Hellsten S, Lindholm K, Mikulowski P, Tribukait B. Flow DNA analysis of the characterization of carcinoma of the renal pelvis and ureter. Cancer 1989;64:2141–5.

53. Osathanondh V, Potter EL. II. Renal pelvis, calyces, and papillae. Arch Pathol 1963;76:277–89.

54. Petronic VJ, Burkurov NS, Djokic MR, et al. Balkan endemic nephropathy and papillary transitional cell tumors of the renal pelvis and ureters. Kidney Int 1991;34(Suppl):S77–9.

55. Pitts WR Jr, Muecke EC. A 20-year experience with ileal conduits: the fate of the kidneys. J Urol 1979: 122:154–7.

56. Ravich A. Neurofibroma of the ureter: report of a case with operation and recovery. Arch Surg 1935;30:442–8.

57. Ross DG, D'Amato NA. Papillary mucinous cystadenoma of probable renal pelvic origin in a horseshoe kidney. Arch Pathol Lab Med 1985;109:954–5.

58. Rushton HG, Sens MA, Garvin AJ, Turner WR Jr. Primary leiomyosarcoma of the ureter: a case report with electron microscopy. J Urol 1983;129:1045–6.

59. Saad SM, Hanafy HM. Bilharzial (schistosomal) ureteritis cystica. Urology 1974;4:261–6.

60. Tajima Y, Aizawa M. Unusual renal pelvic tumor containing transitional cell carcinoma, adenocarcinoma, and sarcomatoid elements (so-called sarcomatoid carcinoma of the renal pelvis): a case report and review of the literature. Acta Pathol Jpn 1988;38:805–14.

61. Tapper D, Folkman J. Lymphoid depletion in ileal loops: mechanism and clinical implications. J Pediatr Surg 1976;11:871–80.

62. Uchida M, Watanabe H, Mishina T, Shimada N. Leiomyoma of the renal pelvis. J Urol 1981;125:572–4.

63. Uhlir K. Hemangioma of the ureter. J Urol 1973; 110.047–9.

64. Vahlensieck W Jr, Riede U, Wimmer B, Ihling C. Beta-human chorionic gonadotropin-positive extragonadal germ cell neoplasia of the renal pelvis. Cancer 1991;67:3146–9.

65. Weinberg AG, Currarino G, Hurt GE Jr. Botryoid Wilms' tumor of the renal pelvis. Arch Pathol Lab Med 1984;108:147–8.

66. Wolgel CD, Parris AC, Mitty HA, Schapira HE. Fibroepithelial polyp of renal pelvis. Urology 1982;19:436–9.

67. Wolinska WH, Melamed MR. Urinary conduit cytology. Cancer 1973;32:1000–6.

✧✧✧

Index*

*Numbers in boldface indicate table and figure pages.

✧✧✧